Dietary Zn and Human Health

Dietary Zn and Human Health

Special Issue Editor

Elad Tako

MDPI • Basel • Beijing • Wuhan • Barcelona • Belgrade

MDPI

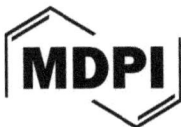

Special Issue Editor
Elad Tako
Cornell University
USA

Editorial Office
MDPI
St. Alban-Anlage 66
Basel, Switzerland

This is a reprint of articles from the Special Issue published online in the open access journal *Nutrients* (ISSN 2072-6643) from 2017 to 2018 (available at: http://www.mdpi.com/journal/nutrients/special_issues/dietary_Zn_human_health)

For citation purposes, cite each article independently as indicated on the article page online and as indicated below:

LastName, A.A.; LastName, B.B.; LastName, C.C. Article Title. *Journal Name* **Year**, *Article Number, Page Range.*

ISBN 978-3-03897-019-4 (Pbk)
ISBN 978-3-03897-020-0 (PDF)

Contents

About the Special Issue Editor

Elad Tako holds degrees in animal science (B.S.), endocrinology (M.S.), and physiology/nutrigenomics (Ph.D.), with previous appointments at the Hebrew University of Jerusalem, North Carolina State University, and Cornell University. As a Research Physiologist with USDA/ARS, Dr. Tako's research focuses on various aspects of trace mineral deficiencies, emphasizing molecular, physiological and nutritional factors and practices that influence the intestinal micronutrient absorption. With over 100 peer-reviewed publications and presentations, he leads a research team focused on understanding the interactions between dietary factors, physiological and molecular biomarkers, the microbiome, and intestinal functionality. His research accomplishments include the development of the Gallus gallus intra-amniotic administration procedure, and establishing recognized approaches for using animal models within mineral bioavailability and intestinal absorption screening processes. He has also developed a zinc status physiological blood biomarker (red blood cell Linoleic Acid:Dihomo--Linolenic Acid Ratio), and molecular tissue biomarkers to assess the effect of dietary mineral deficiencies on intestinal functionality, and how micronutrients dietary deficiencies alter gut microbiota composition and function.

Preface to "Dietary Zn and Human Health"

The importance of micronutrients in health and nutrition is undisputable and, among them, zinc is an essential element whose significance to health is increasingly recognized and whose deficiency may play an important role in the appearance of diseases. Zinc is one of the most important trace elements in living organisms with three major biological roles, as catalyst, structural, and regulatory ion. Zinc-binding motifs are found in many proteins encoded by the human genome physiologically, and free zinc is mainly regulated at the single-cell level. Zinc has a critical effect in homeostasis, in immune function, in oxidative stress, in apoptosis, and in aging, and significant disorders of major public health interest are associated with zinc deficiency. In many chronic diseases—including atherosclerosis, several malignancies, neurological disorders, autoimmune diseases, aging, age-related degenerative diseases, and Wilson's disease—concurrent zinc deficiency may complicate the clinical features, affect adversely immunological status, increase oxidative stress, and lead to the generation of inflammatory cytokines. In these diseases, oxidative stress and chronic inflammation may play important causative roles. It is therefore important that the status of zinc is assessed in all cases and zinc deficiency is corrected, since the unique properties of zinc may have significant therapeutic benefits in these diseases.

Zinc deficiency is a common ailment predicted to affect 17% of the world's population. Deficiency of zinc is a major cause of early childhood morbidity and mortality. Globally, zinc deficiency is widespread, particularly in rural and developing regions where populations consume cereal-based diets and have less opportunities for diet diversification; however, its presence is also detected in prosperous areas where diets are unbalanced, contributing to "hidden hunger". Although whole blood, plasma, and urine zinc decrease in severe zinc deficiency, accurate assessment of zinc status, especially in mild to moderate deficiency, is difficult as studies with these biomarkers are often contradictory and inconsistent. Hence, considering the complexity of zinc metabolism and absorption, the assessment of marginal zinc status is problematic as there is no universally accepted single measure to assess zinc status. As was indicated by the World Health Organization (WHO), the need to develop additional robust indicators of zinc status and to further expand the already known clinical markers, for which limited data of reliability exists, is evident. Functional biomarkers are those indicators which can detect chronic dysfunctions, such as mild–moderate zinc deficiency, that do not initially present with precise organ pathologies. Functional biomarkers may be well-positioned to indicate zinc deficiency, especially because clinical symptoms are usually absent in mild–moderate zinc deficiency. Due to the paucity of sensitive and specific biological indicators of dietary zinc intake and whole-body zinc status, the WHO has urged further development of Zn indicators, especially those in which a marginal deficiency may be detected. Based upon these recommendations, and in terms of evaluating the efficacy of a zinc intervention (supplement and/or biofortified crop), it is incumbent upon researchers to identify biomarkers which may:

(1) respond solely to dietary zinc depletion and repletion; (2) respond rapidly so that early intervention, if necessary, may be properly initiated; (3) indicate sensitivity to all levels of zinc deficiency, especially mild–moderate; (4) appropriately respond to zinc deficiency in both non-healthy and healthy subjects; and (5) be relatively inexpensive and uncomplicated to use and interpret, especially in field circumstances. Further, it remains a central priority to elucidate what, if any, confounding variables exist which can affect the validity, or at least interpretation of, the purported biomarker. This issue is evident in many of the commonly used biomarkers in which,

for example erythrocyte MT, dietary recall plays an integral role in interpreting the biomarker, yet mistakes in recall are common and can affect the determination of zinc status.

In the current manuscript collection, we present a selection of recent knowledge related to dietary zinc and human health, this includes research that discusses updates on zinc dietary requirements, zinc metabolism, zinc deficiency and metabolic disease and zinc status biomarkers.

Elad Tako
Special Issue Editor

nutrients

MDPI

Review

The Linoleic Acid: Dihomo-γ-Linolenic Acid Ratio (LA:DGLA)—An Emerging Biomarker of Zn Status

Marija Knez [1,2,*], James C. R. Stangoulis [1], Maria Glibetic [2] and Elad Tako [3]

[1] College of Science and Engineering, Flinders University, GPO Box 2100, Adelaide, SA 5001, Australia; james.stangoulis@flinders.edu.au

[2] Centre of Research Excellence in Nutrition and Metabolism, Institute for Medical Research, University of Belgrade, 11000 Belgrade, Serbia; mglibetic@gmail.com

[3] USDA/ARS (US Department of Agriculture, Agricultural Research Service), Robert W. Holley Centre for Agriculture and Health, Cornell University, Ithaca, NY 14853, USA; et79@cornell.edu

* Correspondence: marijaknez186@gmail.com or marija.knez@flinders.edu.au; Tel.: +381-612769849

Received: 28 June 2017; Accepted: 28 July 2017; Published: 1 August 2017

Abstract: Zinc (Zn) deficiency is a common aliment predicted to affect 17% of the world's population. Zinc is a vital micronutrient used for over 300 enzymatic reactions and multiple biochemical and structural processes in the body. Although whole blood, plasma, and urine zinc decrease in severe zinc deficiency, accurate assessment of zinc status, especially in mild to moderate deficiency, is difficult as studies with these biomarkers are often contradictory and inconsistent. Hence, as suggested by the World Health Organization, sensitive and specific biological markers of zinc status are still needed. In this review, we provide evidence to demonstrate that the LA:DGLA ratio (linoleic acid:dihomo-γ-linolenic acid ratio) may be a useful additional indicator for assessing Zn status more precisely. However, this biomarker needs to be tested further in order to determine its full potential.

Keywords: biomarker; Zn; LA:DGLA; Zn status; fatty acid

1. Introduction

Zinc (Zn) deficiency was first described in humans in the early 1960s, in Middle Eastern, male adolescent dwarfs consuming plant-based diets [1]. Subsequently, Zn deficiency has been identified in many other regions of the world, and it became evident that dietary deficiency of Zn in humans is a widespread phenomenon. Today, Zn deficiency affects around 17% of the world's population [2]. During the last 50 years, tremendous advances have been made both in our basic and clinical understanding of Zn metabolism [3]. Major progress has been made in understanding the importance of Zn as a structural and catalytic factor in a wide range of biological reactions, in uncovering the cellular Zn absorption and excretion mechanisms, and in clarifying the activities of major Zn transporters (15 Zip and 10 ZnT transporters) [4,5]. A significant research effort has tried to identify a physiological biomarker that predicts Zn status truthfully, especially in mild to moderate Zn deficiency. However, to this day, we are still without an entirely accurate biomarker of Zn status. In 2009, Lowe and colleagues evaluated 32 biomarkers in their review and identified only three as potentially useful: serum/plasma Zn concentrations, hair Zn concentration, and urinary Zn excretion [6]. Similarly, the BOND (Biomarkers of Nutrition for Development) Zinc Expert Panel recommended the following zinc biomarkers for use: dietary intakes, plasma/serum Zn concentrations, and stunting [7]. Last year, an update on Zn biomarkers was provided, recognizing a few as emerging biomarkers that require further investigation: Zn-dependent proteins, taste acuity, oxidative stress, and DNA integrity [8].

This review is a summary of research related to the LA:DGLA ratio (linoleic acid:dihomo-γ-linolenic acid ratio) as a novel biomarker of Zn status. We describe the chemical structure and function of the Δ6 desaturase enzyme, outline the current knowledge related to the role of Zn in desaturase activity and fatty acid metabolism, and provide recent data that demonstrates the usefulness of the LA:DGLA ratio to be used as a potentially new biomarker of Zn status. Lastly, we allude to further research needed on this topic.

2. The Limitations of the Currently Used Biomarkers: "Emerging" Biomarkers

All of the currently accepted and commonly used biomarkers of Zn status have certain limitations. Serum/plasma Zn, hair Zn concentration, and urinary Zn levels tend to fall in severe Zn depletion [9]. However, while plasma Zn concentration responds to altered intake over a short period of time, low plasma Zn concentrations do not remain constant for an extended period due to the homeostatic mechanisms that act to maintain plasma zinc concentration within the physiologic range; by maintaining losses via the GI (gastrointestinal) tract and kidneys [6]. Similarly, dietary Zn intake very often is not correlated with plasma zinc status, and does not realistically reflect the nutritional state of an individual [7,10–12]. For example, unchanged plasma/serum Zn concentrations were observed with intakes as low as 2.8 mg kg^{-1} to as high as 40 mg kg^{-1}, showing the limitation of plasma Zn status to reliably present the dietary Zn intake [13,14]. Serum Zn levels tend to rise and then fall after a meal [15].

While urinary Zn decreases under severe Zn deficiency [16], the precise evaluation of Zn status in mild to moderate Zn deficiency is challenging, as studies with this biomarker give inconsistent and conflicting results [6]. Urinary Zn has been shown to be a poor indicator of early stage Zn deficiency [14,16].

Recently, a few studies provided some evidence to support the effectiveness of hair Zn concentrations in predicting the Zn status of individuals [17–19]. The hair Zn biomarker has some advantages, such as low cost and viability; however, hair zinc still lacks sufficient evidence towards validity as a method to assess Zn status [8,20]. Finally, the reliability of all currently used biomarkers under infection and inflammatory conditions is intricate [6,7]. Plasma Zn concentration can fall as a result of factors not related to Zn status or dietary Zn intake, i.e., infections, inflammation, trauma, and stress [7].

An indicator that truthfully represents Zn status under various physiological conditions in humans is still missing [7]. The role of Zn in various processes and pathways in the body is multifaceted, and this may indicate that one single biomarker may never be sufficiently sensitive and that we need to use a spectrum of Zn biomarkers to be able to precisely differentiate between various Zn deficiency states.

Emerging biomarkers are defined as 'biomarkers for which there is some theoretical basis of a relationship to zinc intake or status, but the testing is insufficient to confirm the relation' [8]. Currently, nail Zn concentration, Zn-dependent proteins, oxidative stress, DNA integrity, and taste acuity are placed in the group of emerging biomarkers [8]. However, for many of the newly identified biomarkers, insufficient evidence is available to demonstrate their true potential and further studies are needed to confirm which ones can be used as biomarkers of Zn status. In this review, we provide the existing evidence to show that the LA:DGLA ratio is likewise an emerging biomarker of Zn status that needs to be assessed further.

3. Delta 6 Desaturase: Structure, Regulation, and Function

Delta 6 desaturase (Δ6 desaturase, D6D or Δ-6-desaturase) is a membrane-bound desaturase enzyme required for the synthesis of polyunsaturated fatty acids (PUFA). The enzyme is molecularly identical across all living organisms. Δ6 desaturase is widely expressed in human tissues, in the liver, the membrane of red blood cells, lung, and heart, with the highest levels being present in the brain [21,22].

Linoleic acid (LA) is an essential omega 6 ($n = 6$) fatty acid that cannot be synthetized in the human body and must be obtained from the diet to ensure the appropriate development of various cells throughout the body [23]. It is the most abundant PUFA in human tissues [24]. LA is a metabolic precursor of dihomo-γ-linolenic acid (DGLA) (Figure 1). Δ6 desaturases are rate-limiting enzymes in the synthesis of PUFA, responsible for conversion of LA to DGLA, and the enzyme catalyzes the addition of a double bond at the sixth carbon-carbon bond position from the carboxylic acid end in fatty acids [22,25].

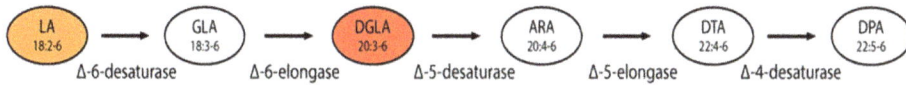

Figure 1. Desaturases involved in the biosynthesis of omega 6 polyunsaturated fatty acids. LA: linoleic acid; GLA: γ-linoleic acid; DGLA: dihomo-γ-linolenic acid; ARA: arachidonic acid; DTA: docosatetraenoic acid; DPA: docosapentaenoic acid. Δ6 desaturase is responsible for the formation of the carbon-carbon double bonds, and the function of an elongase is to lengthen fatty acid chains by the addition of two carbon units. LA (18:2-6) is desaturated by a Δ6 desaturase, introducing a D6 double bond into the substrate, giving γ-linolenic acid (GLA, 18:3-6). GLA is then elongated by a Δ6 elongase to dihomo-γ-linolenic acid (DGLA, 20:3-6). Modified from: Meesapyodsuk & Qiu, 2012 [25].

The first Δ6 desaturase gene was cloned in 1993 from a cyanobacterium, *Synechocystis* [26]. Subsequently, desaturases have been identified and characterized from a wide range of species, and in 1997 the first eukaryotic Δ6 desaturase gene was cloned [27,28]. Mammalian Δ6 desaturase encoded gene is a protein made of a cytochrome b5-like domain, attached to the N-terminus of the main desaturation domain, and a histidine motif, located on a desaturation domain at the C-terminus [29]. The histidine sequence is made of three highly conserved histidine-rich motifs, i.e., HX3-4H, HX2-3HH, and H/QX2-3HH (Figure 2). The first histidine of the third motif is commonly substituted by glutamine [27]. The conversion of glutamine back to histidine results in the loss of activity, suggesting that the process might be very important not only for the structural configuration of desaturases, but also for their activity [30]. The gene coding for Δ6 production is located on human chromosome 11 (11q12.2-13.1), and is made of 12 exons and 11 introns [31].

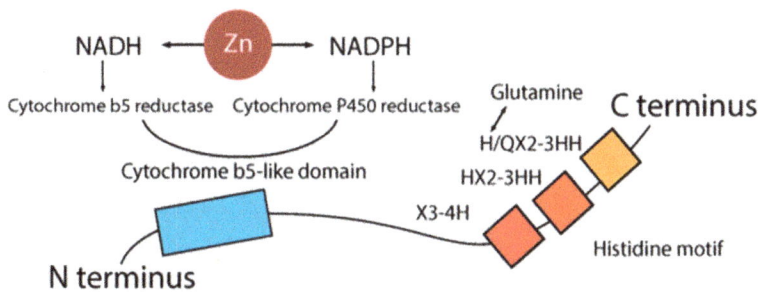

Figure 2. Schematic presentation of the structure of a Δ6 desaturase enzyme. A cytochrome b5-like domain is attached to the N-terminus and a histidine motif is located at the C-terminus. The histidine sequence is made of three histidine-rich motifs. The first histidine of the third motif is often replaced by glutamine. NADPH reductase has a Zn-dependent activity. NADH: nicotinamide adenine dinucleotide hydride; NADPH: nicotinamide adenine dinucleotide phosphate-oxidase.

To date, there has been limited information available on how the expression of the Δ6 desaturase is regulated. Some scientists believe that the regulation is achieved by the feedback control of the transcriptional regulation of fatty acid desaturase genes, mediated through signaling pathways activated by sensors embedded in cellular membranes, in response to environmental factors [32]. There is also some evidence showing that Δ6 desaturase enzymatic activity may be determined by tissue-specific mechanisms that involve both pre- and post-translational events [25].

NADPH reductase is important in the action of the Δ6 desaturase and is a Zn-dependent enzyme [33–35]. Typically, the Zn atom is bound to three or four ligands, which are composed of amino acids residues with histidine being the most frequent, followed by glutamic acid, aspartic acid, and cysteine [36]. Finally, the mutation of the cytochrome b5 domain is critical for the activity of Δ6 desaturases [37,38].

4. The Role of Zn in the Regulation of Δ6 Desaturase Activity and Fatty Acid Metabolism

Zn is an essential component of many enzymes and constitutes a part of their prostetic group [39]. It is present in DNA and RNA polymerases, dehydrogenases, and desaturases, regulating their functions via its catalytic, structural, or regulatory role. Over the years it has been noted that Zn is an important co-factor for the metabolism of fatty acids [40]. Zn is also necessary for at least two stages in essential fatty acid (EFA) metabolism; the conversion of linoleic acid to γ-linolenic acid, and the mobilization of dihomo-γ-linolenic acid (DGLA) to arachidonic acid [41]. Zinc has an effect on Δ6 desaturase itself [41], and affects linoleic acid absorption [42]. Once it was identified that Zn and essential fatty acid deficiencies give similar symptoms, a close association between fatty acid metabolism and Zn status was proposed [41,43,44].

Over the years, a number of studies have demonstrated an effect of Zn deficiency on the metabolism of essential fatty acids by impaired Δ6 desaturation activity [34,42,44–46]. On the other hand, there are a few studies completed in early 1990 that showed no role of Zn in fatty acid desaturation [47–51].

The effect of Zn deficiency on Δ5 and Δ6 activity was initially investigated by a number of groups in the early 1980s [42,45,52]. The findings were consistent, proving the reduced activity of Δ6 desaturase during Zn deficiency. Ayala and Branner [42] used male weaning Wistar rats and examined the influence of Zn on desaturating enzymes of liver and testes microsomes and their impact on fatty acid and lipid alterations of the tissues. The rats were fed Zn-adequate (55 ppm of Zn) or Zn-deficient diets (1.2 ppm of Zn) for 60 days. The progress of the effect of Zn deficiency was notable; Zn deficiency induced a decrease of essential fatty acids of the linoleic family in plasma after only 18 days, which indicates that Zn deficiency causes a rapid change in desaturase activity [42]. The activities of both desaturases were affected by Zn deficiency, but to a different degree. The same level of Zn deficiency caused a 45% reduction in Δ6 activity, while Δ5 was almost completely attenuated [42].

Similar findings were provided by Cunnane and Wahle [53] when it was shown that Zn modulates linoleic acid metabolism in rat mammary glands, modifying the Δ6 desaturation of microsomes. Specifically, 38 Sprague-Dawley rats were fed either a purified Zn-supplemented or a Zn-deficient diet for six weeks. The effects of Zn deficiency on the fatty acid composition of plasma lipids and microsomes of liver, intestine, and testes were studied. Among the polyunsaturated fatty acids, DGLA was significantly reduced by the Zn-deficient diet. Interestingly, the activity of Δ6 activity in liver microsomes was decreased by 25%, while the Δ5 desaturation was reduced by 53% in Zn-depleted rats. In addition, hypertriglyceridemia was observed in the serum of Zn-deficient rats. This study demonstrated that Zn supplementation returned serum triglycerides to normal levels, which shows a strong physiological interaction between Zn and EFAs (essential fatty acids) and confirms that Zn deficiency is responsible for the defects in desaturation [54].

Ten years later, studies completed by Eder and Kirchgessner [44,55,56] provided somewhat contradictory results, demonstrating that Zn deficiency does not affect Δ5 and Δ6 desaturation. The experiments were conducted using various types of dietary fats, including coconut, sunflower, or linseed oil. The proposition was that the activities of Δ5 and Δ6 desaturase depend on the type of dietary fat consumed. Diets rich in fats with high levels of polyunsaturated fatty acids suppress activities of desaturases, while fat free diets significantly raise the activities of these desaturases.

Later in 1995, the authors suggested that one reason for the contradiction between the findings might be the experimental design used in the studies, where the effects of Zn deficiency on desaturase activity was misperceived by a low food intake. After that, the role of Zn in desaturase activity was examined by a serious of experiments with Zn-deficient rats using a force-feeding technique that ensures identical food intake [44]. Δ5 and Δ6 desaturation was investigated in the presence of Zn deficiency in force-fed rats by previously raising the levels of enzymes by feeding a fat-free diet [44]. Zn-deficient rats fed a diet consisting of 5% safflower oil had lower levels of total PUFA than the corresponding rats fed a Zn-adequate diet. The authors clearly demonstrated the role of Zn in Δ5 and Δ6 desaturation in subjects with adequate food and energy intake. Similarly, in subjects with a low-fat intake (fat-free diets), the effect of Zn deficiency on Δ6 desaturation activity was even more pronounced, with a significantly lower activity of the enzyme being observed [44].

In 1999, Waldhauser and colleagues [57] looked at the ratio between *n*-3 PUFA and *n*-6 PUFA in zinc-deficient animals. Four groups of rats were fed zinc-deficient (0.5 mg Zn kg^{-1}) or zinc-adequate (45 mg Zn kg^{-1}) diets with either olive oil or linseed oil as the source of fat. To ensure an adequate food intake, the rats were force-fed by gastric tube over a period of 13 days. The study confirmed that Zn deficiency influences the metabolic balance between *n*-3 and *n*-6 PUFA, whereas saturated and MUFA (monounsaturated fatty acids) seem to remain unaffected by Zn deficiency. In the rats that were fed linseed oil, zinc deficiency caused a marked increase in the ratio between *n*-3 and *n*-6 polyunsaturated fatty acids in liver phospholipids, particularly in phosphatidylcholine. In contrast, in the rats that were fed olive oil, Zn deficiency had only slight effects on the fatty acid composition of the liver phospholipids. Therefore, this study confirms the previous results demonstrating that the effects of Zn deficiency on lipid metabolism may be influenced by the type of dietary fat. However, it must be noted that only hepatic Δ6 desaturase enzymatic activity may be reliant upon the composition of dietary fat [58]. This is not applicable to all other tissues. While, the consumption of an essential fatty acid-deficient diet is paralleled by a similar increase in the hepatic abundance of Δ6 desaturase mRNA and the increase in hepatic Δ6 desaturase activity [21], Δ6 desaturase activity was very low in non-hepatic tissues [58,59].

It seems that the potential role of dietary fat on desaturase activity, under relevant conditions, is only related to hepatic tissue. Similarly, in situations when EFA deficiency is of dietary origin, there is an increased attempt to synthetize more linoleic acid, so Δ6 desaturase activity is increased. However, when EFA deficiency is metabolic (as in Zn deficiency) Δ6 activity is inhibited [60]. Finally, increased Δ6 desaturase activity will not necessarily lead to the elevated metabolizing of linoleic acid and its conversion to DGLA. Below, we summarize the findings that confirm the interaction between Zn deficiency and the metabolism of linoleic acid via desaturase enzymes:

1. Zn may have a role in the absorption of linoleic acid. Lower levels of Zn produce lower levels of linoleic acid [60].
2. Zn has a role in relation to the NADH-NADPH cycle (Figure 2) [35].
3. Cytochrome P-450 activity is significantly reduced under Zn deficiency [34].
4. Zn deficiency reduces the availability of linoleic acid metabolites γ-linolenic and arachidonic acid [52,61].
5. Zn deficiency decreases the mobilization of DGLA from tissue stores [62].
6. Zn is needed in the formation of GLA and in the mobilization of DGLA [41].
7. EFA supplementation worsens the effect of Zn deficiency [43,52,63].
8. Zn deficiency decreases the esterification of essential fatty acids into phospholipids [46].
9. During Zn deficiency, linoleic acid accumulates in tissues when EFA supplements are administered [63].
10. Zn deficiency results in a higher concentration of linoleic and a lower concentration of arachidonic acid in tissue phospholipids [34].
11. Zn-deficient subjects have an increased β-oxidation of linoleic acid, resulting in decreased amounts of linoleic acid available to be metabolized into arachidonic acid [64].
12. The most important EFA functions are carried out by molecules downstream of GLA [41].

13. In animals exposed to diets deficient in essential fatty acids, the characteristic symptoms develop much more rapidly if the diets are also deficient in Zn [43,65].

14. The inhibition of the desaturases by Zn deficiency is so strong that it causes a more rapid decline in tissue arachidonic acid and docosahexaenoic acid than does the direct dietary deficiency of all the omega 6 or omega 3 polyunsaturated fatty acids [64].

15. Enzymes involved in prostaglandin synthesis are also Zn-dependent, and defects in prostaglandin synthesis are observed under Zn deficiency [52].

In summary, Zn has both a direct role in the modulation of desaturase activities involved in the fatty acid metabolism and an indirect effect on fatty acids by influencing their absorption, oxidation, and incorporation [34]. Zn deficiency causes inconsistencies in the ratio of desaturase substrates and products, and linoleic acid (LA) and dihomo-γ-linolenic acid (DGLA), respectively (Figure 1). The most important EFA functions are carried out by molecules downstream of GLA. The Δ6-catalyzed step required for the transformation of LA to DGLA is generally the highest flux pathway, so an elevation in the LA:DGLA ratio could be a sensitive marker for Zn deficiency.

5. The LA:DGLA Ratio as a Biomarker of Zn Status, Current Evidence

In 2014, the concept of the essential role of Zn for Δ6 desaturase activity was reinvented. For the first time, Reed et al. [66] tested and implemented a previously unexplored biomarker of zinc status related to erythrocyte Δ6 desaturation, the LA:DGLA ratio. By using the chicken (*Gallus gallus*) as a model, the authors evaluated the sensitivity of the erythrocyte LA:DGLA ratio to changes in supplemental Zn intake. A significant negative correlation was found between dietary Zn deficiency and the LA:DGLA ratio.

The *Gallus gallus* has a similar membrane fatty acid composition to mammals [67] and is highly sensitive to dietary Zn manipulations [66,68–70], which makes it a potentially ideal animal model for exploring changes in the production of essential fatty acids in relation to Zn nutrition. In the original study, birds were fed either a Zn-adequate control diet ($42.3 \ \mu g \ Zn \ g^{-1}$) or a Zn-deficient diet ($2.5 \ \mu g \ Zn \ g^{-1}$). Diets had identical FA (fatty acids) content/profile. The body weight, feed consumption, Zn intake, and serum Zn concentrations of the birds were measured weekly, showing higher values of all parameters in the Zn control versus the Zn-deficient diet group of birds ($p < 0.05$). There was a relative increase in gene expression of the cytokines: tumor necrosis factor alpha (TNF-α), interleukin 1 beta (IL-1β), and interleukin-6 (IL-6) in the control group. Other assessed parameters included metal transporters (i.e., ZnT1, ZnT5, ZnT7, Zip6, Zip9); transcription factor: nuclear factor kappa B (NF-κB); brush border enzymes: aminopeptidase, sucrose-isomaltase, Na+K+ATPase, sodium glucose transport protein 1 (SGLT-1), and binding metallothionein-4 protein (MT4). These parameters were found to not be significantly different between the groups. However, the expression of hepatic Δ6 desaturase was significantly higher in the control group ($p < 0.001$). Accordingly, the LA:DGLA ratio was noticeably elevated in the low Zn compared to the control Zn group ($22.6 \pm 0.5\%$ and $18.5 \pm 0.5\% \ w/w$, respectively, $p < 0.001$). This study demonstrated that the erythrocyte LA:DGLA is able to differentiate zinc status between zinc-adequate and zinc-deficient subjects. Furthermore, variations in the LA:DGLA ratio were noticeable within seven days, signifying that this biomarker can show changes in the dietary Zn status quickly and that it may be able to detect early stages of Zn deficiency that usually, due to the lack of obvious signs and symptoms, pass unrecognized.

This proposed biomarker has been evaluated further in humans [71]. A study was completed on healthy human volunteers, 25–55 years of age. The content of plasma phospholipid LA, DGLA, and changes in the LA:DGLA ratio were compared to the dietary Zn intake and plasma Zn status in human subjects. Participants were separated into two groups based on dietary Zn intakes, assessed using three 24-h recall questionnaires provided on three non-consecutive days. There were no statistically significant differences in the dietary intake of LA and PUFA among the groups of participants. Plasma phospholipid fatty acid analysis was conducted by gas chromatography, and plasma analysis of minerals was conducted by atomic absorption spectrometry.

In addition, the study assessed correlations of plasma Zn and the LA:DGLA ratio with various biochemical, anthropometrical, and hematological parameters. It was shown that while the plasma Zn concentrations of participants remained unchanged (most likely due to the good homeostatic regulation), there was a statistically significant difference in DGLA production and the LA:DGLA ratio between the groups ($p < 0.05$). The concentration of plasma DGLA was decreased and the LA:DGLA ratio was increased in people with lower dietary Zn intakes. Besides, docosatetraenoic acid (22:4n-6; D5D) was also lower in the group of people with lower dietary Zn intake.

Finally, the efficacy of the LA:DGLA ratio to predict the Zn status of subjects consuming a wheat-based diet, a diet more representative of a diet of the target Zn-deficient populations, was recently evaluated in vivo by using the *Gallus gallus* model [72]. Two groups of birds ($n = 15$) were fed two different diets, a "high-Zn" diet (46.5 ppm Zn) and a "low-Zn" diet (32.8 ppm Zn), for six weeks. Dietary zinc intake, body weight, serum zinc, and the erythrocyte fatty acid profile were assessed. Serum zinc concentrations were greater in the high-Zn group ($p < 0.05$). Similarly, the concentration of Zn in tissues (feather and nail) was higher in the high-Zn group of birds as opposed to the birds fed a low-Zn diet ($p < 0.05$). Duodenal mRNA expression of various Zn transporters (i.e., Zip4, Zip6, Zip9, ZnT1, Znt5 and Znt7) demonstrated a higher mean value in the tissues collected from the birds fed a low-Zn diet ($n = 15$, $p < 0.05$). The measurements of hepatic Δ6 desaturase expression showed significant differences between the groups, with a higher mean value in birds fed high-Zn diets. The LA:DGLA ratio was higher in the low-Zn group of birds at all time points measured (weeks 2, 4, and 6). Once more, the LA:DGLA ratio responded to changes in dietary Zn intake. Even though both groups of birds were fed Zn-deficient diets, with only 14 ppm differential in dietary Zn content, still the LA:DGLA ratio differentiated clearly between the groups, which demonstrates the sensitivity of the biomarker to change in accordance with dietary Zn intake.

6. Conclusions and Recommendations for Further Research

The evidence provided in this review demonstrate the potential of the LA:DGLA ratio to be used as an additional biomarker of Zn status in humans. To date, research shows that the LA:DGLA ratio corresponds to dietary Zn manipulations, both in animals and humans. This biomarker should be tested and evaluated further to illuminate its full potential. This review provides some evidence to justify the requirements for further research.

Well-controlled human dietary intervention trials are needed to examine the sensitivity of this biomarker in larger healthy cohorts, as well as in Zn-deficient populations. Hence, additional research is needed to elucidate any potential limitations of this biomarker, i.e., the effect of inflammatory conditions and infection states on this biomarker. Similarly, the enzymatic activity of hepatic desaturases should be compared to the expression and activity of Δ6 desaturases in non-hepatic tissues in order to determine the exact role of dietary fats in Δ6 desaturase activity. Additional studies are needed to clarify the potential impact of other nutrient deficiencies on the LA:DGLA ratio, in particular the effect of iron and copper deficiencies. The effectiveness of the LA:DGLA ratio, in relation to Zn status and Zn bioavailability over time, requires further investigation. The kinetics of other desaturase enzymes in relation to Zn intake should also be tested (i.e., Δ5 desaturase). Finally, the modifications of Zn-dependent proteins and genes at the main sites of Zn absorption, namely, in the small intestine, in relation to Zn intake and the LA:DGLA ratio need to be tested and evaluated further.

Acknowledgments: Australian Postgraduate Award Scholarship was provided to the principle author. The financing organization had no role in the design, analysis or writing of this article.

Author Contributions: Marija Knez conducted the literature search, synthetized information, and wrote the manuscript and had primary responsibility for the final content. James C. R. Stangoulis, Maria Glibetic revised the final version of the paper. Elad Tako proofread the paper and provided constructive advice. All authors have proofread the manuscript and approved the final version of the paper.

Conflicts of Interest: The authors declare no conflict of interest.

References

1. Prasad, A.S.; Schulert, A.R.; Miale, A.; Farid, Z.; Sanstead, H.H. Zinc and iron deficiencies in male subjects with dwarfism and hypogonadism but without ancylostomiasis, schistosomiasis or severe anemia. *Am. J. Clin. Nutr.* **1963**, *12*, 437–444. [PubMed]
2. Wessells, K.R.; Brown, K.H. Estimating the global prevalence of zinc deficiency: Results based on zinc availability in national food supplies and the prevalence of stunting. *PLoS ONE* **2012**. [CrossRef] [PubMed]
3. Prasad, A.S. Discovery of human zinc deficiency: 50 years later. *J. Trace Elem. Med. Biol.* **2012**, *26*, 66–69. [CrossRef] [PubMed]
4. Cousins, R.J.; Liuzzi, J.P.; Lichten, L.A. Mammalian zinc transport, trafficking, and signals. *J. Biol. Chem.* **2006**, *281*, 24085–24089. [CrossRef] [PubMed]
5. King, J.C.; Cousins, R.J. Zinc. In *Modern Nutrition in Health and Disease*, 10th ed.; Shils, M.E., Shike, M., Eds.; Lippincott Williams and Wilkins: Baltimore, MD, USA, 2006; pp. 271–285.
6. Lowe, N.M.; Fekete, K.; Decsi, T. Methods of assessment of zinc status in humans: A systematic review. *Am. J. Clin. Nutr.* **2009**, *89*, 2040S–2051S. [CrossRef] [PubMed]
7. King, J.C.; Brown, K.H.; Gibson, R.S.; Krebs, N.F.; Lowe, N.M.; Siekmann, J.H.; Raiten, D.J. Biomarkers of nutrition for development (bond)-zinc review. *J. Nutr.* **2016**. [CrossRef] [PubMed]
8. Lowe, N.M. Assessing zinc in humans. *Curr. Opin. Clin. Nutr. Metab. Care* **2016**, *16*, 321–327. [CrossRef] [PubMed]
9. Lowe, N.M.; Dykes, F.C.; Skinner, A.L.; Patel, S.; Warthon-Medina, M.; Decsi, T.; Fekete, K.; Souverein, O.W.; Dullemeijer, C.; Cavelaars, A.E.; et al. Eurreca-estimating zinc requirements for deriving dietary reference values. *Crit. Rev. Food Sci. Nutr.* **2013**, *53*, 1110–1123. [CrossRef] [PubMed]
10. Bailey, A.L.; Maisey, S.; Southon, S.; Wright, A.J.A.; Finglas, P.M.; Fulcher, R.A. Relationships between micronutrient intake and biochemical indicators of nutrient adequacy in a 'free-living' elderly UK population. *Br. J. Nutr.* **1997**, *77*, 225–242. [CrossRef] [PubMed]
11. Paknahad, Z.; Mahdavi, R.; Mahboob, S.; Ghaemmaghami, S.J.; Omidvar, N. Iron and zinc nutritional and biochemical status and their relationship among child bearing women in marand province. *Pak. J. Nutr.* **2007**, *6*, 672–675. [CrossRef]
12. Sian, L.; Mingyan, X.; Miller, L.V.; Tong, L.; Krebs, N.F.; Hambidge, K.M. Zinc absorption and intestinal losses of endogenous zinc in young chinese women with marginal zinc intakes. *Am. J. Clin. Nutr.* **1996**, *63*, 348–353. [PubMed]
13. Bui, V.Q.; Marcinkevage, J.; Ramakrishnan, U.; Flores-Ayala, R.C.; Ramirez-Zea, M.; Villalpando, S.; Martorell, R.; DiGirolamo, A.M.; Stein, A.D. Associations among dietary zinc intakes and biomarkers of zinc status before and after a zinc supplementation program in guatemalan schoolchildren. *Food Nutr. Bull.* **2013**, *34*, 143–150. [PubMed]
14. Johnson, P.E.; Hunt, C.D.; Milne, D.B.; Mullen, L.K. Homeostatic control of zinc metabolism in men: Zinc excretion and balance in men fed diets low in zinc. *Am. J. Clin. Nutr.* **1993**, *57*, 557–565. [PubMed]
15. Iskra, M.; Majewski, W. Copper and zinc concentrations and the activities of ceruloplasmin and superoxide dismutase in atherosclerosis obliterans. *Biol. Trace Elem. Res.* **2000**, *73*, 55–65. [PubMed]
16. King, J.C.; Shames, D.M.; Woodhouse, L.R. Zinc homeostasis in humans. *J. Nutr.* **2000**, *130*, 1360S–1366S. [PubMed]
17. De Gier, B.; Mpabanzi, L.; Vereecken, K.; van der Werff, S.D.; D'Haese, P.C.; Fiorentino, M.; Khov, K.; Perignon, M.; Chamnan, C.; Berger, J.; et al. Height, zinc and soil-transmitted helminth infections in schoolchildren: A sdudy in cuba and cambodia. *Nutrients* **2015**, *7*, 3000–3010. [PubMed]
18. Gao, S.; Tu, D.N.; Li, H.; Cao, X.; Jiang, J.X.; Shi, Y.; Zhou, X.Q.; You, J.B. Relationship betwen zinc and the growth and development of young children. *Genet. Mol. Res.* **2015**, *14*, 9730–9738. [PubMed]
19. Koç, E.R.; Ilhan, A.; Zübeyde, A.; Acar, B.; Gürler, M.; Altuntaş, A.; Karapirli, M.; Bodur, A.S. A comparison of hair and serum trace elements in patients with alzheimer disease and healthy participants. *J. Med. Sci.* **2015**, *45*, 1034–1039.
20. Gmoshinskiĭ, I.V.; Munkhuu, B.; Mazo, V.K. Trace elements in human nutrition: Biological indices of zinc insufficiency. *Vopr. Pitan.* **2006**, *75*, 4–11. [PubMed]
21. Cho, H.P.; Nakamura, M.T.; Clarke, S.D. Cloning, expression, and nutritional regulation of the mammalian Δ-6 desaturase. *J. Biol. Chem.* **1999**, *274*, 471–477. [PubMed]

22. Nakamura, M.T.; Nara, T.Y. Structure, function, and dietary regulation of Δ6, Δ5, and Δ9 desaturases. *Ann. Rev. Nutr.* **2004**, *24*, 345–376. [CrossRef] [PubMed]
23. Ratnayake, W.M.; Galli, C. Fat and fatty acid terminology, methods of analysis and fat digestion and metabolism: A background review paper. *Ann. Nutr. Metab.* **2009**, *55*, 8–43. [CrossRef] [PubMed]
24. Kris-Etherton, P.M.; Hecker, K.D.; Binkoski, A.E. Polyunsaturated fatty acids and cardiovascular health. *Nutr. Rev.* **2004**, *62*, 414–426. [CrossRef] [PubMed]
25. Meesapyodsuk, D.; Qui, X. The front-end desaturase: Structure, function, evolution and biotechnological use. *Lipids* **2012**, *47*, 227–237. [CrossRef] [PubMed]
26. Reddy, A.S.; Nuccio, M.L.; Gross, L.M.; Thomas, T.L. Isolation of a Δ6-desaturase gene from the cyanobacterium *Synechocystis* sp. Strain PCC 6803 by gain-of-function expression in *Anabaena* sp. strain PCC 7120. *Plant Mol. Biol.* **1993**, *22*, 293–300. [CrossRef] [PubMed]
27. Sayanova, O.; Smith, M.A.; Lapinskas, P.; Stobart, A.K.; Dobson, G.; Christie, W.W.; Shewry, P.R.; Napier, J.A. Expression of a borage desaturase cDNA containing an N-terminal cytochrome b_5 domain results in the accumulation of high levels of Δ6-desaturated fatty acids in transgenic tobacco. *Proc. Natl. Acad. Sci. USA* **1997**, *94*, 4211–4216. [CrossRef] [PubMed]
28. Thomas, T.L.; Reddy, A.S.; Nuccio, M.; Nunberg, A.N.; Freyssinet, G. Production of Gamma-Linolenic Acid by a Delta6-Desaturase. U.S. Patent CA2207906 A1, 11 July 1997; Volume 4, pp. 736–866.
29. Lee, J.M.; Lee, H.; Kang, H.; Park, J.W. Fatty acid desaturases, polyunsaturated fatty acid regulation, and biotechnological advances. *Nutrients* **2016**. [CrossRef] [PubMed]
30. Sayanova, O.; Beaudoin, F.; Libisch, B.; Castel, A.; Shewry, P.R.; Napier, J.A. Mutagenesis and heterologous expression in yeast of a plant Δ6-fatty acid desaturase. *J. Exp. Bot.* **2001**, *52*, 1581–1585. [CrossRef] [PubMed]
31. Los, D.; Murata, N. Structure and expression of fatty acid desaturases. *Lipids Lipid Metab.* **1998**, *1*, 3–15. [CrossRef]
32. Aguilar, P.S.; de Mendoza, D. Control of fatty acid desaturation: A mechanism conserved from bacteria to humans. *Mol. Microbiol.* **2006**, *62*, 1507–1514. [CrossRef] [PubMed]
33. Chvapil, M.; Ludwig, J.C.; Sipes, I.G.; Halladay, S.C. Inhibition of NADPH oxidation and related drug oxidation in liver microsomes by zinc. *Biochem. Pharmacol.* **1976**, *25*, 1787–1791. [CrossRef]
34. Cunnane, S.C.; Krieger, I. Long chain fatty acids in serum phospholipids in acrodermatitis enteropathica before and after zinc treatment: A case report. *J. Am. Coll. Nutr.* **1988**, *7*, 249–255. [CrossRef] [PubMed]
35. Ludwig, J.C.; Misiorowski, R.L.; Chvapil, M.; Seymour, M.D. Interaction of zinc irons with electron carrying NADPH and NADH. *Chem. Biol. Interact.* **1980**, *30*, 25–34. [CrossRef]
36. Vallee, B.L.; Falchuk, K.H. The biochemical basis of zinc physiology. *Physiol. Rev.* **1993**, *73*, 79–118. [PubMed]
37. Guillou, H.; D'Andrea, S.; Rioux, V.; Barnouin, R.; Dalaine, S.; Pedrono, F.; Jan, S.; Legrand, P. Distinct roles of endoplasmic reticulum cytochrome b5 and fused cytochrome b5-like domain for rat Δ6-desaturase activity. *J. Lipid Res.* **2004**, *45*, 32–40. [CrossRef] [PubMed]
38. Sayanova, O.; Beaudoin, F.; Libisch, B.; Shewry, P.; Napier, J. Mutagenesis of the borage Δ6 fatty acid desaturase. *Biochem. Soc. Trans.* **2000**, *28*, 636–638. [CrossRef] [PubMed]
39. Sharif, R.; Thomas, P.; Zalewski, P.; Fenech, M. The role of zinc in genomic stability. *Mutat. Res.* **2012**, *733*, 111–121. [CrossRef] [PubMed]
40. Arnold, E.; Pinkham, M.S.; Votolato, N. Does zinc moderate essential fatty acid and amphetamine treatment of attention deficit hyperactivity disorder? *J. Child Adolesc. Pcychopharmacol.* **2000**, *10*, 111–117. [CrossRef] [PubMed]
41. Horrobin, D.F.; Cunnane, S.C. Interactions between zinc, essential fatty acids and prostaglandins: Relevance to acrodermatitis enteropathica, total parenteral nutrition, the glucagonoma syndrome, diabetes, anorexia nervosa and sickle cell syndrome. *Med. Hypotheses* **1980**, *6*, 277–296. [CrossRef]
42. Ayala, S.; Brenner, R.R. Essential fatty acid status in zinc deficiency. Effect on lipid and fatty acid composition, desaturation activity and structure of microsomal membranes of rat liver and testes. *Acta Physiol. Lat. Am.* **1983**, *33*, 193–204. [PubMed]
43. Bettger, W.J.; Reeves, P.G.; Moscatelli, E.A.; Reynolds, G.; O'Dell, B.L. Interaction of zinc and essential fatty acids in the rat. *J. Nutr.* **1979**, *109*, 480–488. [PubMed]
44. Eder, K.; Kirchgessner, M. Zinc deficiency and activities of lipogenic and glycolytic enzymes in liver of rats fed coconut oil or linseed oil. *Lipids* **1995**, *30*, 63–69. [CrossRef] [PubMed]

45. Clejan, S.; Castro-Magana, M.; Collip, P.J.; Jonas, E.; Maddalah, V.T. Effects of zinc deficiency and castration on fatty acid composition and desaturation in rats. *Lipids* **1982**, *17*, 129–135. [CrossRef] [PubMed]

46. Cunnane, S.C.; Horrobin, D.F.; Manku, M.S. Essential fatty acids in tissue phospholipids and triglycerides of the zinc-deficient rat. *Exp. Biol. Med.* **1984**, *177*, 441–446. [CrossRef]

47. Eder, K.; Kirchgessner, M. Zinc deficiency and the desaturation of linoleic acid in rats force-fed fat-free diets. *Biol. Trace Elem. Res.* **1996**, *54*, 173–183. [CrossRef] [PubMed]

48. Fogerty, A.C.; Ford, G.L.; Dreosti, I.E.; Tinsley, I.J. Zinc deficiency and fatty acid composition of tissue lipids. *Nutr. Rep. Int.* **1985**, *32*, 1009–1019.

49. Kramer, T.R.; Priske-Anderson, M.; Johnson, S.B.; Holman, A.T. Influence of reduced food intake on polyunsaturated fatty acid metabolism in zinc-deficient rats. *J. Nutr.* **1984**, *114*, 1224–1230. [PubMed]

50. Kudo, N.; Nakagawa, Y.; Waku, K. Effects of zinc deficiency on the fatty acid composition and metabolism in rats fed a fat-free diet. *Biol. Trace Elem. Res.* **1990**, *24*, 49–60. [CrossRef] [PubMed]

51. Roth, H.P.; Kirchgessner, M. Influence of zinc deficiency on the osmotic fragility of erythrocyte membranes of force-fed rats. *J. Trace Elem. Electrolytes* **1994**, *1*, 46–50.

52. Cunnane, S.C.; Huang, Y.S. Incorporation of dihomogamma linolenic acid into tissue lipids in zinc deficiency. In *V International Confernce on Prostaglandins*; Fondazione Giovanni Lorenzini: Florence, Italy, 1982.

53. Cunnane, S.C.; Wahle, K.W. Zinc deficiency increases the rate of delta 6 desaturation of linoleic acid in rat mammary tissue. *Lipids* **1981**, *16*, 771–774. [CrossRef] [PubMed]

54. Cunnane, S.C.; Wahle, K.W. Differential effects of zinc deificiency on delta 6 desaturase activity and fatty acid composition of various tissues in lactating rats. In *XII International Congress on Nutrition*; Nutrition Today: San Diego, CA, USA, 1981.

55. Eder, K.; Kirchgessner, M. The effect of isolated zinc deficiency on parameters of lipid and protein metabolism in rats fed a diet with coconut oil or fish oil. *J. Trace Elem. Electrolytes* **1994**, *11*, 55–60.

56. Eder, K.; Kirchgessner, M. Dietary fat influences the effect of zinc deficiency on liver lipids and faty acids in rats force-fed equal quantities of diet. *J. Nutr.* **1994**, *124*, 1917–1924. [PubMed]

57. Waldhauser, K.; Eder, K.; Kirchgessner, M. The activity of hepatic lysophospholipid acyltransferase in zinc-deficient rats. *J. Anim. Physiol. Anim. Nutr.* **1999**, *81*, 103–112. [CrossRef]

58. Brenner, R.R. *The Role of Fats in Human Nutrition*; Vergroesen, A.J., Crawford, M., Eds.; Academic Press: San Diego, CA, USA, 1989.

59. Scott, B.L.; Bazan, N.G. Membrane docosahexaenoate is supplied to the developing brain and retina by the liver. *Proc. Natl. Acad. Sci. USA* **1989**, *86*, 2903–2907. [CrossRef] [PubMed]

60. Cunnane, S.C. Essential fatty acid/mineral interactions with reference to the pig. In *Fatis in Animal Nutrition*; Wiseman, J., Ed.; Butterworths: London, UK, 1990; pp. 167–185.

61. Hamilton, R.M.; Gillespie, C.T.; Cook, H.W. Relationships between levels of essential fatty acids and zinc in plasma of cystic fibrosis patients. *Lipids* **1981**, *16*, 374–376. [CrossRef] [PubMed]

62. Horrobin, D.F. Loss of delta-6-desaturase activity as a key factor in aging. *Med. Hypotheses* **1981**, *7*, 1211–1220. [CrossRef]

63. Huang, Y.; Cunnane, S.C.; Horrobin, D.F.; Davignon, J. Most biological effects of zinc deficiency corrected by γ-linolenic acid (18:3ω6) but not by linoleic acid (18:2ω6). *Arterosclerosis* **1982**, *41*, 193–207. [CrossRef]

64. Cunnane, S.C.; Yang, J. Zinc deficiency impairs whole-body accumulation of polyunsaturates and increases the utilisation of linoleate for de novo synthesis in pregnant rats. *J. Physiol. Pharmacol.* **1995**, *73*, 1246–1252. [CrossRef]

65. Odutuga, A.A. Effects of low-zinc status and essential fatty acid deficiency on growth and lipid composition of rat brain. *Clin. Exp. Pharmacol. Physiol.* **1982**, *9*, 213–221. [CrossRef] [PubMed]

66. Reed, S.; Qin, X.; Ran-Ressler, R.; Brenna, J.T.; Glahn, R.P.; Tako, E. Dietary zinc deficiency affects blood linoleic acid: Dihomo-gamma-linolenic acid (LA:DGLA) ratio; a sensitive physiological marker of zinc status in vivo (*Gallus gallus*). *Nutrients* **2014**, *6*, 1164–1180. [CrossRef] [PubMed]

67. Hulbert, A.J. Exlaning longevity of different animals: Is membrane fatty acid composition the missing link? *Age* **2008**, *30*, 89–97. [CrossRef] [PubMed]

68. Burrell, A.L.; Dozier, W.A.; Davis, A.J.; Compton, M.M.; Freeman, M.E.; Vendrell, P.F.; Ward, T.L. Responses of broilers to dietary zinc concentrations and sources in relation to environmental implications. *Br. Poult. Sci.* **2004**, *45*, 255–263. [CrossRef] [PubMed]

69. Reed, S.M.; Neuman, H.; Moskovitch, S.; GlSahn, R.P.; Koren, O.; Tako, E. Chronic zinc deficiency alters chick gut microbiota composition and function. *Nutrients* **2015**, *7*, 1–17. [CrossRef] [PubMed]

70. Wang, X.B.; Fosmire, G.J.; Gay, C.V.; Leach, R.M., Jr. Short-term zinc deficiency inhibits chondrocyte proliferation and induces cell apoptosis in the epiphyseal growth plate of young chickens. *J. Nutr.* **2002**, *132*, 665–673. [PubMed]

71. Knez, M.; Stangoulis, J.C.R.; Zec, M.; Debeljak-Martacic, J.; Pavlovic, Z.; Gurinovic, M.; Glibetic, M. An initial evaluation of newly proposed biomarker of zinc status in humans-linoleic acid: Dihomo-γ-linolenic acid (LA:DGLA) ratio. *Clin. Nutr. ESPEN* **2016**, *15*, 85–92. [CrossRef] [PubMed]

72. Knez, M.; Tako, E.; Raymond, P.G.; Kolba, N.; de Courcy Ireland, E.; Stangoulis, J.C.R. The linoleic acid: dihomo-γ-linolenic acid ratio predicts the efficacy of Zn biofortified wheat in *Gallus gallus*. *Nutrients* **2017**. under review.

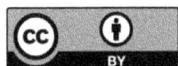

nutrients

MDPI

Article

Chronic High Dose Zinc Supplementation Induces Visceral Adipose Tissue Hypertrophy without Altering Body Weight in Mice

Xiaohua Huang [1,2,†], **Dandan Jiang** [1,†], **Yingguo Zhu** [1], **Zhengfeng Fang** [1], **Lianqiang Che** [1], **Yan Lin** [1], **Shengyu Xu** [1], **Jian Li** [1], **Chao Huang** [3], **Yuanfeng Zou** [3], **Lixia Li** [3], **De Wu** [1,2,*] and **Bin Feng** [1,2,*]

[1] Animal Nutrition Institute, Sichuan Agricultural University, Chengdu 611130, China;
    hxh3028@163.com (X.H.); dandanjiang17@163.com (D.J.); yingguozhu@outlook.com (Y.Z.);
    zfang@sicau.edu.cn (Z.F.); clianqiang@hotmail.com (L.C.); able588@163.com (Y.L.);
    shengyu_x@hotmail.com (S.X.); lijian522@hotmail.com (J.L.)
[2] Key Laboratory of Animal Disease-Resistant Nutrition of Ministry of Education, Sichuan Agricultural
    University, Chengdu 611130, China
[3] College of Veterinary Medicine, Sichuan Agricultural University, Chengdu 611130, China;
    huangchao@sicau.edu.cn (C.H.); yuanfengzou@sicau.edu.cn (Y.Z.); lilixia905@163.com (L.L.)
*   Correspondence: wude@sicau.edu.cn (D.W.); fengbin@sicau.edu.cn (B.F.);
    Tel.: +86-28-8629-0990 (D.W.); +86-28-8629-0922 (B.F.)
†   These authors contributed equally to this work.

Received: 1 September 2017; Accepted: 12 October 2017; Published: 18 October 2017

Abstract: The trace element zinc plays an important role in human life. Zinc deficiency impairs growth, reproduction, metabolism and immunity in both human and animals. Thus, zinc supplementation is recommended in daily life. However, the effect of long-term chronic zinc supplementation on adipose homeostasis has not been well elucidated. In the current study, mice were supplemented with zinc sulfate in the drinking water for 20 weeks. The results suggested that chronic zinc supplementation impaired systemic glucose clearance after exogenous insulin or glucose challenges, as compared to the control mice. Further study revealed that chronic zinc supplementation made no difference to body weight, but increased visceral adipose tissue weight and adipocyte size. In addition, gene expression of leptin and IL6 in the visceral adipose tissue of zinc-supplemented mice were higher than those of control mice. Moreover, serum level of leptin of the zinc-supplemented mice was twice as high as that of the control mice. Besides, phosphorylation level of AKT T308 was attenuated in the perirenal adipose tissue of zinc-supplemented mice. In comparison, the expression of macrophage marker genes and lipogenic genes were not affected by chronic zinc supplementation, but the protein levels of FAS and SCD1 decreased or tended to decrease in the perirenal adipose tissue of zinc-supplemented mice, as compared to the control mice. Our findings suggest that chronic high dose zinc supplementation induces visceral adipose tissue hypertrophy and impairs AKT signaling in perirenal adipose tissue.

Keywords: zinc; visceral adipose tissue; hypertrophy; glucose clearance; leptin; IL6; AKT

1. Introduction

The trace element zinc is essential for human health as it plays an important role in growth, immunity, reproduction, inflammation, metabolism and gastrointestinal function [1–5]. Notably, zinc deficiency induces metabolic diseases, such as non-alcoholic fatty liver disease (NAFLD), insulin resistance, adipose tissue inflammation and hyperglycemia [6–8]. Zinc displays an insulin-like character, which can stimulate cellular insulin signaling [9]. Short-term zinc supplementation reduces blood glucose level in individuals with obesity and type 2 diabetes [10–12], as well as reverses alcohol-induced steatosis [13]. Moreover, it is also reported that zinc stimulates the adipose differentiation of preadipocytes in vitro [14]. Besides, Zhang et al. reported that zinc supplementation induced intramuscular adipocytes content in weaned piglets [15].

Adipose tissue is a storage pool for excess energy, while triglyceride is the major source of energy in adipose tissue [16]. On the one hand, when energy intake is in excess, adipocytes uptake glucose and lipids from the blood stream to synthetize triglyceride, which is subsequently stored in adipocytes, in a process known as lipogenesis. On the other hand, when the body is in a negative energy balance state, triglyceride is mobilized by hormones to release free fatty acid (FFA) and glycerol into the blood stream, which is also known as lipolysis. FFA is subsequently used by the body as an energy source, while glycerol is used for gluconeogenesis [17]. Additionally, adipose tissue is a major endocrine organ, which secretes cytokines and adipokines, including adiponectin, leptin, monocyte chemotactic protein 1 (MCP1), interleukin 6 (IL6) and tumor necrosis factor alpha (TNFα) [18]. Furthermore, adipose tissue is a target organ of insulin, which stimulates the glucose uptake and lipogenesis while inhibiting the lipolysis in adipocytes. Notably, the insulin sensitivity of adipocytes can be regulated by cytokines, trace elements and drugs [19]. Increased lipogenesis or decreased lipolysis results in adipocyte hypertrophy, which subsequently induces the secretion of inflammatory cytokines and impairs insulin sensitivity of adipose tissue [20]. Afterwards, the reduced insulin sensitivity of adipose tissue breaks the balance of systemic glucose metabolism, which manifests as hyperglycemia, insulin resistance and glucose intolerance [21,22].

Lipogenesis is regulated by lipogenic enzymes, such as fatty acid synthase (FAS), stearoyl-CoA desaturase-1 (SCD1) and acetyl-CoA carboxylase 1 (ACC1), whose expression is up-regulated by peroxisome proliferator-activated receptor gamma (PPARγ), CCAAT-enhancer-binding protein alpha (C/BPα) and sterol-regulatory element binding protein (SREBP1). In comparison, hormone-sensitive lipase (HSL) is the rate-limiting enzyme for lipolysis [17,23,24]. In vitro study has revealed that a high zinc level in the medium stimulates the expression of *SREBP1*, *FAS*, *SCD1* and *ACC1* in hepatocytes [25]. Moreover, in vivo study also demonstrates that zinc supplementation for 40 days increases the expression of *PPARγ*, *SREBP1*, *FAS*, *SCD1* and *ACC1*, while decreasing the expression of *HSL* in the intramuscular fat tissue [15]. However, the effects of long-term chronic zinc supplementation on fat metabolism in visceral adipose tissue have not been well elucidated.

In the current study, mice were supplemented with zinc sulfate in the drinking water for over 20 weeks. The results indicated that, as compared to the control group, chronic zinc supplementation increased serum zinc concentration, impaired systemic glucose clearance, increased visceral adipose tissue weight and adipocyte size, as well as stimulated the expression and secretion of leptin in visceral adipose tissue. In addition, phosphorylation level of protein kinase B (AKT) and protein levels of FAS and SCD1 were decreased in the zinc-supplemented perirenal adipose tissue. Our study suggested that long-term chronic over-dosage zinc intake might increase the risk of visceral adipose tissue hypertrophy.

2. Materials and Methods

2.1. Animal Study

Animal study protocol (MICE2015012, 7 October 2015) was reviewed and approved by the Animal Care and Use Committee of Sichuan Agricultural University. All animal procedures were performed according to the National Institutes of Health guide for the care and use of Laboratory animals. 3-week-old C57BL/6 male mice were obtained from Vital River Laboratory Animal Technology Co. Ltd. (Beijing, China). The mice were allowed one week of acclimation in a pathogen- free room at the temperature of 22 °C and the humidity of 60%. Subsequently, they were randomly divided into 2 groups according to similar average body weight. One group was given spring water, and the other was given 30 ppm zinc-supplemented spring water (Supplementary Table S1)

(132.4 mg/L zinc sulfate heptahydrate (Z0251, Sigma, Shanghai, China)). Both groups were fed with normal chow diet according to AIN93, which contained 38.3 ppm zinc (Supplementary Table S1) (Dashuo, Chengdu, China). Mice were free to access water and food. Food intake, water consumption, and body weight were measured every two weeks. At age of 25 weeks, mice were made to fast overnight. Body weight and tail-vein blood glucose levels (Blood glucose strips (5D-2) were purchased from Beijingyicheng, Beijing, China) were measured at 8 a.m. in the next morning. Then, mice were euthanized using carbon dioxide, followed by cervical dislocation. Serum was collected for further analysis. Perirenal and epididymal adipose tissue were rapidly dissected and weighed. One piece of fat tissue was fixed in 10% formalin for H&E, while the remaining was frozen at −80 °C for further analysis.

2.2. Insulin Tolerance Test and Glucose Tolerance Test

For insulin tolerance test (ITT), 20 weeks old mice were deprived of food in the morning. 6 h later, mice were injected intraperitoneally with 0.5 U/kg insulin (Novo Nordisk, Beijing, China). Tail-vein blood glucose levels were measured 0, 15, 30, 45, 60 and 90 min after insulin injection.

For glucose tolerance test (GTT), 23 weeks old mice were deprived of food for 14 h (overnight). The next morning, mice were intraperitoneally injected with 1.5 g/kg dextrose (G7021, Sigma, Shanghai, China). Tail-vein blood glucose levels were measured at 0, 15, 30, 45, 60 and 90 min after dextrose injection.

2.3. Zinc Content Analysis

Zinc contents in the water and feed and copper levels in the serum were measured using the method of flame atomic absorption spectrometry (ContrAA, Analytik Jena, Jena, Germany). Serum zinc concentration was measured with a zinc detection kit (E011, Nanjing Jiancheng Bioengineering Institute, Nanjing, China) according to the manufacturer's instruction.

2.4. Serum Metabolites Profile Analysis

Serum triglyceride and FFA levels were measured on an automatic biochemical analyzer (7020, HITACHI, Tokyo, Japan) with their analysis kits respectively according to the manufacturer's instructions. Triglyceride kit (CH0105151) was purchased from Muccura (Chengdu, China), and FFA kit (GS191Z) was obtained from Beijing Strong Biotechnologies (Beijing, China).

2.5. Serum Hormone Levels Measurement

Serum insulin levels were measured with a mouse insulin ultrasensitive ELISA kit (80-INSMSU, ALPCO, Salem, MA, USA) according to the manufacturer's instruction.

Serum leptin levels were measured with a mouse leptin ELISA kit (ezml-82, Millipore, Billerica, MA, USA) according to the manufacturer's instruction.

Serum IL6 and MCP1 levels were measured with the respected ELISA kits (431301 and 432701, BioLegend, San Diego, CA, USA) according to the manufacturer's instruction.

2.6. Fat Tissue Histology Staining

For H&E staining, fresh fat tissues were fixed in 10% formalin for 48 h, and then dehydrated and embedded in paraffin. Embedded tissues were sliced into 4 μm sections (RM2016, Leica, Shanghai, China). Sections were then dehydrated, stained with hematoxylin for 5 min, washed with ddH$_2$O, and stained with eosin for 2 min. The sections were then dehydrated and mounted with a neutral resin onto slides. Images were captured on a microscope (TS100, Nikon, Tokyo, Japan) with a CCD (DS-U3, Nikon, Tokyo, Japan) using imaging software (NIS-Elements F3.2, Nikon, Tokyo, Japan).

Cell area was measured with the software of ImageJ (National Institutes of Health, Bethesda, USA). Briefly, 16 images from 4 mice of each group were used for cell area measurement, and 10 cells which stood for the average cell size of each image were used to calculate the average cell size. The cell area of 160 cells in total for each group of each tissue was used for average cell area calculation.

2.7. Cell Culture

Cell culture and adipose differentiation were performed as previously reported [26]. Briefly, 3T3-L1 preadipocytes (CL-173, American Type Culture Collection, Manassas, VA, USA) were cultured in basic medium (DMEM medium (11995040, Gibco, Shanghai, China) supplemented with 10% fetal bovine serum (10099-141, Gibco, Shanghai, China), 100 U/mL penicillin and 100 µg/mL streptomycin (10378016, Gibco) at 37 °C and 5% CO_2. Once 75% confluence was reached, cells were subcultured into 12-well plate at 90% confluence. 2 days after 100% confluence, cells were treated with 1 µg/mL insulin (I5500, Sigma, Shanghai, China), 1 µM dexamethasone (D1881, Sigma, Shanghai, China) and 0.5 mM isobutyl methyl xanthine (IBMX) (I7018, Sigma, Shanghai, China) for 3 days. Cells were then maintained in 1 µg/mL insulin-supplemented basic medium. Medium was freshly changed 3 times in the next days. On day 9, fully differentiated adipocytes were washed 3 times with serum-free DMEM, followed by incubating in serum-free DMEM medium for 14 h. Cells were then treated with 50 µM zinc or the vehicle for 6 h.

2.8. RNA Extraction and Real-Time PCR

RNA extraction and real-time PCR were performed as previously reported [27]. Briefly, 100 mg fat tissue powder was homogenized in 1 mL Trizol Reagent (15596018, Invitrogen, Shanghai, China) and RNA was extracted in accordance with the manufacturer's instruction. The quality of RNA was assessed by agarose gel and the concentration was measured with a spectrophotometer (NanoDrop 2000, Thermo Scientific, Shanghai, China). 1 µg RNA was reverse-transcribed into cDNA with a reverse-transcription PCR kit according to the manufacturer's instructions (RR037A, Takara, Dalian, China). Real-time PCR was conducted on a quantitative-PCR machine (7900HT, ABI, Carlsbad, CA, USA) with Power SYBR Green RT-PCR reagents (4368702, Thermo Fisher Scientific, Shanghai, China). The following reagent amounts were used for each reaction: forward primer, 300 nM; reverse primer, 300 nM; cDNA sample, 20 ng. The conditions used for PCR were: 95 °C for 10 min for 1 cycle, and then 40 cycles of 95 °C for 15 s followed by 60 °C for 1 min. The real time PCR data was analyzed by the 2-delta delta CT method with *β-actin* as the reference. The sequences of the primers are listed below.

β-actin forward GGCTGTATTCCCCTCCATCG and reverse CCAGTTGGTAACAATGCCATGT; *FAS*, forward GGCTCTATGGATTACCCAAGC and reverse CCAGTGTTCGTTCCTCGGA; *SCD1*, forward CCTACGACAAGAACATTCAATCCC and reverse CAGGAACTCAGAAGCCCAAAGC; *CD11c*, forward CTGGATAGCCTTTCTTCTGCTG and reverse GCACACTGTGTCCGAACTCA; *F4/80*, forward TGACTCACCTTGTGGTCCTAA and reverse CTTCCCAGAATCCAGTCTTTCC; *MCP1*, forward TTAAAAACCTGGATCGGAACCAA and reverse GCATTAGCTTCAGATTTACGGGT; *Leptin*, forward GAGACCCCTGTGTCGGTTC and reverse CTGCGTGTGTGAAATGTCATTG; *IL6*, forward TAGTCCTTCCTACCCCAATTTCC and reverse TTGGTCCTTAGCCACTCCTTC; *Glut4*, forward ACCGGATTCCATCCCACAAG and reverse TCCCAACCATTGAGAAATGATGC; *PPARγ*, forward GGAAGACCACTCGCATTCCTT and reverse TCGCACTTTGGTATTCTTGGAG; *C/EBPα*, forward CAAGAACAGCAACGAGTACCG and reverse GTCACTGGTCAACTCCAGCAC; *SREBP1*, forward AACTGCCCATCCACCGACTC and reverse ATTGATAGAAGACCGGTAGCGC; *ACC1*, forward CGGACCTTTGAAGATTTTGTCAGG and reverse GCTTTATTCTGCTGGGTGAACTCTC; *PLIN*, forward CGTGGAGAGTAAGGATGTCAATG and reverse GGCTTCTTTGGTGCTGTTGTAG; *HSL*, forward TGAAGCCAAAGATGAAGTGAGAC and reverse CTTGACTATGGGTGACGTGTAGAG.

2.9. Western Blot Analysis

Western blot analysis was performed as previously reported [27]. For the preparation of protein lysates, 100 mg fat tissue powder was homogenized in 1 mL cell lysis buffer (P0013C, Beyotime

Biotechnology, Shanghai, China) supplemented with protease inhibitor cocktail (04693132001, Roche, Mannheim, Germany) on a homogenizer. The concentration of protein in the supernatant was measured with a BCA Protein Assay Kit (23250, Thermo, Shanghai, China). 100 µg protein was used to prepare an electrophoresis sample with loading buffer (1610747, BioRad, Shanghai, China) in a volume of 30 µL for each sample. Proteins were separated on 12% polyacrylamide gel, and then transferred onto PVDF membranes (1620177, BioRad, Shanghai, China). The membranes were blocked in 1% BSA/1 × TBST for 1 h at room temperature, followed by incubation with the appropriate primary antibodies (1 µg/mL) overnight. pAKT T308 (4056), AKT (9272), PPARγ (2443), pHSL (3891), SCD1 (2794) and tubulin (3873) antibodies were obtained from Cell Signaling Technology (Shanghai, China); HSL (sc-74489) and FAS (sc-48357) antibody was obtained from Santa Cruz (Shanghai, China). After thorough washing, membranes were incubated with appropriate horseradish peroxidase-linked secondary antibodies (7074 and 7076, CST) (1:2000 dilution in 5% milk/1 × TBST) for 1 h. After further thorough washing, protein signals were detected by ECL western blotting detection reagent (1705060, BioRad, Shanghai, China) on a Molecular Imager ChemiDoc XRS+ System (BioRad). Blots were quantified with ImageJ software (National Institutes of Health).

2.10. Statistical Analysis

Data were analyzed using the SAS 9.3 software (SAS Institute Inc., Cary, NC, USA). The normality and homogeneity of variances of data were firstly tested with univariate test. Independent t-test was used to compare the difference between two groups with normal distribution data, while non-Gaussian and heterogeneous data were analyzed using non-parametric analysis. One-way repeated measures ANOVA was used to analyze the statistical difference of water consumption, food intake, GTT and ITT; one-way ANOVA was applied to analyze the effect of zinc sulfate on gene expression in 3T3-L1 adipocytes, when two-way ANOVA was used to analyze the effect of insulin and zinc on AKT phosphorylation in 3T3-L1 adipocytes. Post-hoc analysis was then applied. Results were presented as mean ± SEM. Statistical significance was determined at $P < 0.05$.

3. Results

3.1. Chronic Zinc Supplementation Induced Glucose Intolerance

To investigate the effect of long-term chronic zinc supplementation on adipose metabolism, mice were supplemented with zinc sulfate in the drinking water for 20 weeks. Results showed that zinc-supplemented mice had comparable water consumption and food intake to those of control mice during the experimental period, except that zinc-supplemented mice consumed more water at the age of 9 than the control mice ($P = 0.0226$) (Supplementary Figure S1A,B and Tables S2 and S3). As was expected, serum zinc concentration in zinc-supplemented mice was significantly higher than that in the control mice ($P = 0.0017$) (Figure 1A and Supplementary Table S4). At the same time, serum copper levels were similar between the zinc-supplemented group and control group, while the zinc/copper ratio was higher in the zinc-supplemented mice than that in the control mice ($P = 0.0462$) (Supplementary Figure S1C,D and Table S4). Blood glucose level was then measured, which revealed that zinc-supplemented mice had similar blood glucose levels to the control mice at both fed and fasting state (Supplementary Figure S2A,B and Table S5). Moreover, serum insulin remained unchanged in zinc-supplemented mice compared with that in the control mice (Supplementary Figure S2C and Supplementary Table S6). However, zinc-supplemented mice had higher blood glucose levels after 6 h fasting and 45 min of exogenous insulin challenge, as compared to the control mice ($P = 0.0174$ and $P = 0.0429$) (Figure 1B and Supplementary Table S7). In addition, zinc-supplemented mice had slower glucose clearance rate ($P = 0.0318$) and higher blood glucose levels 30 and 90 min after exogenous glucose administration ($P = 0.0278$ and $P = 0.0131$) (Figure 1C and Supplementary Table S8). These data indicated that chronic high dose zinc supplementation in the drinking water did not affect basal blood glucose or insulin levels, but impaired systemic glucose clearance rate after exogenous insulin and glucose challenge.

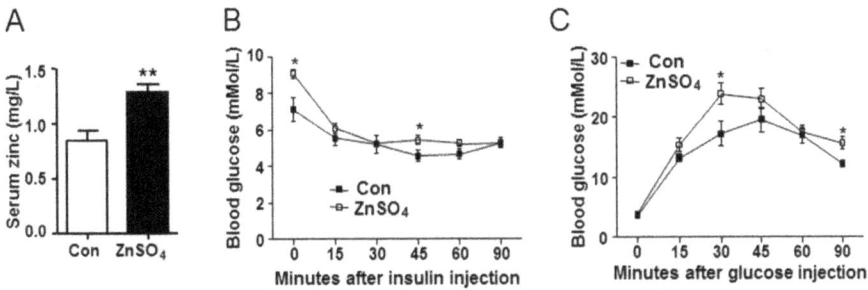

Figure 1. Chronic zinc supplementation impaired systemic insulin sensitivity and glucose clearance. (**A**) Serum zinc levels ($N = 8$ for each group) ($P = 0.0017$); (**B**) Insulin tolerance test ($P_{zinc} = 0.1007$; $P_{time} < 0.0001$; $P_{zincXtime} = 0.0012$; $P_0 = 0.0174$; $P_{45} = 0.0429$) ($N = 7$ for each group); (**C**) Glucose tolerance test ($P_{zinc} = 0.0318$; $P_{time} < 0.0001$; $P_{zincXtime} = 0.0621$; $P_{30} = 0.0278$; $P_{90} = 0.0131$) ($N = 7$ for each group). Data were shown as mean $\pm$ SEM. Con, control group; ZnSO$_4$, zinc sulfate-supplemented group. * $P < 0.05$, ** $P < 0.01$ ZnSO$_4$ vs. Con.

3.2. Chronic Zinc Supplementation Induced Visceral Adipose Tissue Hypertrophy

Effects of zinc supplementation on body weight and tissue weight was subsequently examined. Results showed that zinc-supplemented mice had similar body weight to that of control mice during the experiment and at the time of harvest (Supplementary Figure S2D, Figure 2A and Supplementary Tables S9 and S10). Further study indicated that liver weight and subcutaneous adipose tissue weight were not altered by zinc supplementation, as compared to those of the control (Supplementary Figure S2E,F and Table S10). However, the weight of perirenal adipose tissue was increased by 60% in the zinc-supplemented mice, while that of epididymal adipose tissue tended to increase by 26%, relative to those in the control mice ($P = 0.0143$ and $P = 0.0767$) (Figure 2B,C and Supplementary Table S10). Similar results were obtained in a repeated experiment with another cohort of mice (data not shown).

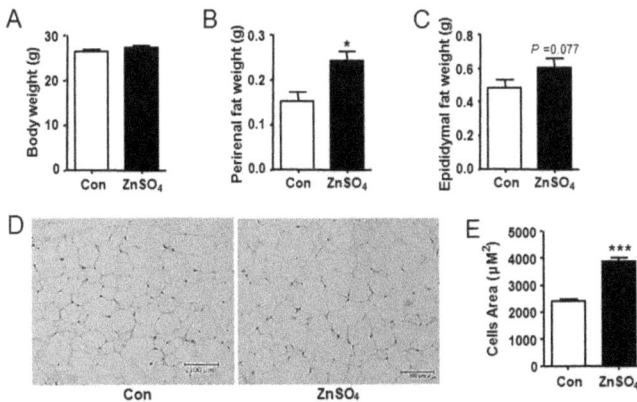

Figure 2. *Cont.*

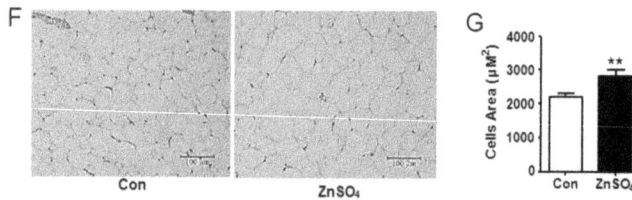

Figure 2. Chronic zinc supplementation induced visceral adipose tissue hypertrophy. (A) Body weight
(N = 8 for each group); (B) The weight of perirenal adipose tissue (N = 8 for each group) (P = 0.0143);
(C) The weight of epididymal adipose tissue (N = 8 for each group); (D) H&E staining images for
perirenal fat pad; (E) Adipocyte size of perirenal adipose tissue (N = 160 cells from 4 mice for each
group) (P < 0.0001); (F) H&E staining images for epididymal fat pad; (G) Adipocyte size of epididymal
adipose tissue (N = 160 cells from 4 mice for each group) (P = 0.0012). Scale bars were equal to 100 μm.
Data were shown as mean ± SEM. Con, control group; ZnSO₄, zinc sulfate-supplemented group.
* P < 0.05, ** P < 0.01, *** P < 0.001 ZnSO₄ vs. Con.

Both enlargement of adipocyte size and increase in adipocyte number result in adipose tissue
hypertrophy. Thus, H&E staining was thereby performed to analyze the cell morphology, the results
of which indicated that the adipocyte sizes of zinc-treated mice increased by 60% and 25% in perirenal
fat tissue and epididymal fat tissue respectively, compared with those in the control mice ($P < 0.0001$
and $P = 0.0012$) (Figure 2D–G and Supplementary Table S11). These data demonstrated that chronic
zinc supplementation induced visceral adipose tissue hypotrophy at least partially through enlarging
adipocyte size in lean mice.

3.3. Chronic Zinc Supplementation Stimulated the Expression and Secretion of Leptin in Visceral Adipose Tissue

The expression of adipokine and cytokine genes in the adipose tissue were analyzed.
Results indicated that both the expression of *leptin* and *IL6* were increased in the perirenal and
epididymal adipose tissue of zinc-supplemented mice as compared to those in the control mice
($P = 0.0329$, $P = 0.0297$, $P = 0.0328$ and $P = 0.0482$) (Figure 3A,B and Supplementary Figure S3A,B
and Tables S12 and S13). Moreover, serum levels of leptin and IL6 were subsequently analyzed,
the results of which showed that serum leptin level of zinc-supplemented mice was twice as high as
that of the control mice ($P = 0.0420$) (Figure 3C and Supplementary Table S6). However, serum level of
IL6 remained unchanged (Figure 3D and Supplementary Table S6).

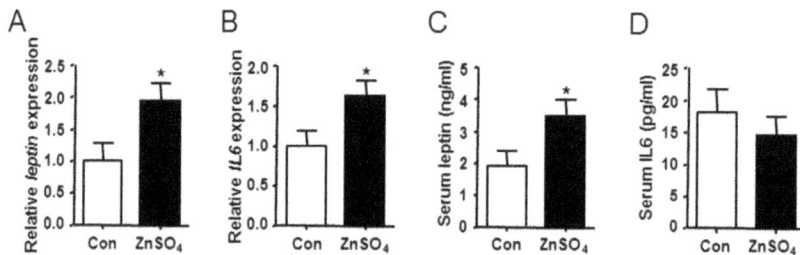

Figure 3. Chronic zinc supplementation stimulated the expression and secretion of leptin in perirenal
adipose tissue. (A) The expression of *leptin* in perirenal adipose tissue (P = 0.0216); (B) The expression
of IL6 in perirenal adipose tissue (P = 0.0297); (C) Serum leptin levels (P = 0.0420); (D) Serum
IL6 levels. N = 8 for each group. Data were shown as mean ± SEM. Con, control group; ZnSO₄,
zinc sulfate-supplemented group. * P < 0.05 ZnSO₄ vs. Con.

The effect of zinc on the expression of *leptin* and *IL6* in cultured adipocytes was also investigated. Results indicated that the expression of *leptin* and *IL6* were also increased by zinc sulfate or zinc chloride in cultured 3T3-L1 adipocytes (Supplementary Figure S4A–D and Tables S14 and S15).

3.4. Chronic Zinc Supplementation Attenuated AKT Phosphorylation in Perirenal Adipose Tissue

AKT signaling in the adipose tissue was subsequently detected. Results illustrated that the phosphorylation level of AKT T308 was outstandingly attenuated in the perirenal adipose tissue of zinc-supplemented mice compared with that of control mice ($P = 0.0040$), while that of AKT S473 remained unchanged (Figure 4A,B and Supplementary Table S16). However, phosphorylation level of either AKT T308 or S473 in the epididymal adipose tissue of zinc-supplemented mice was similar to that of control mice (Supplementary Figure S5A and Table S17). Meanwhile, the effect of zinc supplementation on AKT phosphorylation was also investigated in cultured adipocytes, the results of which revealed that zinc supplementation induced the phosphorylation of both AKT T308 and S473 in cultured adipocytes, both at basal and insulin-stimulating state (Supplementary Figure S5B and Table S18).

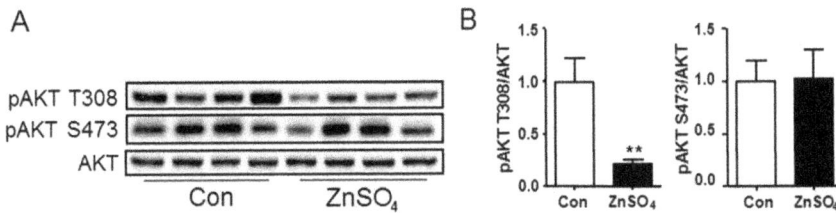

Figure 4. Chronic zinc supplementation attenuated the phosphorylation of AKT in perirenal adipose tissue. (**A**) Western blot bands of phosphorylation AKT and total AKT. Data represented 8 mice of 16 in total; (**B**) The quantification of phosphorylation AKT levels in perirenal adipose tissue ($N = 8$ for each group) ($P = 0.0040$ for pAKT T308). Data were shown as mean $\pm$ SEM. Con, control group; ZnSO$_4$, zinc sulfate-supplemented group. ** $P < 0.05$ ZnSO$_4$ vs. Con.

3.5. Chronic Zinc Supplementation Did Not Alter Macrophage Content in the Adipose Tissue

It was reported that chronic macrophage infiltration induced inflammation and hypertrophy of adipose tissue [28]. Thus, the expression of macrophage marker genes was analyzed, the results of which showed that the expression of *CD11c* and *F4/80* in the visceral adipose tissues of chronic zinc-supplemented mice remained unchanged, as compared to the control mice (Figure 5A, Supplementary Figure S3C and Tables S12 and S13). MCP1 was reported to stimulated adipose tissue to recruit macrophages [28]. However, the expression of *MCP1* in the visceral adipose tissue of zinc-supplemented mice was similar to that of the control mice (Figure 5B and Supplementary Figure S3D and Tables S12 and S13). Further analysis indicated that serum MCP1 level in the zinc-supplemented mice was also comparable to that in the control mice (Figure 5C and Supplementary Table S6). These data demonstrated that chronic zinc supplementation did not alter microphage content in the visceral adipose tissue.

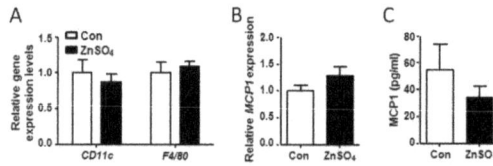

Figure 5. Chronic zinc supplementation did not alter the expression of macrophage marker genes and *MCP1* in perirenal adipose tissue. (**A**) The expression of *CD11c* and *F4/80* in perirenal adipose tissue; (**B**) The expression of *MCP1* in perirenal adipose tissue; (**C**) Serum MCP1 levels. Data were shown as mean ± SEM. Con, control group; ZnSO₄, zinc sulfate-supplemented group.

3.6. The Protein Levels of FAS and SCD1 Were Decreased in the Perirenal Adipose Tissue of Chronic Zinc-Supplemented Mice

As the adipose tissue weight and the adipocyte size were increased in the zinc-supplemented mice, the expression of fat metabolic genes was then investigated. Results suggested that the expression of glucose transporter 4 (*Glut4*), the main regulator for adipocyte glucose uptake, remained unchanged in the perirenal fat and epididymal fat of zinc-supplemented mice, as compared with those of control mice (Figure 6A, Supplementary Figure S6A and Tables S12 and S13). Besides, the expression of lipogenic genes and lipid droplets coating gene were unchanged by zinc supplementation, as compared with those of the control group (Figure 6B,C and Supplementary Figure S6B,C, Tables S12 and S13). Furthermore, protein level of PPAR γ in the perirenal fat tissue remained unchanged by zinc supplementation (Figure 6D and Supplementary Table S16). However, compared with control mice, the protein level of FAS ($P = 0.0006$) was significantly decreased and that of SCD1 ($P = 0.0723$) tended to decrease in the perirenal adipose tissue of zinc supplemented-mice (Figure 6D and Supplementary Table S16). Moreover, protein levels of FAS and SCD1 in epididymal adipose tissue of zinc-supplemented mice were similar to those of the control mice (data not shown).

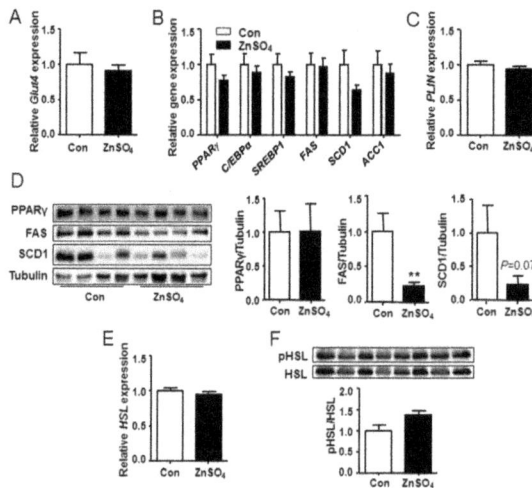

Figure 6. Chronic zinc supplementation did not alter the expression of lipogenic genes but decreased protein levels of FAS and SCD1 in perirenal adipose tissue. (**A**) The expression of *Glut4*; (**B**) The expression of lipogenic genes and their regulatory genes; (**C**) The expression of *PLIN*; (**D**) Protein levels of PPARγ, FAS and SCD1 ($P = 0.0006$ for FAS); (**E**) The expression of *HSL*; (**F**) Phosphorylation levels of HSL. $N = 8$ for each group. Data were shown as mean ± SEM. Western blots represented 8 mice of 16 in total. Con, control group; ZnSO₄, zinc sulfate-supplemented group. ** $P < 0.01$ ZnSO₄ vs. Con.

Both lipolysis and lipogenesis regulate adipose deposition in the adipose tissue [17]. Consequently, gene expression and protein phosphorylation levels of lipolysis regulator HSL were analyzed. Results showed that both gene expression and phosphorylation level of HSL in the visceral adipose tissue of zinc-supplemented mice were similar to those of the control mice (Figure 6E,F and Supplementary Figure S6D,E and Tables S12, S13, S16 and S17). These data indicated that lipolysis might be not affected by chronic zinc supplementation.

3.7. Chronic Zinc Supplementation Did Not Alter the Metabolic Profiles of Serum Lipids

Metabolic profiles of serum lipids were further investigated, which indicated that both serum TAG and serum FFA levels remained unchanged in the zinc-supplemented mice relative to those in the control mice (Figure 7A,B and Supplementary Table S19).

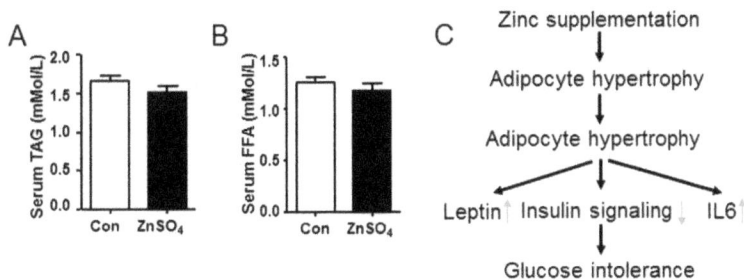

Figure 7. Chronic zinc supplementation did not affect serum levels of triglyceride and free fatty acid. (**A**) Serum triglyceride levels; (**B**) Serum free fatty acid levels; (**C**) The illustration of chronic zinc supplementation inducing adipose tissue hypertrophy. $N = 8$ for each group. Data were shown as mean $\pm$ SEM. Con, control group; ZnSO$_4$, zinc sulfate-supplemented group.

4. Discussion

It is reported that zinc stimulates insulin sensitivity and induces adipogenesis in adipocytes. However, it is shown in the current study that long-term chronic zinc supplementation in the drinking water impairs systemic glucose clearance rate, induces visceral adipocyte tissue hypertrophy and attenuates AKT signaling in perirenal adipose tissue. Meanwhile, zinc supplementation stimulates the expression of *leptin* and *IL6* in visceral adipose tissue while increasing serum leptin level (Figure 7C). Moreover, it is also found that protein levels of FAS and SCD1 are down-regulated in perirenal adipose tissue of chronic zinc-supplemented mice relative to those of control mice, though their gene expression are similar to those of control mice.

4.1. Correlation of Chronic Zinc Supplementation with Systemic Glucose Clearance

It has been reported that diet induced zinc deficiency impairs systemic insulin sensitivity, whereas acute zinc supplementation enhances insulin signaling and glucose deposition [29–31]. However, the study of Kim et al. has reported that zinc supplementation for eight weeks does not improve systemic insulin resistance in humans [32]. Besides, zinc supplementation for four weeks shows no effect on insulin sensitivity in healthy black and white early-adolescent girls [33]. Furthermore, ITT and GTT data of our study suggest that chronic zinc supplementation attenuates systemic insulin sensitivity and glucose clearance (Figure 1B,C). Further study on AKT phosphorylation levels indicates that chronic zinc supplementation attenuates AKT signaling in the perirenal adipose tissue (Figure 4), which may be the reason why chronic zinc supplementation impairs the systemic glucose clearance after exogenous insulin or glucose challenges as compared with the control group. Zinc stimulates insulin signaling in adipocytes (Supplementary Figure S5B), while acute zinc supplementation enhances insulin sensitivity in adipose tissue [31]. Thus, the impaired AKT signaling may be attributed to the secondary effect of adipose tissue hypertrophy (Figure 2). Difference in the effects of zinc supplementation on systemic insulin sensitivity and glucose clearance among different studies may be resulted from the different duration of zinc supplementation.

Increased blood glucose level stimulates the beta islet cells to secret insulin, which subsequently gives rise to insulin signaling in perirenal tissues, such as liver, adipose tissue and muscle. The induced insulin signaling stimulates glycogen synthesis in liver as well as stimulates glucose uptake in adipose tissue and muscle, thus reducing the blood glucose level to a normal level. On the other hand, the secretion of insulin in the beta islet cells is inhibited in the presence of low blood glucose level, whereas the secretion of glucagon is stimulated to induce glycogenolysis and gluconeogenesis. However, the glucose decreasing effect of insulin is diminished when the insulin sensitivity of perirenal tissue is impaired, which results in insulin resistance and hyperinsulinemia [34]. The results of insulin tolerance and glucose intolerance should be at least partially ascribed to the impaired insulin sensitivity of adipose tissue (Figure 1B,C), since the serum insulin levels are similar between the zinc-supplemented mice and the control mice (Figure S2C).

Blood glucose is mainly obtained from glycogenolysis in the first 12 h of fasting, while gluconeogenesis is the major source of blood glucose after 12 h of fasting [35]. Thus, the finding that zinc decreased the blood glucose levels after 6 h of fasting, but not at 14 h of fasting suggests that chronic zinc supplementation may impair glycogenolysis in the liver. However, the exact mechanism needs to be explored in future study.

4.2. Correlation of Chronic Zinc Supplementation with Adipose Accumulation in Visceral Adipose Tissue

Zinc is a stimulator for insulin signaling, which mimics several actions of insulin [31]. Ghosh et al. reported that zinc-chelated vitamin C stimulated the adipogenesis in preadipocytes [14]. In addition, it is demonstrated in the current study that long-term chronic zinc supplementation induces adipose accumulation of the visceral adipose tissue in mice (Figure 2). Zhang et al. reported that dietary zinc supplementation increased intramuscular adipose deposition in piglets, which supports our results [15]. Our data reveals that the expression of glucose transporter gene and lipogenic genes are not affected by chronic zinc supplementation (Figure 6A,B and Supplementary Figure S6A,B). Therefore, the increased adipose accumulation may be independent of lipogenesis at the time of harvest. At the same time, the expression and phosphorylation level of HSL remain unchanged in the visceral adipose tissue of zinc-supplemented mice (Figure 6E,F and Supplementary Figure S6D,E). Consequently, the increased adipose deposition is probably independent of lipolysis. Besides, serum TAG and FFA levels are similar in both control and zinc-supplemented mice (Figure 7), further supporting the observation that lipolysis in the visceral adipose tissue is not altered by chronic zinc supplementation. Thus, the increased adipogenesis at the early stage of zinc supplementation may lead to the hypertrophy of visceral adipose tissue at the late stage of zinc supplementation. Nevertheless, further study is needed to elucidate the exact mechanism by which mice accumulate more visceral adipose tissue than control mice after long-term chronic zinc supplementation.

Compared with control mice, the gene expression of *FAS* and *SCD1* remains unchanged in the chronic zinc-supplemented mice. Therefore, the decreased protein levels of FAS and SCD1 (Figure 6D) may be regulated by chronic high dose zinc supplementation in a post-translational manner. However, the precise mechanism by which chronic high dose zinc supplementation down-regulates the protein levels of FAS and SCD1 in adipose tissue remains to be elucidated in further studies.

4.3. Correlation of Chronic Zinc Supplementation with Adipokines and Cytokines

Leptin is one of the most abundant adipokines secreted by adipocytes [36], which is positively corelated with obesity, diabetes and insulin resistance [37]. The expression of leptin in the visceral adipose tissue, together with the serum leptin level, is remarkably increased in the chronic zinc-supplemented mice (Figure 3A,C). In addition, it is indicated in our in vitro study that zinc also stimulates the expression of leptin in 3T3-L1 adipocytes (Supplementary Figure S4A,B). These findings are supported by the report of Baltaci et al., which demonstrates that zinc deficiency for six weeks leads to decreased plasma leptin level, whereas zinc supplementation for six weeks significantly increases plasma leptin level [38]. In addition, Ott and Shay also reported that zinc deficiency reduced the expression and secretion of leptin in cultured rat adipocytes [39], which was similar to the findings of our study. However, it is also reported in some studies that short-term zinc supplementation reduces serum leptin level, whereas zinc deficiency for three weeks increases circulatory leptin level [7,40]. The contradictory results from different studies may be related to the duration of zinc deficiency or zinc supplementation. However, the exact mechanism by which zinc upregulates the expression of leptin should be elucidated in further studies.

Inflammation impairs the insulin sensitivity of adipose tissue [28,41]. The expression of IL6 is increased in the visceral adipose tissue of chronic zinc-supplemented mice (Figure 3B and Supplementary Figure S3B), which may also give rise to insulin intolerance in zinc-supplemented mice. Furthermore, macrophage infiltration into the adipose tissue also accounts for one of the causes of adipose inflammation and insulin resistance [28,41]. However, our findings demonstrate that chronic zinc supplementation does not alter macrophage content in the adipose tissue (Figure 5). In addition, leptin is reported to be a pro-inflammatory factor, which stimulates the expression of inflammatory factors [42]. This suggests that chronic zinc supplementation may stimulate the expression of inflammation factors (such as IL6) in adipocytes and macrophages through leptin.

Taken together, it is indicated in our study that chronic high dose zinc supplementation will increase the risk of visceral adipose tissue hypertrophy and systemic glucose intolerance. Thus, chronic high dose zinc supplementation may be harmful for health. Therefore, zinc supplementation should be carried out in controlled time and dosage. Moreover, further studies will be focused on the mechanism by which chronic zinc supplementation induces visceral adipose tissue hypertrophy as well as the different effects of short-term and long-term zinc supplementation on fat metabolism.

Supplementary Materials: The following are available online at www.mdpi.com/2072-6643/9/10/1138/s1, Figure S1: Water consumption and food intake of mice during the experiment; Figure S2: Blood glucose levels, body weight and tissue weight; Figure S3: Gene expression in epididymal adipose tissue; Figure S4: Gene expression in 3T3-L1 adipocytes; Figure S5: Phosphorylation levels of AKT in epididymal adipose tissue and 3T3-L1 adipocytes; Figure S6: The expression of fat metabolic genes in epididymal adipose tissue; Table S1: The concentration of zinc in the drinking water; and Tables S2–S19: Data for all the figures.

Acknowledgments: We thank Shiping Bai from Sichuan Agricultural University for the assistance in analyzing zinc and copper contents. Meanwhile, our thanks should also go to Heju Zhong from Sichuan Agricultural University for the help in statistical analysis. This study is supported by Educational Commission of Sichuan Province to B.F. (16ZA0023) and Chang Jiang Scholars Program from Chinese Ministry of Education to D.W. (T2012157). B.F. is a receipt of initial research funding from Sichuan Agricultural University and Thousand Talent Program from Sichuan Province.

Author Contributions: B.F., D.W., X.H. and D.J. conceived and designed the experiments; X.H., D.J., Y.Z., Z.F., L.C., Y.L., S.X. and J.L. performed the experiments; B.F., X.H., D.J., C.H., Y.Z., L.L. and D.W. analyzed the data; B.F. wrote the paper. All authors read and approved the final manuscript.

Conflicts of Interest: The authors declare no conflict of interest.

References

1. Myers, S.; Shastri, M.D.; Adulcikas, J.; Sohal, S.S.; Norouzi, S. Zinc and gastrointestinal disorders: A role for the zinc transporters Zips and ZnTs. *Curr. Pharm. Des.* **2017**, *23*, 2328–2332. [CrossRef] [PubMed]

2. Hojyo, S.; Fukada, T. Roles of Zinc Signaling in the Immune System. *J. Immunol. Res.* **2016**, *2016*, 6762343. [CrossRef] [PubMed]

3. Nissensohn, M.; Sanchez-Villegas, A.; Fuentes Lugo, D.; Henriquez Sanchez, P.; Doreste Alonso, J.; Pena Quintana, L.; Ruano, C.; Lowe, N.L.; Hall Moran, V.; Skinner, A.L.; et al. Effect of Zinc Intake on Growth in Infants: A Meta-analysis. *Crit. Rev. Food Sci. Nutr.* **2016**, *56*, 350–363. [CrossRef] [PubMed]

4. Bonaventura, P.; Benedetti, G.; Albarede, F.; Miossec, P. Zinc and its role in immunity and inflammation. *Autoimmun. Rev.* **2015**, *14*, 277–285. [CrossRef] [PubMed]

5. Cabrera, A.J. Zinc, aging, and immunosenescence: An overview. *Pathobiol. Aging Age Relat. Dis.* **2015**, *5*, 25592. [CrossRef] [PubMed]

6. Zhong, W.; Zhao, Y.; Sun, X.; Song, Z.; McClain, C.J.; Zhou, Z. Dietary zinc deficiency exaggerates ethanol-induced liver injury in mice: Involvement of intrahepatic and extrahepatic factors. *PLoS ONE* **2013**, *8*, e76522. [CrossRef] [PubMed]

7. Liu, M.J.; Bao, S.; Bolin, E.R.; Burris, D.L.; Xu, X.; Sun, Q.; Killilea, D.W.; Shen, Q.; Ziouzenkova, O.; Belury, M.A.; et al. Zinc deficiency augments leptin production and exacerbates macrophage infiltration into adipose tissue in mice fed a high-fat diet. *J. Nutr.* **2013**, *143*, 1036–1045. [CrossRef] [PubMed]

8. Fung, E.B.; Gildengorin, G.; Talwar, S.; Hagar, L.; Lal, A. Zinc status affects glucose homeostasis and insulin secretion in patients with thalassemia. *Nutrients* **2015**, *7*, 4296–4307. [CrossRef] [PubMed]

9. Cruz, K.J.; Morais, J.B.; de Oliveira, A.R.; Severo, J.S.; Marreiro, D.D. The Effect of Zinc Supplementation on Insulin Resistance in Obese Subjects: A Systematic Review. *Biol. Trace Elem. Res.* **2017**, *176*, 239–243. [CrossRef] [PubMed]

10. Umrani, R.D.; Paknikar, K.M. Zinc oxide nanoparticles show antidiabetic activity in streptozotocin-induced Type 1 and 2 diabetic rats. *Nanomed. Lond.* **2014**, *9*, 89–104. [CrossRef] [PubMed]

11. Shan, Z.; Bao, W.; Zhang, Y.; Rong, Y.; Wang, X.; Jin, Y.; Song, Y.; Yao, P.; Sun, C.; Hu, F.B.; et al. Interactions between zinc transporter-8 gene (SLC30A8) and plasma zinc concentrations for impaired glucose regulation and type 2 diabetes. *Diabetes* **2014**, *63*, 1796–1803. [CrossRef] [PubMed]

12. Khan, M.I.; Siddique, K.U.; Ashfaq, F.; Ali, W.; Reddy, H.D.; Mishra, A. Effect of high-dose zinc supplementation with oral hypoglycemic agents on glycemic control and inflammation in type-2 diabetic nephropathy patients. *J. Nat. Sci. Biol. Med.* **2013**, *4*, 336–340. [CrossRef] [PubMed]

13. Kang, X.; Zhong, W.; Liu, J.; Song, Z.; McClain, C.J.; Kang, Y.J.; Zhou, Z. Zinc supplementation reverses alcohol-induced steatosis in mice through reactivating hepatocyte nuclear factor-4alpha and peroxisome proliferator-activated receptor-alpha. *Hepatology* **2009**, *50*, 1241–1250. [CrossRef] [PubMed]

14. Ghosh, C.; Yang, S.H.; Kim, J.G.; Jeon, T.I.; Yoon, B.H.; Lee, J.Y.; Lee, E.Y.; Choi, S.G.; Hwang, S.G. Zinc-chelated Vitamin C Stimulates Adipogenesis of 3T3-L1 Cells. *Asian-Australas. J. Anim. Sci.* **2013**, *26*, 1189–1196. [CrossRef] [PubMed]

15. Zhang, H.B.; Wang, M.S.; Wang, Z.S.; Zhou, A.M.; Zhang, X.M.; Dong, X.W.; Peng, Q.H. Supplementation dietary zinc levels on growth performance, carcass traits, and intramuscular fat deposition in weaned piglets. *Biol. Trace Elem. Res.* **2014**, *161*, 69–77. [CrossRef] [PubMed]

16. Sun, K.; Kusminski, C.M.; Scherer, P.E. Adipose tissue remodeling and obesity. *J. Clin. Invest.* **2011**, *121*, 2094–2101. [CrossRef] [PubMed]

17. McTernan, P.G.; Harte, A.L.; Anderson, L.A.; Green, A.; Smith, S.A.; Holder, J.C.; Barnett, A.H.; Eggo, M.C.; Kumar, S. Insulin and rosiglitazone regulation of lipolysis and lipogenesis in human adipose tissue in vitro. *Diabetes* **2002**, *51*, 1493–1498. [CrossRef] [PubMed]

18. Kuryszko, J.; Slawuta, P.; Sapikowski, G. Secretory function of adipose tissue. *Pol. J. Vet. Sci.* **2016**, *19*, 441–446. [CrossRef] [PubMed]

19. Guilherme, A.; Virbasius, J.V.; Puri, V.; Czech, M.P. Adipocyte dysfunctions linking obesity to insulin resistance and type 2 diabetes. *Nat. Rev. Mol. Cell Biol.* **2008**, *9*, 367–377. [CrossRef] [PubMed]

20. Lee, B.C.; Lee, J. Cellular and molecular players in adipose tissue inflammation in the development of obesity-induced insulin resistance. *Biochim. Biophys. Acta* **2014**, *1842*, 446–462. [CrossRef] [PubMed]

21. Kim, S.M.; Lun, M.; Wang, M.; Senyo, S.E.; Guillermier, C.; Patwari, P.; Steinhauser, M.L. Loss of white adipose hyperplastic potential is associated with enhanced susceptibility to insulin resistance. *Cell Metab.* **2014**, *20*, 1049–1058. [CrossRef] [PubMed]

22. Landgraf, K.; Rockstroh, D.; Wagner, I.V.; Weise, S.; Tauscher, R.; Schwartze, J.T.; Loffler, D.; Buhligen, U.; Wojan, M.; Till, H.; et al. Evidence of early alterations in adipose tissue biology and function and its association with obesity-related inflammation and insulin resistance in children. *Diabetes* **2015**, *64*, 1249–1261. [CrossRef] [PubMed]

23. White, U.A.; Stephens, J.M. Transcriptional factors that promote formation of white adipose tissue. *Mol. Cell. Endocrinol.* **2010**, *318*, 10–14. [CrossRef] [PubMed]

24. Chen, Q.; Wang, T.; Li, J.; Wang, S.; Qiu, F.; Yu, H.; Zhang, Y.; Wang, T. Effects of Natural Products on Fructose-Induced Nonalcoholic Fatty Liver Disease (NAFLD). *Nutrients* **2017**, *9*, 96. [CrossRef] [PubMed]

25. Li, X.; Guan, Y.; Shi, X.; Ding, H.; Song, Y.; Li, C.; Liu, R.; Liu, G. Effects of high zinc levels on the lipid synthesis in rat hepatocytes. *Biol. Trace Elem. Res.* **2013**, *154*, 97–102. [CrossRef] [PubMed]
26. Feng, B.; Jiao, P.; Helou, Y.; Li, Y.; He, Q.; Walters, M.S.; Salomon, A.; Xu, H. Mitogen-activated protein kinase phosphatase 3 (MKP-3)-deficient mice are resistant to diet-induced obesity. *Diabetes* **2014**, *63*, 2924–2934. [CrossRef] [PubMed]
27. Feng, B.; Huang, X.; Jiang, D.; Hua, L.; Zhuo, Y.; Wu, D. Endoplasmic Reticulum Stress Inducer Tunicamycin Alters Hepatic Energy Homeostasis in Mice. *Int. J. Mol. Sci.* **2017**, *18*, 1710. [CrossRef]
28. Feng, B.; Jiao, P.; Nie, Y.; Kim, T.; Jun, D.; van Rooijen, N.; Yang, Z.; Xu, H. Clodronate liposomes improve metabolic profile and reduce visceral adipose macrophage content in diet-induced obese mice. *PLoS ONE.* **2011**, *6*, e24358. [CrossRef] [PubMed]
29. Marchesini, G.; Bugianesi, E.; Ronchi, M.; Flamia, R.; Thomaseth, K.; Pacini, G. Zinc supplementation improves glucose disposal in patients with cirrhosis. *Metabolism* **1998**, *47*, 792–798. [CrossRef]
30. Quarterman, J.; Mills, C.F.; Humphries, W.R. The reduced secretion of, and sensitivity to insulin in zinc-deficient rats. *Biochem. Biophys. Res. Commun.* **1966**, *25*, 354–358. [CrossRef]
31. Shisheva, A.; Gefel, D.; Shechter, Y. Insulinlike effects of zinc ion in vitro and in vivo. Preferential effects on desensitized adipocytes and induction of normoglycemia in streptozotocin-induced rats. *Diabetes* **1992**, *41*, 982–988. [CrossRef] [PubMed]
32. Kim, J.; Lee, S. Effect of zinc supplementation on insulin resistance and metabolic risk factors in obese Korean women. *Nutr. Res. Pract.* **2012**, *6*, 221–225. [CrossRef] [PubMed]
33. Lobene, A.J.; Kindler, J.M.; Jenkins, N.T.; Pollock, N.K.; Laing, E.M.; Grider, A.; Lewis, R.D. Zinc Supplementation Does Not Alter Indicators of Insulin Secretion and Sensitivity in Black and White Female Adolescents. *J. Nutr.* **2017**, *147*, 1296–1300. [CrossRef] [PubMed]
34. Samuel, V.T.; Shulman, G.I. Mechanisms for insulin resistance: Common threads and missing links. *Cell* **2012**, *148*, 852–871. [CrossRef] [PubMed]
35. Rothman, D.L.; Magnusson, I.; Katz, L.D.; Shulman, R.G.; Shulman, G.I. Quantitation of hepatic glycogenolysis and gluconeogenesis in fasting humans with 13C NMR. *Science* **1991**, *254*, 573–576. [CrossRef] [PubMed]
36. Stofkova, A. Leptin and adiponectin: From energy and metabolic dysbalance to inflammation and autoimmunity. *Endocr. Regul.* **2009**, *43*, 157–168. [CrossRef] [PubMed]
37. DePaoli, A.M. 20 years of leptin: Leptin in common obesity and associated disorders of metabolism. *J. Endocrinol.* **2014**, *223*, T71–T81. [CrossRef] [PubMed]
38. Baltaci, A.K.; Mogulkoc, R.; Halifeoglu, I. Effects of zinc deficiency and supplementation on plasma leptin levels in rats. *Biol. Trace Elem. Res.* **2005**, *104*, 41–46. [CrossRef]
39. Ott, E.S.; Shay, N.F. Zinc deficiency reduces leptin gene expression and leptin secretion in rat adipocytes. *Exp. Biol. Med.* **2001**, *226*, 841–846. [CrossRef]
40. Argani, H.; Mahdavi, R.; Ghorbani-haghjo, A.; Razzaghi, R.; Nikniaz, L.; Gaemmaghami, S.J. Effects of zinc supplementation on serum zinc and leptin levels, BMI, and body composition in hemodialysis patients. *J. Trace Elem. Med. Biol.* **2014**, *28*, 35–38. [CrossRef] [PubMed]
41. Xu, H.; Barnes, G.T.; Yang, Q.; Tan, G.; Yang, D.; Chou, C.J.; Sole, J.; Nichols, A.; Ross, J.S.; Tartaglia, L.A.; et al. Chronic inflammation in fat plays a crucial role in the development of obesity-related insulin resistance. *J. Clin. Invest.* **2003**, *112*, 1821–1830. [CrossRef] [PubMed]
42. Abella, V.; Scotece, M.; Conde, J.; Pino, J.; Gonzalez-Gay, M.A.; Gomez-Reino, J.J.; Mera, A.; Lago, F.; Gomez, R.; Gualillo, O. Leptin in the interplay of inflammation, metabolism and immune system disorders. *Nat. Rev. Rheumatol.* **2017**, *13*, 100–109. [CrossRef] [PubMed]

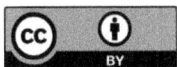

nutrients

MDPI

Article

Intrauterine Zn Deficiency Favors Thyrotropin-Releasing Hormone-Increasing Effects on Thyrotropin Serum Levels and Induces Subclinical Hypothyroidism in Weaned Rats

Viridiana Alcántara-Alonso [†], Elena Alvarez-Salas [†], Gilberto Matamoros-Trejo and Patricia de Gortari *

Molecular Neurophysiology Laboratory, Department of Neurosciences Research,
National Institute of Psychiatry Ramon de la Fuente Muñiz, Calzada México-Xochimilco 101,
Col. San Lorenzo Huipulco, Mexico City C.P. 14370, Mexico; viridiana15kr@hotmail.com (V.A.-A.);
alvareze@imp.edu.mx (E.A.-S.); gilmtrejo@yahoo.com.mx (G.M.-T.)
* Correspondence: gortari@imp.edu.mx; Tel.: +52-55-4160-5056
† These authors contributed equally to this work.

Received: 28 August 2017; Accepted: 11 October 2017; Published: 18 October 2017

Abstract: Individuals who consume a diet deficient in zinc (Zn-deficient) develop alterations in hypothalamic-pituitary-thyroid axis function, i.e., a low metabolic rate and cold insensitivity. Although those disturbances are related to primary hypothyroidism, intrauterine or postnatal Zn-deficient adults have an increased thyrotropin (TSH) concentration, but unchanged thyroid hormone (TH) levels and decreased body weight. This does not support the view that the hypothyroidism develops due to a low Zn intake. In addition, intrauterine or postnatal Zn-deficiency in weaned and adult rats reduces the activity of pyroglutamyl aminopeptidase II (PPII) in the medial-basal hypothalamus (MBH). PPII is an enzyme that degrades thyrotropin-releasing hormone (TRH). This hypothalamic peptide stimulates its receptor in adenohypophysis, thereby increasing TSH release. We analyzed whether earlier low TH is responsible for the high TSH levels reported in adults, or if TRH release is enhanced by Zn deficiency at weaning. Dams were fed a 2 ppm Zn-deficient diet in the period from one week prior to gestation and up to three weeks after delivery. We found a high release of hypothalamic TRH, which along with reduced MBH PPII activity, increased TSH levels in Zn-deficient pups independently of changes in TH concentration. We found that primary hypothyroidism did not develop in intrauterine Zn-deficient weaned rats and we confirmed that metal deficiency enhances TSH levels since early-life, favoring subclinical hypothyroidism development which remains into adulthood.

Keywords: Zn deficiency; TRH; TSH; subclinical hypothyroidism

1. Introduction

Zinc (Zn) deficiency is a public health problem due to its increasing prevalence not only in underdeveloped countries but also in first world countries [1–3]. Gestating and lactating women are the most affected groups [4], leading to Zn malnutrition in their offspring. This impairs fetal development due to the metal's involvement in a wide diversity of cellular processes: differentiation, reproduction, metabolism and neurogenesis [5].

Given that Zn is the cofactor of a wide number of enzymes, deficiency of the metal alters their activity with severe consequences in children and adults health [6]. For example, Zn-deficient animals and humans present growth retardation, cold sensitivity and decreased metabolic rate [7], which are alterations associated with primary hypothyroidism (low thyroid hormone (TH) levels). Moreover,

Zn deficiency is also related to psychiatric disturbances such as depression, anxiety, schizophrenia, attention deficit hyperactivity disorder and epilepsy [8–11].

The hypothalamic-pituitary-thyroid (HPT) axis is regulated by a negative feedback loop, in such a way that during primary hypothyroidism the decreased TH serum levels lead to an increased release of thyrotropin (TSH) from the adenohypophysis (AH) and to a high synthesis and release of the hypothalamic peptide thyrotropin-releasing hormone (TRH) into the portal blood in order to activate the HPT axis.

There is controversy about the effects of Zn deficiency on HPT axis. Some authors support the development of subclinical hypothyroidism [12,13], while others describe the occurrence of a primary one [14,15]. A previous study from our laboratory in adult rats subjected to intrauterine or postnatal Zn deficiency, showed an increase in serum TSH levels but unchanged T_3 or T_4 concentration [16], which argues against primary hypothyroidism as the main alteration of the HPT axis in Zn deficiency. Furthermore, these animals maintained a low body weight as adults, which is not compatible with low circulating TH levels [15,16].

In order to disentangle this controversy, in a previous study we analyzed the effects of a Zn-deficient diet on the activity of a metalloprotease called pyroglutamyl aminopeptidase II (PPII) present in the AH and the mediobasal hypothalamus (MBH) [17–20], along with its repercussion in the function of the HPT axis of gestating and lactating rats and in their adult offspring [16]. The high specificity of PPII in degrading the hypothalamic peptide TRH when released from the median eminence into the portal blood, as well as its positive regulation by TH levels, has indicated that the activity of this enzyme is part of the negative feedback control of the HPT axis exerted by low TH levels, that would allow a more effective stimulation of TSH release by TRH [21]. However, there is a TH-independent down-regulation of adenohypophyseal PPII activity in intrauterine and postnatal Zn-deficient adult rats and in the MBH in whole-life malnourished weanling and adult animals [16]. This supports the fact that low enzyme activity by itself may be responsible for a greater stimulation of TSH release and serum concentration [16].

Nevertheless, we still have not ruled out if intrauterine Zn deficiency induces an earlier decrease in T_3 and T_4 serum concentration since weaning, which could be reducing PPII activity and thus increasing TSH levels previous to our measurements in ten-week old adults. This will be arguing against a PPII regulation only by Zn, supporting that the high TSH concentration observed in Zn-deficient adults results from a previous primary hypothyroidism.

Thus, we here analyzed adenohypophyseal PPII activity, TSH and TH serum levels, as well as TRH concentration in the median eminence of intrauterine Zn-deficient weanling pups. Our findings supported that PPII activity might be modulated independently of the changes in TH levels since weaning. This is relevant to explain the TSH rise when TH concentration is in normal levels as in the subclinical hypothyroidism induced by Zn deficiency. Moreover, since chronic high TSH serum levels are associated with increased lipolysis, low body weight and growing rate, our results help to solve the contradiction of the low body weight maintained by Zn malnourishment in adult animals even when T_3 and T_4 levels do not change.

2. Materials and Methods

2.1. Animals and Diets

All procedures described in the present study were approved by the Ethics Committee and Project Commission of the INPRFM, which follows the regulations established in the Mexican Official Norm for the use and care of laboratory animals (NOM-062-ZOO-1999).

Ten nulliparous female and six male adult (220–270 g) Wistar rats were obtained from the INPRFM's animal housing. They were housed in groups (2–3 animals per cage) and allowed to acclimatize to the facilities. They were provided with food (Lab rodent diet #5001, PMI feeds, St. Louis, MO, USA) and tap water ad libitum, and kept in controlled light conditions (lights on from 7:00 to

19:00) and temperature (24 ± 1 °C). After one week of habituation, animals were mated (1–2 females per male) and divided into two groups: control group (C) (*n* = 3 females, 2 males) receiving a diet with 20 ppm of Zn (Purina Mills, LLC/PMI Nutrition International Co., Richmond, IN, USA) and deficient (D) group (*n* = 7 females, 4 males), which received a diet with 2 ppm of Zn (Purina Mills, LLC/PMI Nutrition International Co., Richmond, IN, USA). This Zn content in the diet is known to be sufficient to decreased serum Zn levels after 7 weeks [16]. Except for their Zn content, both diets were the same regarding nutrient composition (19% proteins; 10% lipids; 61% carbohydrates); both groups had ad libitum access to food and distilled water. The mating period lasted 10 days and pregnancy was confirmed by identifying a 10% increase of the initial female body weight (b.w.). Pregnant dams were individually housed throughout gestation and lactation periods and maintained under the same C or D diet. After pregnancy completion, the body weight of the pups was registered at 2, 7, 14 and 21 days of age. At 21 days of age, weaned pups from C (*n* = 6) or D (*n* = 6) dams, were sacrificed by decapitation. Brain and AH were rapidly removed and frozen at −70 °C. Blood was collected and centrifuged at 3000 × *g* for 30 min at 4 °C. Serum was obtained, aliquoted and kept at −70 °C until analysis.

2.2. TRH Content in Median Eminence (ME)

Medial basal hypothalamus (MBH) was hand-dissected from frozen brains using Paxinos and Watson Rat Brain Atlas [22]. This region contains the median eminence (ME) (known to be outside the blood brain barrier (BBB)). In order to obtain the MBH, a coronal slice was cut between the coordinates −1.2 to −3.6 mm from bregma, then ME was removed with a scalpel in the ventral part of the slice.

TRH extraction from tissue and the following radioimmunoassay (RIA) were both performed as previously described [23]. TRH content was determined using a previously characterized antibody [24]. The MEs of the pups were homogenized by sonication in 20% acetic acid and centrifuged at 12,000× *g* for 15 min at 4 °C. A 30 μL aliquot of supernatant was kept for protein quantification. The supernatant was obtained and then extracted with 100% methanol and evaporated. Pellets were diluted in RIA buffer (50 mM NaPO$_4$ buffer, pH 7.4, containing 0.25% bovine serum albumin (BSA) RIA grade (Sigma-Aldrich, St. Louis, MO, USA), 150 mM NaCl and 0.02% sodium azide (Sigma-Aldrich, St. Louis, MO, USA). Then, a TRH antibody (1:10^6 dilution) and ^{125}I-TRH (5000 cpm) were added. After 36 h of incubation, samples were precipitated with 100% ethanol and centrifuged at 12,000× *g* for 5 min at 4 °C). Supernatant was evaporated in a concentrator (Vacufuge Eppendorf, Brinkmann Instruments, Westbury, NY, USA), and tubes read for 1 min in a radiation counter (LKB Wallace Minigamma Counter, Mount Waverley, Victoria, Australia). A standard curve and an internal standard of hypothalamic extract were included in every assay and parallelism with the curve was verified. Limit of detection was 20 pg, inter and intra-assay variation was 4% and 8%, respectively. Results are expressed in ng TRH/mg protein.

2.3. PPII Specific Activity

PPII activity in AH was measured as previously described [16]. Briefly, each AH was homogenized by sonication in 200 μL of 50 mM NaPO$_4$ buffer pH 7.5, and centrifuged at 2600× *g* for 15 min at 4 °C. PPII activity was measured in supernatants by using 400 μM pGlu-His-Pro-β-naphtylamine (βNA) (Bachem, Torrance, CA, USA) as substrate, an excess of dipeptidylaminopeptidase IV (EC 3.4.14.15) (Sigma-Aldrich, St. Louis, MO, USA), 0.2 mM *N*-ethylmaleimide (Sigma, St. Louis, MO, USA), an inhibitor of pyroglutamyl peptidase I (EC 3.4.19.3), and 0.2 mM bacitracin (Sigma-Aldrich, St. Louis, MO, USA) an inhibitor of prolyl oligopeptidase (EC 3.4.21.26); in a total volume of 250 μL. Samples were incubated at 37 °C, 50 μL were withdrawn every 60 min and the reaction stopped with 50 μL 100% methanol. Aliquots were diluted to 400 μL with 50% methanol in buffer, before detecting βNA with a fluorometer (Perkin Elmer LS50, Waltham, MA, USA) (excitation 335 nm, emission 410 nm) from a standard curve of βNA (Sigma-Aldrich, St. Louis, MO, USA). A 30 μL aliquot of supernatant was kept for protein quantification. The activity was linear with the time elapsed and referred to supernatant protein content.

2.4. Protein Determination

Protein content in AH and ME was determined in 30 µL of homogenate, by digesting with 1 N NaOH for 24 h at room temperature (RT) and protein concentration quantified by folin-phenol reagent method [25].

2.5. Serum Hormones' Determination

TSH determination was performed by RIA using the NIDDK (National Hormone and Pituitary Program) protocol and materials. We used 50 µL of serum in duplicate, samples were diluted 1:3 in RIA buffer (50 mM $NaPO_4$, pH 7.5; 150 mM NaCl, 0.25% BSA, 50 mM EDTA), and antibody raised in rabbit against TSH (1:375,000) was added. After 18–24 h incubation at RT, ^{125}I-TSH was added (10,000 cpm), followed by 18–24 h incubation at RT. The secondary antibody (goat anti rabbit IgG) was added in 1:40 dilution in PBS (50 mM $NaPO_4$, pH 7.5, 150 mM NaCl) plus 2% normal rabbit serum and incubated for 2 h at RT. After adding polyethylene glycol (0.04 g PEG/mL RIA buffer), samples were centrifuged at $5000\times g$ for 30 min at 4 °C. Supernatant was aspirated and tubes read for 1 min in a radiation counter (LKB Wallace Minigamma Counter, Mount Waverley, Victoria, Australia). Limit of detection: 5 pg, 13% inter-assay, 6% intra-assay variability.

Five µL of serum were used to determine corticosterone in duplicate (dilution 1:1000) considering the mean as one determination using ICN Biomedicals kit (Aurora, OH, USA). Limits of sensitivity: corticosterone: 20 ng/mL. Intra-assay variability: 7%, inter-assay variability: 8%.

T_4 and T_3 were determined in 100 and 25 µL of serum, respectively, using commercial RIA kits (Coat-A-Count Solid-Phase ^{125}I RIA. Total T3 DPC TKT31, Total T4 DPC TKT41, Los Angeles, CA, USA) and following manufacturer's instructions (analytical sensitivity: T_3, 7 ng/dL and T_4, 0.25 µg/dL; inter-assay variability: T_3, T_4 < 15%, and intra-assay variability T_3, T_4 < 9%).

Leptin was determined in order to evaluate if our early-life diet manipulation influences energy balance regulation and satiety. Leptin was measured colorimetrically with a commercially available kit (Merck Rat Leptin ELISA kit, Life Science Merck, Darmstadt, Hesse, Germany using 25 µL of serum diluted 1:4 with an assay buffer and following the manufacturer's instructions (limit of detection: 4.76 pg/mL; inter-assay variability (8%), intra-assay variability (7%)).

2.6. Statistical Analysis

Body weight changes between control and Zn-deficient pups during lactation were analyzed by repeated measures ANOVA. Kolmogorov-Smirnov tests for normality were used for each of the biochemical variables (PPII specific activity in AH, TRH ME content, TSH, corticosterone, T_3, T_4 and leptin serum levels) and then Mann-Whitney U tests were performed in order to identify the statistical differences of these variables between groups. A $p < 0.05$ was considered as statistically significant. A variable interdependence between TRH content and leptin serum levels was analyzed given the positive effect of leptin on TRH synthesis and release [26,27]. A correlation coefficient with magnitude ≥ 0.8 was considered as strong correlation.

3. Results

3.1. Body Weight

Body weight at birth was similar between control and Zn-deficient animals; however from post-natal day 7 and until post-natal day 21, the body weight of deficient pups was 30% lower on average, when compared to control offspring (100%). Repeated measures ANOVA showed an effect of treatment ($F_{(1,30)} = 26.548$ $p < 0.001$); time ($F_{(3,30)} = 219.015$ $p < 0.0001$) and interaction between variables ($F_{(3,30)} = 22.509$ $p < 0.0001$) (Figure 1).

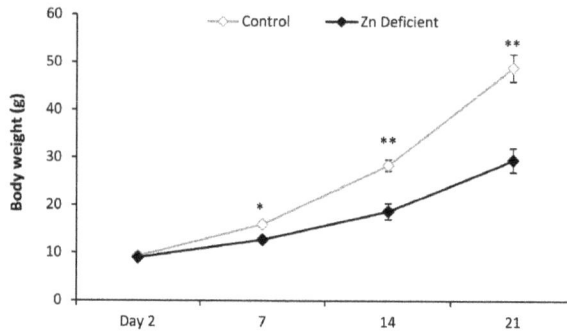

Figure 1. Body weight of control and zinc-deficient (Zn-deficient) pups during lactation period. Values are the mean ± standard error of mean (SEM) of grams of body weight, (n = 6/group). Fisher's post-hoc test showed significant differences: * $p < 0.01$, ** $p < 0.001$ vs. control group.

3.2. Biochemical Determinations

Adenohypophyseal PPII specific activity of Zn-deficient pups showed a trend to decrease, but there was no statistically significant difference between groups (Zn-deficient = 472.5 ± 67 pmol of βNA min/mg of protein vs. controls = 631.2 ± 194 pmol of βNA/min/mg of protein). TRH content of ME in the Zn-malnourished group decreased to 4.7 ± 1.8 ng of TRH/mg protein, when compared to control values: 22.36 ± 6.2 ng of TRH/mg protein. Low accumulation of TRH in the synaptic terminals of hypothalamic paraventricular neurons (median eminence) is associated with a high release of the peptide into the portal blood, mainly because the antibody used is able to detect changes in TRH concentration only in the intracellular compartment.

Increased TSH serum levels in Zn-deficient pups confirmed the enhanced release of TRH: the Zn-deficient group presented TSH levels of 2.32 ± 0.2 ng/dL, whereas those of the controls were: 1.66 ± 0.1 ng/dL. Mann-Whitney U-test for TRH showed a U = 42 equivalent to a Z = −2.6 with a p value < 0.01 and that of TSH was U = 40 equivalent to a Z = −2.714 with a p value < 0.01 (Figure 2).

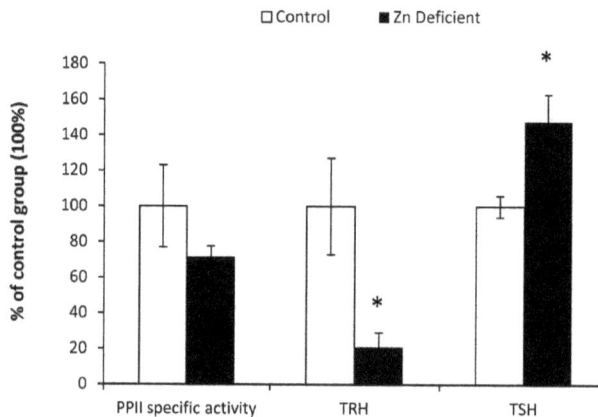

Figure 2. Adenohypophyseal pyroglutamyl aminopeptidase II (PPII) specific activity, median eminence thyrotropin-releasing hormone (TRH) content and thyrotropin (TSH) serum levels of Zn-deficient and control pups at weaning. Control values for PPII specific activity: 631.2 ± 194 pmol βNA/min/mg prot; TRH: 22.36 ± 6.2 ngTRH/mg proteins; TSH: 1.66 ± 0.1 ng/dL. Values are the mean ± SEM of percentage of control values (=100%), (n = 6/group).* $p < 0.01$ vs. controls.

Zn deficiency did not affect T_3, T_4 or corticosterone serum levels.

In contrast, circulatory leptin levels decreased to $43.5 \pm 7\%$ compared to those of controls (100%); Mann-Whitney U analysis for leptin showed a value for U = 15 that is equivalent to a $Z = -2.021$ with a p value < 0.05 (Table 1). We observed a strong positive linear correlation between median eminence TRH and leptin serum concentration ($n = 8$ rats; correlation coefficient = 0.825; $Z = 2.62$; $p < 0.01$).

Table 1. Hormones serum concentrations of Zn-deficient and control pups at weaning.

Group	T_3 (ng/dL)	T_4 (µg/dL)	Leptin (ng/mL)	Corticosterone (ng/mL)
Control	8.17 ± 0.15	8.5 ± 1	4.3 ± 0.8	149 ± 19
Zn-deficient	7.35 ± 0.49	8.86 ± 1.1	1.86 ± 0.2 *	99 ± 17

Values are the mean $\pm$ SEM ($n = 4$–6/group); * $p < 0.05$ vs. control group.

4. Discussion

In this study, TH levels of Zn-deficient rats were normal, thus intrauterine metal malnourishment failed to induce primary hypothyroidism since weaning. This was in agreement with the unchanged levels of T_3 and T_4 observed in adult rats subjected to Zn deficiency during the prenatal and postnatal periods. Overall, these findings supported the conclusion that high TSH levels and the development of subclinical hypothyroidism in adults [16] and weanling rats, are not a response to low T_3, but to other factors that we discuss below.

The weight loss at weaning observed in the offspring of dams eating a Zn-deficient diet could be associated to the increase in TSH serum concentration, even when TH did not increase. TSH receptors have been identified in adipocytes and its activation by TSH increases lipid degradation [28,29]. It is well known that high levels of TSH have a down-regulatory effect on its receptors in the thyroid cell [30,31], which may account for the thyroid's lack of response to the TSH released, thus T_3 and T_4 serum concentration did not change in Zn-deficient pups.

Given that body weight of Zn-deficient animals was similar to that of controls at birth, it is likely that dams in the malnourished group compensated Zn availability for the offspring by homeostatic adjustments, at the expense of their own metal content in bone and muscle [32,33] and also, by delivering small litters. The lower body weight in the first week of life seemed also to be a consequence of the known anorexic effect of Zn deficiency [34]. Weanling pups from Zn-deficient dams have a reduction of 40% milk intake on average [35]. We did not evaluate milk consumption since this is a rather stressful procedure, but in our previous study, we describe a decreased food intake in prenatally and postnatally Zn-deficient rats after weaning [16]. This anorexic effect along with the high TSH concentration contributed to the weight loss of malnourished pups.

It was noteworthy that the evident low body weight of Zn-deficient pups was not able to reduce HPT axis activity and to decrease TH levels as has been proposed [36,37]. In contrast, our data supported that hypothalamic neurons are firstly responding to low nutrient availability and as a consequence, metabolic rate is adjusted through HPT axis function modulation. For example, negative energy balance decelerates HPT axis and lipids waste in adults, but in weanling rats such adaptation is not successful [38]. Similarly, in this study, the low Zn intake seemed to activate TRH release from the ME (discussed below) and to increase TSH serum levels, with no abatement of the metabolic rate.

The high TSH serum levels found in Zn-deficient weanling rats was coincident with that previously found in prenatally or postnatally deficient adults [16]. TSH release is known to result from a high release of its secretagogue TRH, or, by a low concentration of TH. In the first case, TRH by activating its receptor (TRH-R1) expressed in thyrotrophs, leads to an enhanced TSH release [39,40]. In the second case, the low concentration of T_3 favors the detachment of a nuclear thyrotropin receptor (TR) from the TSH gene promoter, in such a way that the expression of the hormone is uninhibited [41].

In this study the effect of low TH concentration appears not to be responsible for the increase in TSH serum levels of Zn-deficient animals. This result argues against the proposed primary hypothyroidism and slow growth induced by low Zn dietary content [15] and, against the decreased Zn concentrations in individuals with primary hypothyroidism [42].

Therefore, a more plausible explanation for the increased circulation of TSH was that the ME nerve terminals of Zn-deficient pups maintained a high TRH concentration in the portal blood. Indeed, pups showed low TRH levels in the tissue containing the nerve terminals from the hypothalamic paraventricular nucleus (PVN) cells. That can be interpreted as a high release given that the titer of the antibody used allows for the quantification of the peptide concentration only in the intracellular compartment, which is greater than that of the extracellular one [43]. When TRH levels decay in the ME along with a high concentration of TSH in serum, then an increased release of the peptide can be assumed.

Trying to identify which factors might be involved in the higher release of hypophysiotropic TRH, we analyzed leptin and corticosterone serum levels, which respectively decrease and increase in a negative energy balance. Both are modulators of TRH synthesis in the hypothalamus [26]. Indeed we found decreased leptin serum levels in Zn-deficient animals, which should be decreasing the function of HPT axis as an advantageous adaptation to their low body weight and reduced energy reservoirs. In contrast and as previously mentioned, a high release of TRH was observed along with increased TSH serum levels that led to further energy utilization; thus we assumed that leptin signaling was impaired in Zn-deficient group.

The shift between leptin/corticosterone levels during fasting elevates the activity of type-2 deiodinase, an enzyme residing in the ependymal cells of the third ventricle that is able to increase T_3 hypothalamic concentration, which in turn down-regulates TRH expression and release [44], and also would decrease TSH serum levels. However, a Zn-deficient diet did not increase circulating corticosterone in pups. Thus, it is unlikely that alterations found in HPT axis were stress mediated. It is possible that an unchanged type-2 deiodinase activity was not able to reduce TRH expression, avoiding the inhibitory effect of this enzyme on the metabolic rate. Association between high TRH release with activation of its mRNA expression is assumed after observing the coordination of those processes in PVN TRHergic neurons by stimuli, such as suction in lactating rats [45], cold [45,46] and dehydration-induced anorexia [47].

TRH release is modulated by glutamate, of which neurotransmission is altered by brain Zn availability. Zn is able to directly and specifically inhibit responses of glutamate by altering the NMDA receptors [48–50]. Thus, low Zn levels might be activating the glutamate receptors expressed in TRHergic neurons [51] and stimulating the release of peptides, inducing different behavioral outcomes [52,53], although this deserves further study.

The other direct effect that Zn deficiency could have to induce the greater actions of TRH on the AH of weaned offspring was the down-regulation of PPII specific activity (the TRH-degrading enzyme) that we have already observed in the MBH of malnourished pups [16]. Low PPII activity most likely decreased TRH degradation and contributed to the greater TRH effect on AH and on TSH release of Zn-deficient pups by enhancing the peptide content in the portal blood and its access to thyrotrophs.

Even when it is known that TH exerts a positive regulation of PPII, its decreased activity in the MBH could not be attributed to T_3 or T_4 given that these hormones did not change, but instead it can be attributed to the low Zn availability. This is supported by the Zn dependence of PPII activity that has already proven to be modulated by dietary Zn in adults, as happens for other enzymes, such as alcohol dehydrogenase of the liver [54], alkaline phosphatase [55] and angiotensin-converting enzyme [56–58].

In contrast to what we observed in the MBH (in pups and adults in our previous study) and in AH (adults) [16], we did not find a down-regulation of PPII activity in the AH of Zn-deficient weanling pups, which supports a tissue and age specific effect of metal availability on enzyme function. The ontogeny of hypothalamic PPII activity reveals a maximum functionality at postnatal day 8 [59]. By this time, the BBB had already developed in a Zn-deficient environment, avoiding Zn entry through its transporters present in this barrier [60] and affecting PPII activity in the MBH [16]. Moreover, PPII is more active in the hypothalamus when compared to the AH [59], therefore a higher supply of Zn may be required in this brain region in order to assure enzyme activity. On the other hand, Zn-deficient dams might still be able to provide sufficient Zn for PPII activity to function in the AH.

5. Conclusions

We conclude that the subclinical hypothyroidism associated with Zn deficiency in adults [12,13,61] is developed at least after weaning; that this is not due to an early decrease in TH serum levels at weaning; and thus, that the increased TSH concentration is not a response to a primary hypothyroidism.

Our data better support the conclusion that Zn deficiency has a direct effect on TRH release, along with a decreased degrading activity of MBH PPII since weaning and later in the AH, which favored TRH stimulation of its receptor in the thyrotrophs inducing a high release of TSH. These elevated TSH levels may be responsible for the low body weight of Zn-deficient pups and may have long lasting effects on animals' health. For example, high TSH is a possible indicator of Zn deficiency and subclinical hypothyroidism that have been associated to a risk of developing overt hypothyroidism [62,63]. Additionally, high circulating TSH levels are related to several comorbidities such as metabolic syndrome, being overweight, insulin resistance, cardiovascular risk, and dyslipidemia, amongst others [64–69].

Acknowledgments: We want to thank Q.F.B. Miguel Cisneros from the Instituto de Biotecnologia UNAM for his technical assistance; also thanks to José Luis Calderón and Raúl Cardoso from the National Institute of Psychiatry for their assistance with drawing work. This study was supported by CONACyT 128316 and 233918 (Patricia de Gortari).

Author Contributions: Viridiana Alcántara-Alonso, Elena Alvarez-Salas and Gilberto Matamoros-Trejo, took care of animals and made the biochemical determinations. Viridiana Alcántara-Alonso, Elena Alvarez-Salas, helped in the interpretation of results and in revising the manuscript. Patricia de Gortari designed the experiments, interpreted the results and wrote the manuscript.

Conflicts of Interest: Authors declare that there is no conflict of interest that could be perceived as prejudicing the impartiality of the reported research.

References

1. Duque, X.; Flores-Hernandez, S.; Flores-Huerta, S.; Mendez-Ramirez, I.; Munoz, S.; Turnbull, B.; Martinez-Andrade, G.; Ramos, R.I.; Gonzalez-Unzaga, M.; Mendoza, M.E.; et al. Prevalence of anemia and deficiency of iron, folic acid, and zinc in children younger than 2 years of age who use the health services provided by the Mexican Social Security Institute. *BMC Public Health* **2007**, *7*, 345. [CrossRef] [PubMed]
2. Villalpando, S.; Garcia-Guerra, A.; Ramirez-Silva, C.I.; Mejia-Rodriguez, F.; Matute, G.; Shamah-Levy, T.; Rivera, J.A. Iron, zinc and iodide status in Mexican children under 12 years and women 12–49 years of age. A probabilistic national survey. *Salud Publica Mex.* **2003**, *45*, S520–S529. [CrossRef] [PubMed]
3. Caulfield, L.E.; Zavaleta, N.; Shankar, A.H.; Merialdi, M. Potential contribution of maternal zinc supplementation during pregnancy to maternal and child survival. *Am. J. Clin. Nutr.* **1998**, *68*, 499S–508S. [PubMed]
4. Shapira, N. Prenatal nutrition: A critical window of opportunity for mother and child. *Womens Health* **2008**, *4*, 639–656. [CrossRef] [PubMed]
5. Nuttall, J.R.; Supasai, S.; Kha, J.; Vaeth, B.M.; Mackenzie, G.G.; Adamo, A.M.; Oteiza, P.I. Gestational marginal zinc deficiency impaired fetal neural progenitor cell proliferation by disrupting the ERK1/2 signaling pathway. *J. Nutr. Biochem.* **2015**, *26*, 1116–1123. [CrossRef] [PubMed]
6. Golub, M.S.; Gershwin, M.E.; Hurley, L.S.; Saito, W.Y.; Hendrickx, A.G. Studies of marginal zinc deprivation in rhesus monkeys. IV. Growth of infants in the first year. *Am. J. Clin. Nutr.* **1984**, *40*, 1192–1202. [PubMed]
7. Kralik, A.; Eder, K.; Kirchgessner, M. Influence of zinc and selenium deficiency on parameters relating to thyroid hormone metabolism. *Horm. Metab. Res.* **1996**, *28*, 223–226. [CrossRef] [PubMed]
8. Amani, R.; Saeidi, S.; Nazari, Z.; Nematpour, S. Correlation between dietary zinc intakes and its serum levels with depression scales in young female students. *Biol. Trace Elem. Res.* **2010**, *137*, 150–158. [CrossRef] [PubMed]

9. Russo, A.J. Decreased zinc and increased copper in individuals with anxiety. *Nutr. Metab. Insights* **2011**, *4*, 1–5. [CrossRef] [PubMed]

10. Hagmeyer, S.; Haderspeck, J.C.; Grabrucker, A.M. Behavioral impairments in animal models for zinc deficiency. *Front. Behav. Neurosci.* **2014**, *8*, 443. [CrossRef] [PubMed]

11. Seven, M.; Basaran, S.Y.; Cengiz, M.; Unal, S.; Yuksel, A. Deficiency of selenium and zinc as a causative factor for idiopathic intractable epilepsy. *Epilepsy Res.* **2013**, *104*, 35–39. [CrossRef] [PubMed]

12. Napolitano, G.; Palka, G.; Lio, S.; Bucci, I.; De, R.P.; Stuppia, L.; Monaco, F. Is zinc deficiency a cause of subclinical hypothyroidism in Down syndrome? *Ann. Genet.* **1990**, *33*, 9–15. [PubMed]

13. Bucci, I.; Napolitano, G.; Giuliani, C.; Lio, S.; Minnucci, A.; Di, G.F.; Calabrese, G.; Sabatino, G.; Palka, G.; Monaco, F. Zinc sulfate supplementation improves thyroid function in hypozincemic Down children. *Biol. Trace Elem. Res.* **1999**, *67*, 257–268. [CrossRef] [PubMed]

14. Baltaci, A.K.; Mogulkoc, R.; Bediz, C.S.; Kul, A.; Ugur, A. Pinealectomy and zinc deficiency have opposite effects on thyroid hormones in rats. *Endocr. Res.* **2003**, *29*, 473–481. [CrossRef] [PubMed]

15. Jing, M.Y.; Sun, J.Y.; Wang, J.F. The effect of peripheral administration of zinc on food intake in rats fed Zn-adequate or Zn-deficient diets. *Biol. Trace Elem. Res.* **2008**, *124*, 144–156. [CrossRef] [PubMed]

16. Alvarez-Salas, E.; Alcantara-Alonso, V.; Matamoros-Trejo, G.; Vargas, M.A.; Morales-Mulia, M.; de Gortari, P. Mediobasal hypothalamic and adenohypophyseal TRH-degrading enzyme (PPII) is down-regulated by zinc deficiency. *Int. J. Dev. Neurosci.* **2015**, *46*, 115–124. [CrossRef] [PubMed]

17. Czekay, G.; Bauer, K. Identification of the thyrotropin-releasing-hormone-degrading ectoenzyme as a metallopeptidase. *Biochem. J.* **1993**, *290*, 921–926. [CrossRef] [PubMed]

18. O'Connor, B.; O'Cuinn, G. Localization of a narrow-specificity thyroliberin hydrolyzing pyroglutamate aminopeptidase in synaptosomal membranes of guinea-pig brain. *Eur. J. Biochem.* **1984**, *144*, 271–278. [CrossRef] [PubMed]

19. Garat, B.; Miranda, J.; Charli, J.L.; Joseph-Bravo, P. Presence of a membrane bound pyroglutamyl amino peptidase degrading thyrotropin releasing hormone in rat brain. *Neuropeptides* **1985**, *6*, 27–40. [CrossRef]

20. Friedman, T.C.; Wilk, S. Delineation of a particulate thyrotropin-releasing hormone-degrading enzyme in rat brain by the use of specific inhibitors of prolyl endopeptidase and pyroglutamyl peptide hydrolase. *J. Neurochem.* **1986**, *46*, 1231–1239. [CrossRef] [PubMed]

21. Ponce, G.; Charli, J.L.; Pasten, J.A.; Aceves, C.; Joseph-Bravo, P. Tissue-specific regulation of pyroglutamate aminopeptidase II activity by thyroid hormones. *Neuroendocrinology* **1988**, *48*, 211–213. [CrossRef] [PubMed]

22. Paxinos, G.; Watson, C. *The Rat Brain in Stereotaxic Coordinates*, 5th ed.; Elsevier Academic Press: Burlington, MA, USA, 2005.

23. de Gortari, P.; Fernandez-Guardiola, A.; Martinez, A.; Cisneros, M.; Joseph-Bravo, P. Changes in TRH and its degrading enzyme pyroglutamyl peptidase II, during the development of amygdaloid kindling. *Brain Res.* **1995**, *679*, 144–150. [CrossRef]

24. Joseph-Bravo, P.; Charli, J.L.; Palacios, J.M.; Kordon, C. Effect of neurotransmitters on the in vitro release of immunoreactive thyrotropin-releasing hormone from rat mediobasal hypothalamus. *Endocrinology* **1979**, *104*, 801–806. [CrossRef] [PubMed]

25. Lowry, O.; Rosebrough, N.; Farr, A.; Randall, R. Protein measurement with the Folin phenol reagent. *J. Biol. Chem.* **1951**, *193*, 265–275. [PubMed]

26. Coppola, A.; Meli, R.; Diano, S. Inverse shift in circulating corticosterone and leptin levels elevates hypothalamic deiodinase type 2 in fasted rats. *Endocrinology* **2005**, *146*, 2827–2833. [CrossRef] [PubMed]

27. Pekary, A.E.; Sattin, A.; Blood, J. Rapid modulation of TRH and TRH-like peptide release in rat brain and peripheral tissues by leptin. *Brain Res.* **2010**, *1345*, 9–18. [CrossRef] [PubMed]

28. Endo, T.; Ohta, K.; Haraguchi, K.; Onaya, T. Cloning and functional expression of a thyrotropin receptor cDNA from rat fat cells. *J. Biol. Chem.* **1995**, *270*, 10833–10837. [CrossRef] [PubMed]

29. Endo, T.; Kobayashi, T. Expression of functional TSH receptor in white adipose tissues of hyt/hyt mice induces lipolysis in vivo. *Am. J. Physiol. Endocrinol. Metab.* **2012**, *302*, E1569–E1575. [CrossRef] [PubMed]

30. Denereaz, N.; Lemarchand-Beraud, T. Severe but not mild alterations of thyroid function modulate the density of thyroid-stimulating hormone receptors in the rat thyroid gland. *Endocrinology* **1995**, *136*, 1694–1700. [CrossRef] [PubMed]

31. Singh, S.P.; McDonald, D.; Hope, T.J.; Prabhakar, B.S. Upon thyrotropin binding the thyrotropin receptor is internalized and localized to endosome. *Endocrinology* **2004**, *145*, 1003–1010. [CrossRef] [PubMed]

32. Donangelo, C.M.; King, J.C. Maternal zinc intakes and homeostatic adjustments during pregnancy and lactation. *Nutrients* **2012**, *4*, 782–798. [CrossRef] [PubMed]

33. Masters, D.G.; Keen, C.L.; Lonnerdal, B.; Hurley, L.S. Release of zinc from maternal tissues during zinc deficiency or simultaneous zinc and calcium deficiency in the pregnant rat. *J. Nutr.* **1986**, *116*, 2148–2154. [PubMed]

34. Levenson, C.W. Zinc regulation of food intake: New insights on the role of neuropeptide Y. *Nutr. Rev.* **2003**, *61*, 247–249. [PubMed]

35. Chowanadisai, W.; Kelleher, S.L.; Lonnerdal, B. Maternal zinc deficiency raises plasma prolactin levels in lactating rats. *J. Nutr.* **2004**, *134*, 1314–1319. [PubMed]

36. Blake, N.G.; Eckland, D.J.; Foster, O.J.; Lightman, S.L. Inhibition of hypothalamic thyrotropin-releasing hormone messenger ribonucleic acid during food deprivation. *Endocrinology* **1991**, *129*, 2714–2718. [CrossRef] [PubMed]

37. Van Haasteren, G.A.; Linkels, E.; van, T.H.; Klootwijk, W.; Kaptein, E.; de Jong, F.H.; Reymond, M.J.; Visser, T.J.; de Greef, W.J. Effects of long-term food reduction on the hypothalamus-pituitary-thyroid axis in male and female rats. *J. Endocrinol.* **1996**, *150*, 169–178. [CrossRef] [PubMed]

38. de Gortari, P.; Gonzalez-Alzati, M.E.; Cisneros, M.; Joseph-Bravo, P. Effect of fasting on the content of thyrotropin-releasing hormone and its RNAm in the central nervous system and pyroglutamyl peptidase II activity in the anterior pituitary of post-weaned and adult rats. *Nutr. Neurosci.* **2000**, *3*, 255–265. [CrossRef]

39. Geras, E.J.; Gershengorn, M.C. Evidence that TRH stimulates secretion of TSH by two calcium-mediated mechanisms. *Am. J. Physiol.* **1982**, *242*, E109–E114. [PubMed]

40. Nillni, E.A. Regulation of the hypothalamic thyrotropin releasing hormone (TRH) neuron by neuronal and peripheral inputs. *Front. Neuroendocrinol.* **2010**, *31*, 134–156. [CrossRef] [PubMed]

41. Dyess, E.M.; Segerson, T.P.; Liposits, Z.; Paull, W.K.; Kaplan, M.M.; Wu, P.; Jackson, I.M.; Lechan, R.M. Triiodothyronine exerts direct cell-specific regulation of thyrotropin-releasing hormone gene expression in the hypothalamic paraventricular nucleus. *Endocrinology* **1988**, *123*, 2291–2297. [CrossRef] [PubMed]

42. Baltaci, A.K.; Mogulkoc, R. Leptin, NPY, Melatonin and Zinc Levels in Experimental Hypothyroidism and Hyperthyroidism: The Relation to Zinc. *Biochem. Genet.* **2017**, *55*, 223–233. [CrossRef] [PubMed]

43. Mendez, M.; Joseph-Bravo, P.; Cisneros, M.; Vargas, M.A.; Charli, J.L. Regional distribution of in vitro release of thyrotropin releasing hormone in rat brain. *Peptides* **1987**, *8*, 291–298. [CrossRef]

44. Diano, S.; Naftolin, F.; Goglia, F.; Horvath, T.L. Fasting-induced increase in type II iodothyronine deiodinase activity and messenger ribonucleic acid levels is not reversed by thyroxine in the rat hypothalamus. *Endocrinology* **1998**, *139*, 2879–2884. [CrossRef] [PubMed]

45. Uribe, R.M.; Redondo, J.L.; Charli, J.L.; Joseph-Bravo, P. Suckling and cold stress rapidly and transiently increase TRH mRNA in the paraventricular nucleus. *Neuroendocrinology* **1993**, *58*, 140–145. [CrossRef] [PubMed]

46. Zoeller, R.T.; Rudeen, P.K. Ethanol blocks the cold-induced increase in thyrotropin-releasing hormone mRNA in paraventricular nuclei but not the cold-induced increase in thyrotropin. *Brain Res. Mol. Brain Res.* **1992**, *13*, 321–330. [CrossRef]

47. Jaimes-Hoy, L.; Joseph-Bravo, P.; de Gortari, P. Differential response of TRHergic neurons of the hypothalamic paraventricular nucleus (PVN) in female animals submitted to food-restriction or dehydration-induced anorexia and cold exposure. *Horm. Behav.* **2008**, *53*, 366–377. [CrossRef] [PubMed]

48. Peters, S.; Koh, J.; Choi, D.W. Zinc selectively blocks the action of N-methyl-D-aspartate on cortical neurons. *Science* **1987**, *236*, 589–593. [CrossRef] [PubMed]

49. Mayer, M.L.; Vyklicky, L., Jr. The action of zinc on synaptic transmission and neuronal excitability in cultures of mouse hippocampus. *J. Physiol.* **1989**, *415*, 351–365. [CrossRef] [PubMed]

50. Amico-Ruvio, S.A.; Murthy, S.E.; Smith, T.P.; Popescu, G.K. Zinc effects on NMDA receptor gating kinetics. *Biophys. J.* **2011**, *100*, 1910–1918. [CrossRef] [PubMed]

51. Wittmann, G.; Lechan, R.M.; Liposits, Z.; Fekete, C. Glutamatergic innervation of corticotropin-releasing hormone- and thyrotropin-releasing hormone-synthesizing neurons in the hypothalamic paraventricular nucleus of the rat. *Brain Res.* **2005**, *1039*, 53–62. [CrossRef] [PubMed]

52. Takeda, A.; Itoh, H.; Yamada, K.; Tamano, H.; Oku, N. Enhancement of hippocampal mossy fiber activity in zinc deficiency and its influence on behavior. *Biometals* **2008**, *21*, 545–552. [CrossRef] [PubMed]

53. Doboszewska, U.; Szewczyk, B.; Sowa-Kucma, M.; Noworyta-Sokolowska, K.; Misztak, P.; Golebiowska, J.; Mlyniec, K.; Ostachowicz, B.; Krosniak, M.; Wojtanowska-Krosniak, A.; et al. Alterations of Bio-elements, Oxidative, and Inflammatory Status in the Zinc Deficiency Model in Rats. *Neurotox. Res.* **2016**, *29*, 143–154. [CrossRef] [PubMed]

54. Kawashima, Y.; Someya, Y.; Sato, S.; Shirato, K.; Jinde, M.; Ishida, S.; Akimoto, S.; Kobayashi, K.; Sakakibara, Y.; Suzuki, Y.; et al. Dietary zinc-deficiency and its recovery responses in rat liver cytosolic alcohol dehydrogenase activities. *J. Toxicol. Sci.* **2011**, *36*, 101–108. [CrossRef] [PubMed]

55. Cho, Y.E.; Lomeda, R.A.; Ryu, S.H.; Sohn, H.Y.; Shin, H.I.; Beattie, J.H.; Kwun, I.S. Zinc deficiency negatively affects alkaline phosphatase and the concentration of Ca, Mg and P in rats. *Nutr. Res. Pract.* **2007**, *1*, 113–119. [CrossRef] [PubMed]

56. Dahlheim, H.; White, C.L.; Rothemund, J.; von Lutterotti, N.; Jacob, I.C.; Rosenthal, J. Effect of zinc depletion on angiotensin I-converting enzyme in arterial walls and plasma of the rat. *Miner. Electrolyte Metab.* **1989**, *15*, 125–129. [PubMed]

57. White, C.L.; Pschorr, J.; Jacob, I.C.; von Lutterotti, N.; Dahlheim, H. The effect of zinc in vivo and in vitro on the activities of angiotensin converting enzyme and kininase-I in the plasma of rats. *Biochem. Pharmacol.* **1986**, *35*, 2489–2493. [CrossRef]

58. Reeves, P.G.; O'Dell, B.L. An experimental study of the effect of zinc on the activity of angiotensin converting enzyme in serum. *Clin. Chem.* **1985**, *31*, 581–584. [PubMed]

59. Vargas, M.A.; Herrera, J.; Uribe, R.M.; Charli, J.L.; Joseph-Bravo, P. Ontogenesis of pyroglutamyl peptidase II activity in rat brain, adenohypophysis and pancreas. *Dev. Brain Res.* **1992**, *66*, 251–256. [CrossRef]

60. Takeda, A. Zinc homeostasis and functions of zinc in the brain. *Biometals* **2001**, *14*, 343–351. [CrossRef] [PubMed]

61. Licastro, F.; Mocchegiani, E.; Zannotti, M.; Arena, G.; Masi, M.; Fabris, N. Zinc affects the metabolism of thyroid hormones in children with Down's syndrome: Normalization of thyroid stimulating hormone and of reversal triiodothyronine plasmic levels by dietary zinc supplementation. *Int. J. Neurosci.* **1992**, *65*, 259–268. [CrossRef] [PubMed]

62. Franklyn, J.A. The thyroid—Too much and too little across the ages. The consequences of subclinical thyroid dysfunction. *Clin. Endocrinol.* **2013**, *78*, 1–8. [CrossRef] [PubMed]

63. Parle, J.V.; Franklyn, J.A.; Cross, K.W.; Jones, S.C.; Sheppard, M.C. Prevalence and follow-up of abnormal thyrotrophin (TSH) concentrations in the elderly in the United Kingdom. *Clin. Endocrinol.* **1991**, *34*, 77–83.

64. Mueller, A.; Schofl, C.; Dittrich, R.; Cupisti, S.; Oppelt, P.G.; Schild, R.L.; Beckmann, M.W.; Haberle, L. Thyroid-stimulating hormone is associated with insulin resistance independently of body mass index and age in women with polycystic ovary syndrome. *Hum. Reprod.* **2009**, *24*, 2924–2930. [CrossRef] [PubMed]

65. Yu, Q.; Wang, J.B. Subclinical Hypothyroidism in PCOS: Impact on Presentation, Insulin Resistance, and Cardiovascular Risk. *Biomed. Res. Int.* **2016**, *2016*, 2067087. [CrossRef] [PubMed]

66. Unal, E.; Akin, A.; Yildirim, R.; Demir, V.; Yildiz, I.; Haspolat, Y.K. Association of Subclinical Hypothyroidism with Dyslipidemia and Increased Carotid Intima-Media Thickness in Children. *J. Clin. Res. Pediatr. Endocrinol.* **2017**, *9*, 144–149. [CrossRef] [PubMed]

67. Decandia, F. Risk factors for cardiovascular disease in subclinical hypothyroidism. *Ir. J. Med. Sci.* **2017**. [CrossRef] [PubMed]

68. Zhou, J.B.; Li, H.B.; Zhu, X.R.; Song, H.L.; Zhao, Y.Y.; Yang, J.K. Subclinical hypothyroidism and the risk of chronic kidney disease in T2D subjects: A case-control and dose-response analysis. *Medicine* **2017**, *96*, e6519. [CrossRef] [PubMed]

69. Rahbar, A.R.; Kalantarhormozi, M.; Izadi, F.; Arkia, E.; Rashidi, M.; Pourbehi, F.; Daneshifard, F.; Rahbar, A. Relationship between Body Mass Index, Waist-to-Hip Ratio, and Serum Lipid Concentrations and Thyroid-Stimulating Hormone in the Euthyroid Adult Population. *Iran. J. Med. Sci.* **2017**, *42*, 301–305. [PubMed]

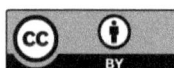

nutrients

MDPI

Article

Zinc Supplementation Improves Glucose Homeostasis in High Fat-Fed Mice by Enhancing Pancreatic β-Cell Function

Vinícius Cooper-Capetini [1], Diogo Antonio Alves de Vasconcelos [1], Amanda Roque Martins [1], Sandro Massao Hirabara [2], José Donato Jr. [1], Angelo Rafael Carpinelli [1] and Fernando Abdulkader [1,*]

[1] Department of Physiology and Biophysics, Institute of Biomedical Sciences, University of São Paulo, São Paulo 05508-000, Brazil; viniciuscapetini@gmail.com (V.C.-C.); diogovasconcelos13@yahoo.com.br (D.A.A.d.V.); amandamartins@usp.br (A.R.M.); jdonato@icb.usp.br (J.D.); angelo@icb.usp.br (A.R.C.)

[2] Institute of Physical Activity Sciences and Sports, Cruzeiro do Sul University, São Paulo 01506-000, Brazil; sandro.hirabara@gmail.com

*   Correspondence: fkader@icb.usp.br; Tel.: +55-11-3091-7286; Fax: +55-11-3091-7285

Received: 15 August 2017; Accepted: 3 October 2017; Published: 20 October 2017

Abstract: Zinc is an essential component of the insulin granule and it possibly modulates insulin secretion and signaling. Since insulin resistance is a hallmark in the development of type 2 diabetes mellitus, this study aimed at investigating if zinc supplementation is able to improve glucose tolerance and β-cell function in a model of insulin resistance. Male C57BL/6 mice were distributed in four groups according to the diet: normal fat (NF); normal fat supplemented with $ZnCl_2$ (NFZ); high-fat (HF); and, high-fat chow supplemented with $ZnCl_2$ (HFZ). Intraperitoneal glucose (ipGTT) and insulin (ipITT) tolerance, glycemia, insulinemia, HOMA-IR, and HOMA-β were determined after 15 weeks in each diet. Glucose-stimulated insulin secretion (GSIS) was investigated in isolated islets. The insulin effect on glucose uptake, metabolism, and signaling was investigated in soleus muscle. $ZnCl_2$ did not affect body mass or insulin sensitivity as assessed by ipITT, HOMA-IR, muscle glucose metabolism, and Akt and GSK3-β phosphorylation. However, glucose tolerance, HOMA-β, and GSIS were significantly improved by $ZnCl_2$ supplementation. Therefore, $ZnCl_2$ supplementation improves glucose homeostasis in high fat-fed mice by a mechanism that enhances β-cell function, rather than whole-body or muscle insulin sensitivity.

Keywords: zinc; diabetes mellitus; insulin; insulin resistance

1. Introduction

Diabetes mellitus is a growing public health problem affecting approximately 9% of the adult population worldwide [1]. While type 1 diabetes mellitus (T1DM) predominantly results from autoimmune destruction of pancreatic β-cells, with little or no insulin synthesis, type 2 diabetes mellitus (T2DM) develops due to the installation of insulin resistance in target tissues (reviewed in [2]), and high circulating insulin levels. This condition in the long-term can lead to a progressive exhaustion and ultimate destruction of the β-cells [3]. Currently, the treatment of T2DM is based on lifestyle modification, in addition to the administration of oral antihyperglycemic drugs or, in later stages, insulin treatment. However, an ancillary effect of zinc supplementation has been previously proposed to treat T2DM and its complications. Those studies have reported better glycemic control associated with the administration of this mineral [4–6], suggesting that zinc is a potential therapeutic agent for the treatment of diabetes.

In the secretory granules of β-cells, insulin is associated with zinc in a stoichiometry of two zinc ions to six molecules of insulin. This combination stabilizes and prevents the degradation of insulin hexamers, protecting this hormone from the action of proteolytic enzymes [7]. In β-cells, the level of zinc appears to mediate various signaling pathways, suggesting that this mineral can act as a signaling molecule. In addition, zinc can also be a regulator of cellular metabolism [8], having antioxidant and anti-apoptotic effects. These effects occur via an enhancement in the cytosolic copper-zinc superoxide dismutase activity, metallothionein overexpression, or the inhibition of caspases and xanthine oxidase [9]. Additionally, zinc is an essential part of zinc finger-based transcription factors, such as transcription factor teashirt zinc finger homeobox 1 (Tshz1) and GLIS family zinc finger 3 (Glis3). The deficiency of these transcription factors is associated with the development of diabetes mellitus (DM) [10,11]. Therefore, an imbalance in the homeostatic control of zinc in these cells could cause significant damage in insulin secretion [12].

The effect of zinc on peripheral insulin sensitivity has also aroused the interest of many researchers. This mineral appears to be involved in insulin receptor signal transduction [13,14]. Zinc supplementation improves insulin sensitivity in adipocytes by activating hormone signaling pathways. Therefore, this mineral has insulin-mimetic effects [15,16], leading to the translocation of GLUT-4-containing vesicles to the plasma membrane [14]. Although it has been widely known that skeletal muscle is the predominant site of insulin-mediated glucose uptake [17,18] and that abnormalities in the insulin receptor signaling pathway in this tissue are associated with insulin resistance [19,20], there is little information about the metabolic effects of zinc on the insulin-signaling pathway in the skeletal muscle in DM.

While several studies have reported the participation of zinc in the synthesis and secretion of insulin, and on the control of insulinemia and glycemia [12,14,15], it is still unclear whether these positive effects on glycemic control in diabetic patients could be associated with an improvement in insulin secretion or sensitivity. The understanding of the molecular mechanisms of the action of zinc in DM would contribute to the development of targeted therapies and direct future research. In that regard, we have investigated in this study the effect of $ZnCl_2$ in the control of insulin secretion and glycemia in a mouse model of glucose intolerance induced by high-fat chow. The results will be important to understand if the supplementation with $ZnCl_2$ prevents or delays the manifestation of T2DM.

2. Materials and Methods

2.1. Animals, Treatments and Monitoring

After 11 days of weaning, male C57BL/6 mice were weighed and randomly divided into four experimental groups with the following dietary treatments for 15 weeks: (1) Normal-Fat chow (NF); (2) Normal-Fat chow, Zinc-supplemented (NFZ), in which the animals received normal-fat chow and supplementation with 20 mM $ZnCl_2$ in water; (3) High-Fat chow (HF); and, (4) High-Fat chow, Zinc-supplemented (HFZ), that received high-fat chow and supplementation with 20 mM $ZnCl_2$. The animals were maintained under controlled environmental conditions and had free access to chow and water (pH 5.0). The chow was adapted from the guidelines of the American Institute of Nutrition [21]. Pork lard was added in the high-fat chow in substitution to cornstarch. The normal-fat chow consisted of 69.9% carbohydrates, 10% fat, and 20.1% proteins. In contrast, the high-fat chow had 60% of its energetic value composed of fats, 19.9% carbohydrates, and 20.1% proteins. All of the procedures with animals were previously approved by the IACUC of the Institute of Biomedical Sciences, University of São Paulo, São Paulo, Brazil.

2.2. Glucose Tolerance and Insulin Sensitivity Tests

In the 14th week of treatment, animals were submitted to intraperitoneal glucose tolerance test (ipGTT) and insulin (ipITT). After 6 h of food restriction, animals had their glycemia measured by glucometer FreeStyle Lite® (Abbott, Alameda, CA, USA), through blood sample collection from the tail, before (0 min) and 15, 30, 60, 90, and 120 min after an intraperitoneal administration of saline solution (0.9% NaCl) containing 20% glucose (at a dose of 1 mg glucose/g body weight). Then, the area under the curve (AUC) was calculated with the obtained values. The ipITT was performed 48 h after the ipGTT; after 4 h of food deprivation, animals had their glycemia measured using the same blood glucometer, before (0 min) and after 5, 10, 15, 20, 30, 40, and 60 min of the intraperitoneal administration of insulin Humulin® (0.75 U/kg) (Lilly France, Fegersheim, FRA) [22]. The glucose decay constant rate (k_{ITT}) was calculated as the slope of the linear regression of glucose concentration from 5 to 15 min after insulin administration [23].

2.3. Serum Measurements

After 15 weeks of treatment and 8h-fasting, animals were euthanized by cervical dislocation followed by decapitation. Serum samples were obtained for the measurement of glucose concentration using a glucose oxidase colorimetric kit (Liquiform®, Labtest, Lagoa Santa, MG, Brazil). Serum insulin concentration was determined by radioimmunoassay or by ELISA (Rat/Mouse Insulin Assay EZRMI-13K, Millipore Corporation, Billerica, MA, USA).

The tissue sensitivity to insulin and the functional capacity of pancreatic β-cell function to secrete insulin were assessed by homeostasis model assessment (HOMA). The fasting glycemia and insulinemia values were used to calculate the insulin sensitivity index (HOMA-IR) and the secretory capacity of the β-cell (HOMA-β), using the following equations: (a) HOMA$-$IR = glucose × insulin ÷ 22.5; and, (b) HOMA$-$β = 20 × insulin ÷ (glucose $-$ 3.5), respectively [24].

2.4. Pancreatic Islet Isolation and Glucose-Stimulated Insulin Secretion (GSIS) Determination

Islets were isolated by digesting the pancreas with type IV collagenase solution (Sigma, St. Louis, MO, USA) (0.68 mg/mL) in Hanks' buffer (in mM: NaCl 137, KCl 5, CaCl$_2$ 1, MgSO$_4$ 1, Na$_2$HPO$_4$ 0.3, KH$_2$PO$_4$ 0.4, NaHCO$_3$ 4; pH 7.4) [25]. Islets were then hand-picked in Hanks' buffer and groups of 5 islets, in triplicate, were pre-incubated in Krebs-Henseleit buffer (NaCl 115, CaCl$_2$ 1, NaHCO$_3$ 24, KCl 5, MgCl$_2$ 1; pH 7.4 with 95% O$_2$: 5% CO$_2$), supplemented with 0.2% bovine serum albumin (BSA) w/v and 5.6 mM glucose, at 37 °C for 30 min. After pre-incubation, the solution was discarded and the islets were incubated for 1 h at 37 °C with the same buffer supplemented with 2.8 or 16.7 mM glucose. After glucose stimulation, the supernatant was retrieved and the total insulin content of the islets was extracted using an ethanol–water–HCl solution (52:17:1 v/v). Both supernatant and content samples were then frozen at -20 °C and subsequently assayed for insulin by radioimmunoassay.

2.5. Soleus Muscle Incubation and Protein Extraction

Soleus muscles of both limbs were quickly and carefully isolated after euthanasia, weighed, fixed in stainless steel staples maintaining the resting tension, and pre-incubated for 30 min, with O$_2$/CO$_2$ atmosphere (95%/5%), at 35 °C and 90 oscillations per min, in Krebs-Ringer-bicarbonate buffer (NaCl 118.5, NaHCO$_3$, KCl 3.6, MgSO$_4$ 0.5, CaCl$_2$ 1.5, pH 7.4), containing 5.6 mM glucose and 1% BSA. Following the pre-incubation period, muscles were incubated for 20 min in the same conditions, in the presence or absence of 7 nmol/L insulin. Muscles were then homogenized in an appropriate buffer (Tris 100 mM, EDTA 1mM) supplemented with phosphatase (sodium pyrophosphate 10 mM; sodium fluoride 100 mM and sodium orthovanadate 10 mM) and protease inhibitors (PMSF 2 mM and Protease Inhibitor Cocktail®—Thermo Fisher, Chicago, IL, USA). After homogenization, 1% Triton X-100 was added to the homogenates and all samples were kept for 30 min at 4 °C prior to the centrifugation for 20 min at 340× *g* to remove all of the insoluble material. The Bradford method was used to determine the total protein content of the samples. The protein extracts were boiled for 5 min in a water bath and maintained at -80 °C for future analysis by Western blotting.

2.6. Western Blotting

Thirty micrograms of total proteins of soleus muscle were submitted to electrophoretic separation in 12% polyacrylamide gel containing sodium dodecylsulfate (SDS-PAGE 12%) in the Mini-Protean apparatus for minigel (BioRad, Hercules, CA, USA). Electrotransfer of proteins from the gels to nitrocellulose membranes was performed for 1 h at 15 V in a semi-dry apparatus (BioRad, Hercules, CA, USA). The membranes were incubated overnight at 4 °C, under agitation, in TSB (Tris 10 mM and NaCl 1.5 mM—pH 7.6) with 5% BSA to block nonspecific binding of antibodies to the membranes. Then, membranes were incubated overnight at 4 °C with primary antibodies against total Akt (#9272) and GSK3-β (#2710), phospho-Akt (Ser473) (#5473) and phospho-GSK3-β (Ser9) (#9336) (Cell Signaling Technology, Beverly, MA, USA). The antibodies were diluted (1:1000) in TSB with 3% BSA. Following that, membranes were incubated with a secondary HRP-conjugated antibody (Millipore, Temecula, CA, USA) for 60 min at room temperature and then incubated with a solution containing the chemiluminescence reagent (ECL) and exposed to photographic film. The intensity of the colored bands was determined by densitometry using Image Studio Digits 3.1® software (LI-COR Biosciences, Lincoln, NE, USA). Band intensities were normalized to Ponceau staining to determine the relative protein expression [26].

2.7. Glucose Uptake and Metabolism in Isolated Soleus Muscle

Soleus muscles were isolated and pre-incubated, as described previously (Section 2.5). After pre-incubation, muscles were incubated for 1 h in the same conditions, in the presence or absence of 7 nmol/L insulin with the addition of 0.2 µCi/mL of 2-deoxi-[2,6-^{3}H]-D-glucose, 0.3 µCi/mL of [U-^{14}C]-D-glucose (Perkin Elmer, Waltham, MA, USA). A microtube containing 200 µL NaOH 2 M was added into the incubation flask for $^{14}CO_2$ adsorption. After the incubation period, muscles were washed in cold PBS for one minute and then stored at −80 °C for further measurements. The medium used for the muscle incubation was acidified with 5 N HCl and held at 35 °C under constant stirring (180 oscillation per minute), for 1 h. The NaOH solution was then removed for the quantification of the $^{14}CO_2$ released by muscle metabolism and absorbed by this solution. The muscles were digested in 300 µL of 1 M KOH, at 70 °C for 20 min, and 100 µL were reserved for the quantification of the uptake of 2-deoxy-[2,6-^{3}H]-D-glucose. A saturated solution of Na_2SO_4 was added to the remainder for glycogen extraction in ethanolic solution, and then centrifuged at 4 °C for 15 min, at 425× *g*. The supernatant was discarded and the pellet resuspended and quantified for [U-^{14}C]-glycogen synthesis and incorporation of [U-^{14}C]-D-glucose into the muscle [27,28]. The radioactivity was quantified with Tri-Carb® 2810TR counter (Perkin Elmer, Waltham, MA, USA) using a scintillation solution.

2.8. Statistical Analyses

Data (mean ± SEM) were analyzed with Graph Pad Prism6® software (Graph Pad Software, Inc., La Jolla, CA, USA) by Two-way ANOVA following Bonferroni's multiple comparison post-test or by Student's *t* test, when appropriate. A value of $p \leq 0.05$ was considered for statistical differences. Only *p*-values less than 0.05 are reported in the figures.

3. Results

3.1. Body Mass and Intake of Diet, Water and $ZnCl_2$

As expected, animals consuming high-fat chow gained more body mass in relation to those in normal-fat chow ($p < 0.01$) (Figure 1A). $ZnCl_2$ supplementation did not interfere with the body weight gain. The higher body weight in animals fed the high-fat chow was associated with an increased caloric intake, when compared to normal-fat chow ($p < 0.05$) (Figure 1B). Throughout the treatment, $ZnCl_2$-suplemented animals consumed less water than the NF ($p < 0.01$) and HF ($p < 0.05$—Figure 1C) groups. As expected, the $ZnCl_2$ supplementation was reflected in increased Zn^{2+} daily intake in the supplemented groups, while no effect of chow was observed on Zn^{2+} intake (NF = 0.06 ± 0.0;

HF = 0.09 ± 0.0; NFZ = 8.37 ± 0.3; and HFZ = 8.14 ± 0.2 mg Zn/day per animal — n = 30; 2-way ANOVA: chow $p > 0.05$, zinc supplementation $p < 0.001$, interaction $p > 0.05$; Bonferroni's Post Test: NF vs. HF $p > 0.05$, NFZ vs. HFZ $p > 0.05$).

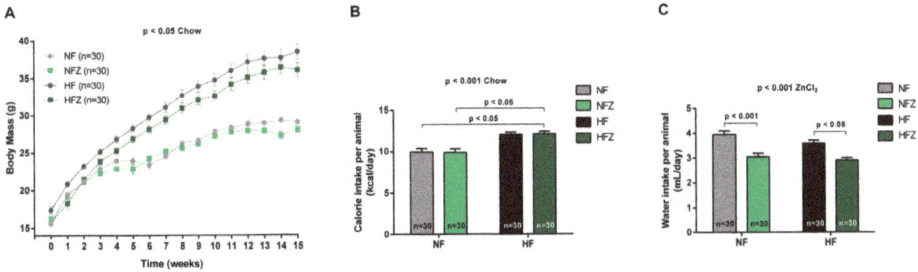

Figure 1. Body mass and caloric, hydric and ZnCl$_2$ intakes. Body weight gain (**A**), calorie intake (**B**) and water intake (**C**) of animals of the NF and HF groups and those supplemented with ZnCl$_2$. Values are means ± S.E.M. Two-way ANOVA: final body mass (chow, $p < 0.01$; zinc, $p > 0.05$; interaction, $p > 0.05$); calorie intake (chow, $p < 0.001$; zinc, $p > 0.05$; interaction, $p > 0.05$); and, water intake (chow, $p > 0.05$; zinc, $p < 0.001$; interaction, $p > 0.05$).

3.2. Glycemia, Insulinemia, Homeostasis Model Assessment, Glucose Tolerance and Insulin Sensitivity

Fifteen weeks in high-fat chow led to hyperglycemia as compared to NF and HFZ groups ($p < 0.05$) and, notably, ZnCl$_2$ supplementation prevented the increase in glycemia induced by high-fat chow (Figure 2A). Basal insulinemia showed no difference between the groups, although a significant effect of the chow was observed in the analysis (Figure 2B).

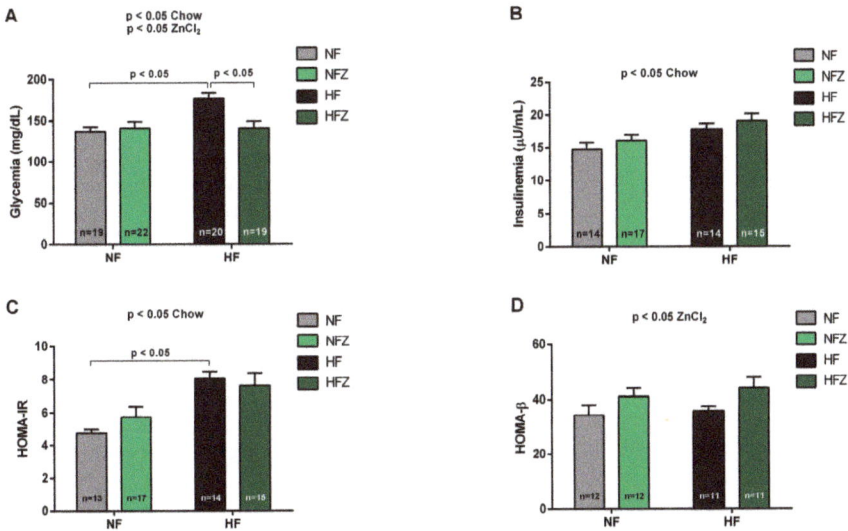

Figure 2. *Cont.*

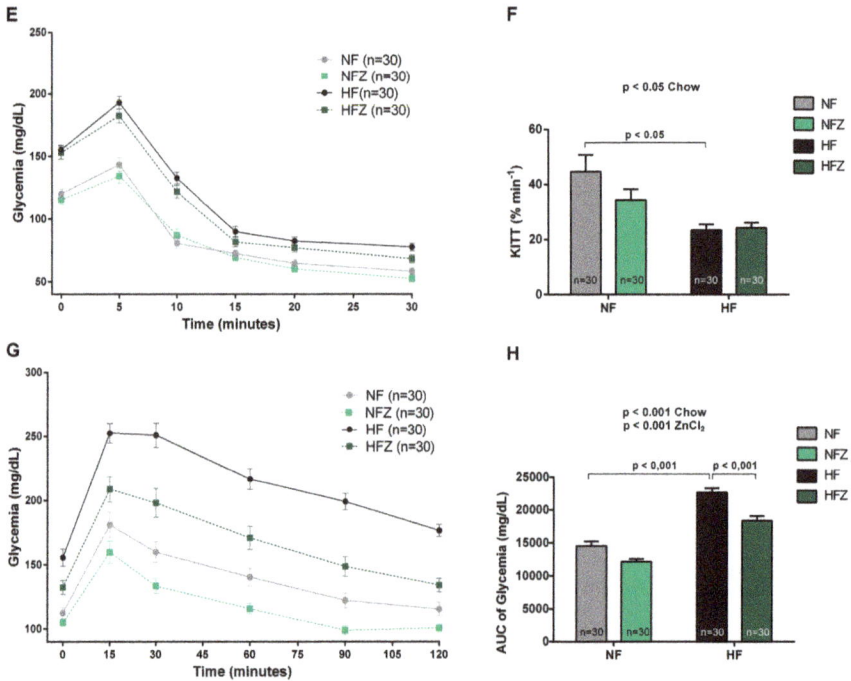

Figure 2. Serum parameters analysis. Glycemia (**A**), insulinemia (**B**), HOMA-IR (**C**), HOMA-β (**D**), ipITT (**E**), k_{ITT} ipGTT (**F**), ipGTT (**G**), and area under the curve (AUC) of ipGTT (**H**). Two-way ANOVA: glycemia (chow, $p < 0.05$; zinc, $p < 0.05$; interaction, $p < 0.05$); insulinemia (chow, $p < 0.05$; zinc, $p > 0.05$; interaction, $p > 0.05$): HOMA-IR (chow, $p < 0.01$; zinc, $p > 0.05$; interaction, $p > 0.05$); HOMA-β (chow, $p > 0.05$; zinc, $p < 0.05$; interaction, $p > 0.05$); k_{ITT} (chow, $p < 0.01$; zinc, $p > 0.05$; interaction, $p > 0.05$); and AUC ipGTT (chow, $p < 0.01$; zinc, $p < 0.01$; interaction, $p > 0.05$).

HOMA-IR and HOMA-β are indices that estimate, respectively, insulin resistance and β-cell secretory function [24]. The results of the HOMA-IR index indicated that high-fat fed groups were more insulin resistant as compared to the NF and NFZ groups ($p < 0.05$), and $ZnCl_2$ supplementation was not able to prevent this dysfunction (Figure 2C). On the other hand, HOMA-β results suggested an improved secretory function of β-cells in $ZnCl_2$-suplemented animals, regardless of the diet ($p < 0.05$) (Figure 2D).

To study in more detail the insulin sensitivity in the experimental groups, an ipITT was performed (Figure 2E). In line with the HOMA-IR results, chronic consumption of high-fat chow significantly reduced the glucose decay constant (k_{ITT}) (Figure 2F), and $ZnCl_2$ supplementation produced no beneficial effects to prevent this insulin resistance. Then, an ipGTT was performed. In contrast to the ipITT results, $ZnCl_2$ supplementation significantly improved the glucose tolerance either in mice consuming low- or high-fat diets. Furthermore, the area under the curve (AUC) (Figure 2G) of glycemia during the ipGTT (Figure 2H) was reduced in the HFZ group ($p < 0.01$), as compared to HF animals. Since the response to the ipGTT relies on endogenous insulin secretion, our findings collectively indicate that $ZnCl_2$ supplementation improves glucose homeostasis via an increased glucose-stimulated insulin secretion.

3.3. Insulin Signaling and Glucose Metabolism in the Soleus Muscle

Previous studies have also described the changes in muscle insulin sensitivity after zinc supplementation [29,30]. Thus, despite no changes in whole-body insulin sensitivity in our zinc-supplemented animals, we further studied if zinc supplementation could affect insulin signaling and metabolism specifically in the skeletal muscle. The content of Akt and GSK3-β proteins in soleus muscle did not change among the groups. Insulin increased the phosphorylation of Akt, but not of phospho-GSK3-β, in the experimental groups. However, supplementation with $ZnCl_2$ did not affect the response to insulin (Figure 3).

When glucose uptake and metabolism were evaluated in soleus muscle, we observed that insulin increased the uptake of 2-deoxy [2,6-3H]-D-glucose (Figure 4A), the incorporation of [U-14C]-D-glucose (Figure 4B) and glycogen synthesis (Figure 4C). On the other hand, high-fat chow reduced soleus glucose uptake, glycogen synthesis, and glucose oxidation (Figure 4). Importantly, zinc intake did not affect these responses, indicating no effect of supplementation directly on glucose metabolism in skeletal muscle.

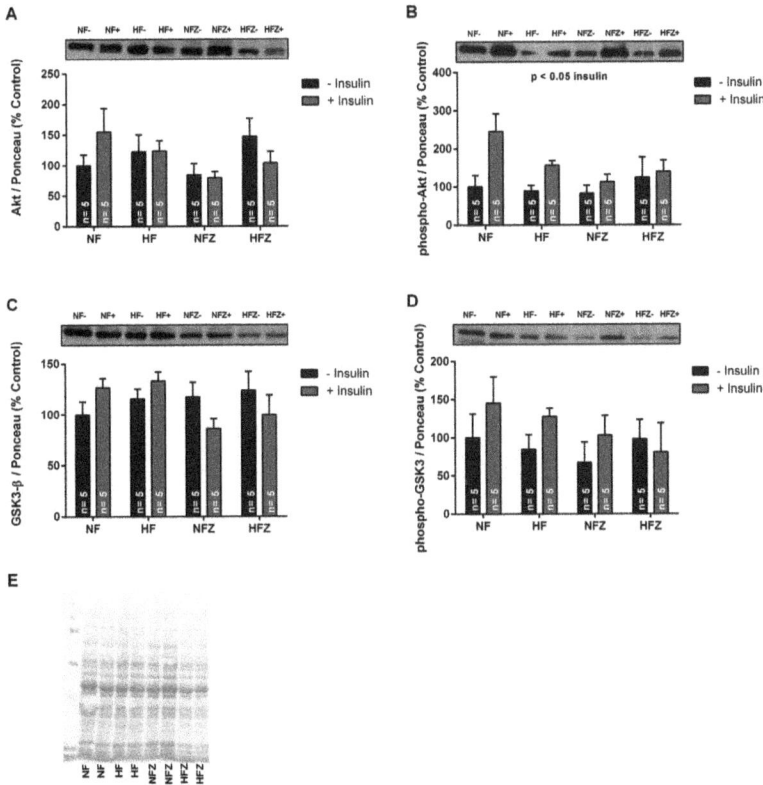

Figure 3. Effect of supplementation with $ZnCl_2$ on the content and phosphorylation of Akt and GSK3-β in soleus muscle. Total Akt (**A**); phospho-Akt (Ser[473]) (**B**); total GSK3-β (**C**); phospho-GSK3- β (Ser[9]) (**D**); ponceau staining used for normalization (**E**). Two-way ANOVA: total Akt (chow, $p > 0.05$; insulin, $p > 0.05$; interaction $p > 0.05$); phospho-Akt (Ser[473]) (chow, $p > 0.05$; insulin, $p < 0.05$; interaction, $p > 0.05$); total GSK3-β (chow, $p > 0.05$; insulin, $p < 0.05$; interaction, $p > 0.05$); and, phospho-GSK3-β (Ser[9]) (chow, $p > 0.05$; insulin, $p > 0.05$; interaction, $p > 0.05$).

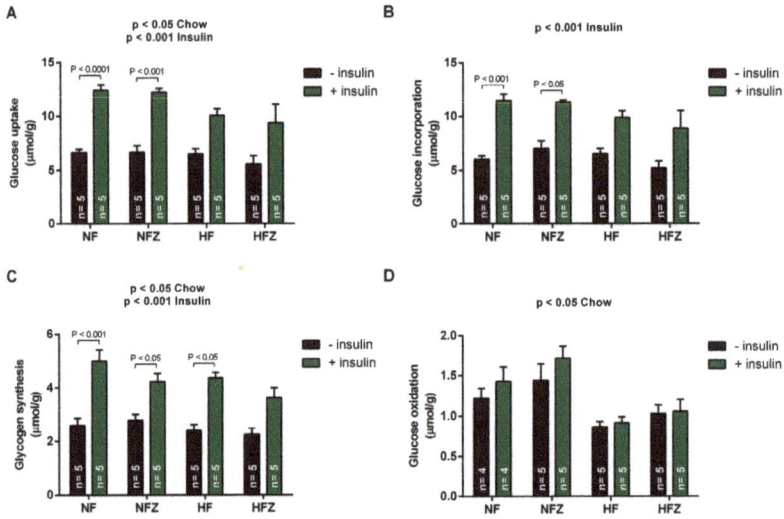

Figure 4. Uptake and metabolism of glucose in the soleus muscle. Glucose uptake (**A**), glucose incorporation (**B**), glycogen synthesis (**C**) and glucose oxidation (**D**) were assessed in the soleus muscle. Two-way ANOVA: glucose uptake (chow, $p < 0.05$; insulin, $p < 0.01$; interaction, $p > 0.05$); glucose incorporation (chow, $p > 0.05$; insulin, $p < 0.01$; interaction, $p > 0.05$); glycogen synthesis (chow, $p < 0.05$; insulin, $p < 0.01$; interaction, $p > 0.05$); and, glucose oxidation (insulin, $p > 0.05$; chow, $p < 0.01$; interaction, $p > 0.05$).

3.4. Glucose-Stimulated Insulin Secretion (GSIS)

To evaluate the effects of zinc supplementation now on β-cell secretory function, we performed incubations of freshly isolated islets from mice of the four experimental groups with different glucose concentrations. Consistent with our previous in vivo results, we observed an enhanced insulin secretion elicited by 16.7 mM glucose in the groups that received $ZnCl_2$ supplementation (Figure 5A right). No effect of the treatments was detected at the low (2.8 mM) glucose concentration (Figure 5A left). The effects of zinc supplementation cannot be explained by changes in the insulin content in the islets, since no significant difference was detected in the islet insulin content among the groups (Figure 5B).

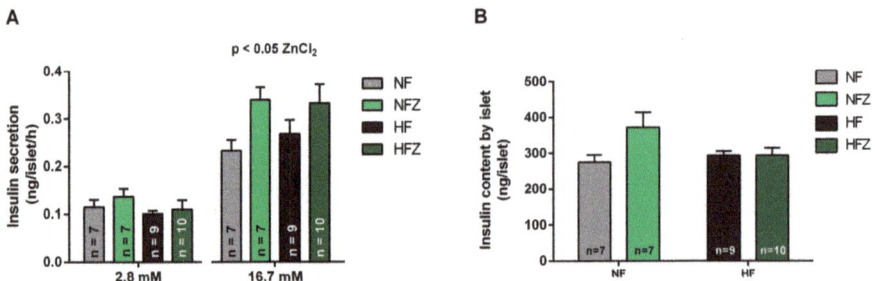

Figure 5. Glucose-stimulated insulin secretion (GSIS) and insulin content of isolated pancreatic islets. Effect of low (2.8 mM) and high (16.7 mM) glucose concentration in insulin secretion (ng/islet/h) (**A**). Islet insulin content (**B**). Two-way ANOVA of the insulin secretion by islets at 16.7 mM glucose (chow, $p > 0.05$; zinc, $p < 0.05$; interaction, $p > 0.05$).

4. Discussion

As expected, high-fat chow used in this study was able to generate an appropriate model of mouse obesity, insulin resistance, and glucose intolerance, which are typical characteristics of T2DM. Supplementation with $ZnCl_2$ was efficient to improve glucose homeostasis in high fat-fed mice. The zinc effects were apparently mediated by a positive effect on β-cell function, improving insulin secretion, instead of affecting body mass, peripheral insulin sensitivity, or muscle glucose uptake, and metabolism (Figure 6).

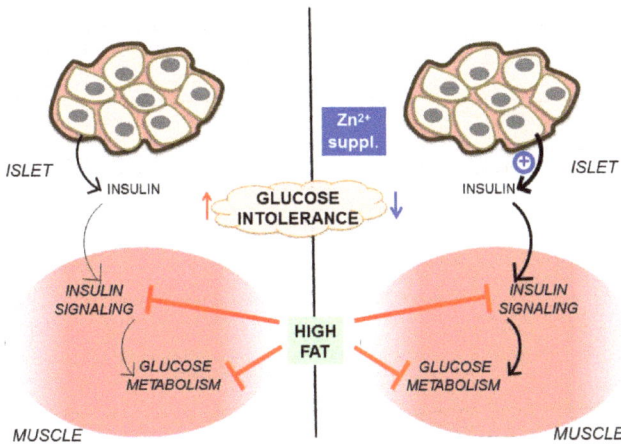

Figure 6. Improvement of glucose homeostasis by zinc supplementation in high fat-fed mice.

Excessive intake of zinc for long periods may interfere with the metabolism of iron and copper, with consequences to the immune system and reducing HDL-cholesterol concentrations [31,32]. Although these biochemical markers were not investigated in the present study, previous studies reported no signs of toxicity or adverse effects in *ob/ob* mice supplemented with 20 mM $ZnCl_2$ in the water for eight weeks [4]. The oral toxicity of $ZnCl_2$ has been observed in rats, when the daily ingestion was administrated in excess (350 mg/kg) [33], but none of the groups supplemented in this study have reached this value. Additionally, zinc supplementation had no effect on body mass gain in the present study. These results are also another evidence of the lack of toxicity in the supplemented dose used. Furthermore, these results also suggest that $ZnCl_2$ supplementation does not interfere with the endocrine and neural control of food intake, energy expenditure, and body mass. Despite it is possible that the $ZnCl_2$ dissolved in water interfered with palatability, since a reduction in water intake was observed in animals receiving supplementation, we believe that this reduced water intake is most probably due to the increased electrolyte drinking in the supplemented animals, and thus a lower fluid intake to sustain whole body fluid and osmolyte balance.

Chronic consumption of a fat rich diet is associated with hyperglycemia and insulin resistance [34,35]. Accordingly, the HF group became hyperglycemic, glucose intolerant, and insulin resistant. Despite some studies have suggested that zinc improves insulin resistance [13,14,36], the results of HOMA-IR, k_{ITT}, muscle expression and phosphorylation of Akt and GSK3-β, and glucose uptake and metabolism in the soleus muscle showed that the $ZnCl_2$ supplementation did not improve diet-induced insulin resistance. In fact, other authors have shown that supplementation with zinc can improve and/or mimic the action of insulin in adipose tissue [15,21], via an increase in glucose transport mediated by PI3-K and Akt [14] and the phosphorylation of GSK3-β [15,36]. However, the contribution of adipose tissue to the whole-body metabolism is limited, particularly when compared to skeletal muscle [37], which is quantitatively the major site of insulin-mediated glucose uptake [38]. Therefore, even if zinc supplementation could have improved glucose uptake in adipose tissue, this effect would possibly not be sufficient to reverse the whole-body insulin resistance induced by high-fat chow. In line with our results, Simon and Taylor [5] did not observe improvement in the tyrosine kinase activity of the insulin receptor in gastrocnemius muscle of *db/db* mice supplemented with 300 ppm of zinc for six weeks, confirming that the insulin resistance in skeletal muscle is not reversed or ameliorated by supplementation with this mineral.

Although insulin resistance was not improved, the supplementation with $ZnCl_2$ increased insulin secretion in islets incubated with 16.7 mM glucose. HOMA-β results were also another evidence of increased efficiency of β-cells in $ZnCl_2$-supplemented animals. The zinc effects on β-cell function were able to improve glucose homeostasis in high fat-fed mice. HFZ group showed a reduced hyperglycemia and a better glucose tolerance, as compared to HF group. Corroborating our results, Chen et al. [4] demonstrated that 20 mM $ZnCl_2$ supplementation in water for eight weeks reduced the glycemia in *ob/ob* mice. Therefore, these results support the hypothesis that $ZnCl_2$ optimized the functioning of the β-cells and consequently improved glycemic control. Also in line with our results, Nygaard et al. [12] showed that $ZnCl_2$ is effective in improving insulin secretion and increasing the expression of zinc transporters ZnT3 and ZnT8 and MT1A in INS-1E cells. The effect in β-cells reported in the present study is apparently a general increase in β-cell function, not a protection against lesion, since zinc supplementation was associated with increased GSIS in both NFZ and HFZ groups, when compared to their respective non-supplemented groups.

Besides increasing GSIS, it is possible that zinc supplementation also decreases the availability of insulin to peripheral tissues, as zinc may increase the activity of the insulin-degrading enzyme (IDE) [39]. The IDE is the major enzyme responsible for insulin degradation in the liver and kidneys [40]. Thus, if IDE enzyme activity was increased in the groups supplemented with zinc, this could explain why we did not observe an effect on fasting insulinemia in these groups. However, zinc-supplemented animals exhibited an unaltered response to insulin infusion and an improved glucose tolerance, which suggest that any potential changes in the activity of IDE did not prevent the insulin effects on target tissues.

Among the possible mechanisms responsible for the β-cell-specific effect of zinc supplementation, one could consider changes promoted by zinc on the expression and/or the maintenance of proteins related to insulin processing in the β-cells, such as zinc transporters, MT, Cu-Zn SOD antioxidant enzyme, and ZnF, Tshz1, and Glis3 [10,14]. The study of the molecular mechanisms of zinc on the expression of these proteins may generate new knowledge about the mechanisms relating to the synthesis, storage, and, mainly, the secretion of insulin. The understanding of the influence of zinc on these mechanisms may allow the development of new therapeutic targets for the treatment of T2DM.

5. Conclusions

The results obtained in this study indicate an improvement in β-cell function and, consequently, in the glycemic control in animals supplemented with $ZnCl_2$. Although the mechanism behind the improvement in β-cells function has not been identified, our findings suggest that supplementation with $ZnCl_2$ can delay the manifestation of T2DM in a mouse model of diet-induced obesity.

Acknowledgments: This work was supported by Coordenação de Aperfeiçoamento de Pessoal de Nível Superior (CAPES), Conselho Nacional de Desenvolvimento Científico e Tecnológico (CNPq) and Fundação de Amparo à Pesquisa do Estado de São Paulo (FAPESP), Brazil. The authors thank Andressa Costa, Juan Pablo Zúñiga-Hertz, Daniel Blanc, Eduardo Rebelato and Pedro Modena for assistance in some experimental procedures and/or analyses, and professors Rui Curi, Silvana Bordin, Ubiratan F. Machado and Fernanda Ortis (Universidade de São Paulo) for critical comments on previous stages of this work.

Author Contributions: V.C.C. carried out experimental design, experimental procedures, data analysis, and paper writing. D.A.A.V. carried out experimental procedures (expression of Akt and GSK3-β in the soleus muscle) and data analysis. A.R.M. and S.M.H. performed experimental procedures (glucose uptake and metabolism in isolated soleus muscle) and data analysis. J.D.J. carried out data analysis and revised the paper. A.R.C. contributed with key reagents and procedures and revised the paper. F.A. carried out experimental design, performed experimental procedures (insulin secretion assays) and revised the paper.

Conflicts of Interest: The authors declare no conflict of interest.

References

1. International Diabetes Federation. IDF Diabetes Atlas-7th Edition-2015. Diabetes Atlas, 7th Ed 2015:1–2. Available online: http://www.diabetesatlas.org/ (accessed 16 November 2016).
2. Halban, P.A.; Polonsky, K.S.; Bowden, D.W.; Hawkins, M.A.; Ling, C.; Mather, K.J.; Powers, A.C.; Rhodes, C.J.; Sussel, L.; Weir, G.C. β-Cell Failure in Type 2 Diabetes: Postulated Mechanisms and Prospects for Prevention and Treatment. *J. Clin. Endocrinol. Metab.* **2014**, *99*, 1983–1992. [CrossRef] [PubMed]
3. Bergman, R.N.; Ader, M.; Huecking, K.; Van Citters, G. Accurate assessment of β-cell function: The hyperbolic correction. *Diabetes* **2002**, *51*, S212–S220. [CrossRef] [PubMed]
4. Chen, M.D.; Liou, S.J.; Lin, P.Y.; Yang, V.C.; Alexander, P.S.; Lin, W.H. Effects of zinc supplementation on the plasma glucose level and insulin activity in genetically obese (ob/ob) mice. *Biol. Trace Elem. Res.* **1998**, *61*, 303–311. [CrossRef] [PubMed]
5. Simon, S.F.; Taylor, C.G. Dietary zinc supplementation attenuates hyperglycemia in db/db mice. *Exp. Biol. Med.* **2001**, *226*, 43–51. [CrossRef]
6. Al-Maroof, R.A.; Al-Sharbatti, S.S. Serum zinc levels in diabetic patients and effect of zinc supplementation on glycemic control of type 2 diabetics. *Saudi Med. J.* **2006**, *27*, 344–350. [PubMed]
7. Emdin, S.O.; Dodson, G.G.; Cutfield, J.M.; Cutfield, S.M. Role of zinc in insulin biosynthesis. *Diabetologia* **1980**, *19*, 174–182. [CrossRef] [PubMed]
8. Sensi, S.L.; Paoletti, P.; Bush, A.I.; Sekler, I. Zinc in the physiology and pathology of the CNS. *Nat. Rev. Neurosci.* **2009**, *10*, 780–791. [CrossRef] [PubMed]
9. Bosco, M.D.; Mohanasundaram, D.M.; Drogemuller, C.J.; Lang, C.J.; Zalewski, P.D.; Coates, P.T. Zinc and zinc transporter regulation in pancreatic islets and the potential role of zinc in islet transplantation. *Rev. Diabet. Stud.* **2010**, *7*, 263–274. [CrossRef] [PubMed]
10. Raum, J.C.; Soleimanpour, S.A.; Groff, D.N.; Coré, N.; Fasano, L.; Garratt, A.N.; Dai, C.; Powers, A.C.; Stoffers, D.A. Tshz1 regulates pancreatic beta cell maturation. *Diabetes* **2015**, *9*, db141443. [CrossRef]
11. Yang, Y.; Chang, B.H.J.; Samson, S.L.; Li M, V.; Chan, L. The Krüppel-like zinc finger protein Glis3 directly and indirectly activates insulin gene transcription. *Nucleic Acids Res.* **2009**, *37*, 2529–2538. [CrossRef] [PubMed]
12. Nygaard, S.B.; Larsen, A.; Knuhtsen, A.; Rungby, J.; Smidt, K. Effects of zinc supplementation and zinc chelation on in vitro β-cell function in INS-1E cells. *BMC Res. Notes* **2014**, *7*, 84. [CrossRef] [PubMed]
13. Haase, H.; Maret, W. Fluctuations of cellular, available zinc modulate insulin signaling via inhibition of protein tyrosine phosphatases. *J. Trace Elem. Med. Biol.* **2005**, *19*, 37–42. [CrossRef] [PubMed]
14. Tang, X.; Shay, N.F. Zinc has an insulin-like effect on glucose transport mediated by phosphoinositol-3-kinase and Akt in 3T3-L1 fibroblasts and adipocytes. *J. Nutr.* **2001**, *131*, 1414–1420. [PubMed]
15. Naito, Y.; Yoshikawa, Y.; Yasui, H. Cellular mechanism of zinchinokitiol complexes in diabetes mellitus. *Bull. Chem. Soc. Jpn.* **2011**, *84*, 298–305. [CrossRef]
16. Nakayama, A.; Hiromura, M.; Adachi, Y.; Sakurai, H. Molecular mechanism of antidiabetic zinc-allixin complexes: Regulations of glucose utilization and lipid metabolism. *J. Biol. Inorg. Chem.* **2008**, *13*, 675–684. [CrossRef] [PubMed]
17. DeFronzo, R.A. Pathogenesis of type 2 diabetes mellitus. *Med. Clin. N. Am.* **2004**, *88*, 787–835. [CrossRef] [PubMed]
18. DeFronzo, R.A. From the triumvirate to the ominous octet: A new paradigm for the treatment of type 2 diabetes mellitus. *Diabetes* **2009**, *58*, 773–795. [CrossRef] [PubMed]
19. Björnholm, M.; Kawano, Y.; Lehtihet, M.; Zierath, J.R. Insulin receptor substrate-1 phosphorylation and phosphatidylinositol 3-kinase activity in skeletal muscle from NIDDM subjects after in vivo insulin stimulation. *Diabetes* **1997**, *46*, 524–527. [CrossRef] [PubMed]
20. Cusi, K.; Maezono, K.; Osman, A.; Pendergrass, M.; Patti, M.E.; Pratipanawatr, T.; DeFronzo, R.A.; Kahn, C.R.; Mandarino, L.J. Insulin resistance differentially affects the PI 3-kinase- and MAP kinase-mediated signaling in human muscle. *J. Clin. Invest.* **2000**, *105*, 311–320. [CrossRef] [PubMed]
21. Reeves, P.G.; Nielsen, F.H.; Fahey, G.C. AIN-93 Purified Diets for Laboratory Rodents: Final Report of the American Institute of Nutrition Ad Hoc Writing Committee on the Reformulation of the AIN-76A Rodent. *Diet. J. Nutr.* **1993**, *123*, 1939–1951. [CrossRef] [PubMed]
22. Bowe, J.E.; Franklin, Z.J.; Hauge-Evans, A.C.; King, A.J.; Persaud, S.J.; Jones, P.M. Assessing glucose homeostasis in rodent models. *J. Endocrinol.* **2014**, *222*, 13–25. [CrossRef] [PubMed]

23. Bonora, E.; Moghetti, P.; Zancanaro, C.; Cigolini, M.; Querena, M.; Cacciatori, V.; Corgnati, A.; Muggeo, M. Estimates of in vivo insulin action in man: Comparison of insulin tolerance tests with euglycemic and hyperglycemic glucose clamp studies. *J. Clin. Endocrinol. Metab.* **1989**, *68*, 374–378. [CrossRef] [PubMed]

24. Matthews, D.R.; Hosker, J.P.; Rudenski, A.S.; Naylor, B.A.; Treacher, D.F.; Turner, R.C. Homeostasis model assessment: insulin resistance and beta-cell function from fasting plasma glucose and insulin concentrations in man. *Diabetologia* **1985**, *28*, 412–419. [CrossRef] [PubMed]

25. Lacy, P.E.; Kostianovsky, M. Method for the isolation of intact islets of Langerhans from the rat pancreas. *Diabetes* **1967**, *16*, 35–39. [CrossRef] [PubMed]

26. Rivero-Gutiérrez, B.; Anzola, A.; Martínez-Augustin, O.; De Medina, F.S. Stain-free detection as loading control alternative to Ponceau and housekeeping protein immunodetection in Western blotting. *Anal. Biochem.* **2014**, *467*, 1–3. [CrossRef] [PubMed]

27. Challiss, R.A.; Lozeman, F.J.; Leighton, B.; Newsholme, E.A. Effects of the beta-adrenoceptor agonist isoprenaline on insulin-sensitivity in soleus muscle of the rat. *Biochem. J.* **1986**, *233*, 377–381. [CrossRef] [PubMed]

28. Crettaz, M.; Prentki, M.; Zaninetti, D.; Jeanrenaud, B. Insulin resistance in soleus muscle from obese Zucker rats. Involvement of several defective sites. *Biochem. J.* **1980**, *186*, 525–534. [CrossRef] [PubMed]

29. Miranda, E.R.; Dey, C.S. Effect of chromium and zinc on insulin signaling in skeletal muscle cells. *Biol. Trace Elem. Res.* **2004**, *101*, 19–36. [CrossRef]

30. Bellomo, E.; Massarotti, A.; Hogstrand, C.; Maret, W. Zinc ions modulate protein tyrosine phosphatase 1B activity. *Metallomics* **2014**, *6*, 1229–1239. [CrossRef] [PubMed]

31. Saper, R.B.; Rash, R. Zinc: An essential micronutrient. *Am. Fam. Phys.* **2009**, *79*, 768–772. [CrossRef]

32. Plum, L.M.; Rink, L.; Hajo, H. The essential toxin: Impact of zinc on human health. *Int. J. Environ. Res. Public Health* **2010**, *7*, 1342–1365. [CrossRef] [PubMed]

33. Lewis, R.J. *Sax's Dangerous Properties of Industrial Materials*, 9th ed.; Wiley-Interscience: Hoboken, NJ, USA, 1996.

34. Burcelin, R.; Crivelli, V.; Dacosta, A.; Roy-Tirelli, A.; Thorens, B. Heterogeneous metabolic adaptation of C57BL/6J mice to high-fat diet. *Am. J. Physiol. Endocrinol. Metab.* **2002**, *282*, E834–E842. [CrossRef] [PubMed]

35. West, D.B.; York, B. Dietary fat, genetic predisposition, and obesity: Lessons from animal models. *Am. J. Clin. Nutr.* **1998**, *67*, 505S–512S. [PubMed]

36. Ilouz, R.; Kaidanovich, O.; Gurwitz, D.; Eldar-Finkelman, H. Inhibition of glycogen synthase kinase-3-beta by bivalent zinc ions: Insight into the insulin-mimetic action of zinc. *Biochem. Biophys. Res. Commun.* **2002**, *295*, 102–106. [CrossRef]

37. Thiebaud, D.; Jacot, E.; DeFronzo, R.A.; Maeder, E.; Jequier, E.; Felber, J.P. The effect of graded doses of insulin on total glucose uptake, glucose oxidation, and glucose storage in man. *Diabetes* **1982**, *31*, 957–963. [CrossRef] [PubMed]

38. DeFronzo, R.A.; Gunnarsson, R.; Bjorkman, O.; Olsson, M.; Wahren, J. Effects of insulin on peripheral and splanchnic glucose metabolism in noninsulin-dependent (type II) diabetes mellitus. *J. Clin. Investig.* **1985**, *76*, 149–155. [CrossRef] [PubMed]

39. Grasso, G.; Pietropaolo, A.; Spoto, G.; Pappalardo, G.; Tundo, G.R.; Ciaccio, C.; Coletta, M.; Rizzarelli, E. Copper(I) and copper(II) inhibit Abeta peptides proteolysis by insulin-degrading enzyme differently: implications for metallostasis alteration in Alzheimer's disease. *Chemistry* **2011**, *17*, 2752–2762. [CrossRef] [PubMed]

40. Bondy, C.A.; Zhou, J.; Chin, E.; Reinhardt, R.R.; Ding, L.; Roth, R.A. Cellular distribution of insulin-degrading enzyme gene expression. Comparison with insulin and insulin-like growth factor receptors. *J. Clin. Investig.* **1994**, *93*, 966–973. [CrossRef] [PubMed]

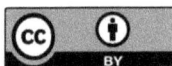

nutrients [MDPI]

Review
Zinc in Wound Healing Modulation

Pei-Hui Lin [1,2,*], Matthew Sermersheim [1,2], Haichang Li [1,2], Peter H. U. Lee [1,2], Steven M. Steinberg [3] and Jianjie Ma [1,2,*]

[1]   Davis Heart and Lung Research Institute, The Ohio State University Wexner Medical Center, Columbus, OH 43210, USA; sermersheim.3@osu.edu (M.S.); Haichang.Li@osumc.edu (H.L.); Peter.Lee@osumc.edu (P.H.U.L.)

[2]   Department of Surgery, Division of Cardiac Surgery, The Ohio State University Wexner Medical Center, Columbus, OH 43210, USA

[3]   Department of Surgery, Division of Trauma, Critical Care and Burn, The Ohio State University Wexner Medical Center, Columbus, OH 43210, USA; Steven.Steinberg@osumc.edu

*   Correspondence: Pei-Hui.Lin@osumc.edu (P.-H.L.); Jianjie.Ma@osumc.edu (J.M.); Tel.: +1-614-292-2802 (P.-H.L.); +1-614-292-3110 (J.M.)

Received: 5 December 2017; Accepted: 21 December 2017; Published: 24 December 2017

Abstract: Wound care is a major healthcare expenditure. Treatment of burns, surgical and trauma wounds, diabetic lower limb ulcers and skin wounds is a major medical challenge with current therapies largely focused on supportive care measures. Successful wound repair requires a series of tightly coordinated steps including coagulation, inflammation, angiogenesis, new tissue formation and extracellular matrix remodelling. Zinc is an essential trace element (micronutrient) which plays important roles in human physiology. Zinc is a cofactor for many metalloenzymes required for cell membrane repair, cell proliferation, growth and immune system function. The pathological effects of zinc deficiency include the occurrence of skin lesions, growth retardation, impaired immune function and compromised would healing. Here, we discuss investigations on the cellular and molecular mechanisms of zinc in modulating the wound healing process. Knowledge gained from this body of research will help to translate these findings into future clinical management of wound healing.

Keywords: inflammation; immune response; anti-oxidant; tissue proliferation; matrix remodelling; TRIM family proteins; matrix metalloproteinase

---

1. Introduction

Wound healing is a physiological response to injury that is essential across all tissue systems. Wound care is a major public health issue. Based on an economic evaluation of 2014 Medicare expenses, the total annual costs of all wound types, such as pressure ulcer, venous ulcers, diabetic foot ulcer, surgical and traumatic wounds and infection, ranged from $USA28.1 to $USA96.8 billion in the United States [1]. The burden of wound treatment remains a significant challenge due to an aging population and increases in diabetes and obesity, conditions that contribute to aberrant wound healing. The underlying complexities of the wound healing process include membrane repair, coagulation, control of inflammation, angiogenesis, cell proliferation, tissue remodelling and scar formation. These cumulative functions are integral for restoring tissue architecture.

Zinc is an essential micronutrient, present at less than 50 mg/kg, in the human body. It is important for human health and disease due to its critical roles in growth and development, bone metabolism, the central nervous system, immune function and wound healing [2]. Zinc is a vital cofactor for the function of more than 10% of proteins encoded by the human genome (~3000 proteins/enzymes) [3,4]. Zinc-dependent proteins play numerous indispensable roles within cells, such as transcriptional regulation, DNA repair, apoptosis [5,6], metabolic processing [7], extracellular matrix (ECM) regulation [8] and antioxidant defence [9].

Low concentration of zinc is found intracellularly across all tissues as a divalent cation incapable of passive diffusion across cell membranes. As such, the cellular homeostasis and bioavailability of zinc is tightly controlled through transcriptional regulation, ion transporters and compartmental stores [10–13]. Metabolically active, labile zinc is present inside cells at pico- to nanomolar concentrations with extracellular concentrations in the sub-micromolar to micromolar range [14]. The zinc transporter protein (ZIP) family zinc uptake/transporter proteins, particularly ZIP4, are responsible for zinc uptake from the extracellular milieu or intracellular vesicles [15]. Cytosolic free zinc ions have recently been identified as secondary messengers, similar to calcium ion transients, capable of interacting with target proteins in order to regulate many signal transduction pathways [16,17]. In this regard, zinc availability and regulation constitute an important component in cell physiology.

A common cause of zinc deficiency is malnutrition. Dietary zinc is absorbed in the small intestines through a carrier-mediated mechanism. Illness/infection and high phytate-containing foods are shown to hinder zinc bioavailability by inhibiting uptake [18,19]. The vast majority of zinc found within the human body is stored in skeletal muscle (60%) but reserves are also found in bone (30%), skin and liver (5%) and other organs (2–3%) [13]. Due to the ubiquitous and multifaceted nature of zinc, the effects of zinc deficiency are widespread and impact many organ systems and tissues. Globally, zinc deficiency is a common plight. This may be the combined result of hereditary or dietary problems and can manifest clinically as many disorders including gastro-intestinal (GI) tract malabsorption syndromes [20], liver and renal diseases [21], aging [22], immune dysfunction [22,23], dermatitis [24], mental and growth retardation [25,26], hypogonadism [27] and impaired wound healing [28].

Studies dating back to 1970 and earlier have shown the importance of zinc concentrations towards healing wounds in patients with thermal injuries or exposure to surgical stress [29]. Zinc is especially important in skin [30]. Skin contains a relatively high (about 5% of body content) zinc content, primarily associated within the epidermis (50–70 µg/g dry weight) [31]. Due to its abundance in the epidermis, mild zinc deficiency is noted to lead to roughened skin and impaired wound healing [32]. Severe zinc deficiency was found to be related to Acrodermatitis enteropathica (AE), a potentially fatal genetic disorder in which individuals are unable to absorb sufficient dietary zinc as a result of mutations in the SLC39A4 gene which encodes hZIP4 [33]. Zinc deficiency associated with AE leads to dermatitis, diarrhoea, secondary bacterial/fungal infections and often mortality in untreated infants. AE patients' symptoms can be dramatically improved via dietary zinc supplements [34].

Zinc deficiency has been linked to delayed wound healing [32,35] and low serum zinc levels have been reported in critically ill patients within Intensive Care Units [36]. Although the benefits of supplemental zinc have been documented in critically ill patients [37], severe burn injury [38,39], subcutaneous abscess, minor surgery [40] and pressure ulcers [41,42], the effects of zinc on wound healing has only been minimally reviewed [32,35].

Wound healing, inflammation and immune response are intimately associated with one another. Over the years zinc has been shown capable of modulating both innate and adaptive immune functions. Zinc alters immune responses in a multitude of ways ranging from myeloid-derived cells and inflammatory signalling to lymphocyte differentiation and antibody production. The ability of zinc to regulate immune homeostasis is a burgeoning field of study and has been extensively reviewed by others [23]. Here, we discuss the contributions of zinc within the wound repair processes with an emphasis on platelet cells and haemostasis, inflammation and host defence, granulation and re-epithelization, ECM remodelling via regulation of matrix metalloproteinases (MMPs) and its association with tripartite motif (TRIM) family proteins in membrane repair and wound healing [43,44]. By identifying roles by which zinc coordinates wound healing, we hope to stimulate further research in tissue repair and regeneration.

2. The Phases of Wound Healing and Zinc's Impact

Wound healing is an intricate and dynamic process which can be subdivided into a series of phases including: (1) coagulating fibrin clot formation (haemostasis, occurs within seconds to 1 h), (2) inflammatory response (within minutes to days), (3) cell proliferation, re-epithelialization, granulation and angiogenesis (begins 18–24 h after wounding and lasts from days to weeks) and (4) matrix remodelling and scar formation (5–7 days after injury and could persist months to years) (Figure 1). As detailed below, these distinct but overlapping phases involve dynamic coordination of soluble mediators (reactive oxygen species (ROS), chemokines, cytokines and growth factors), ECM turnover and cellular cross-talk amongst platelets, infiltrating immune cells, resident keratinocytes, endothelial cells, fibroblasts, epithelial cells and stem cells. Within this section we will closely examine the impact of zinc regulation on wound healing.

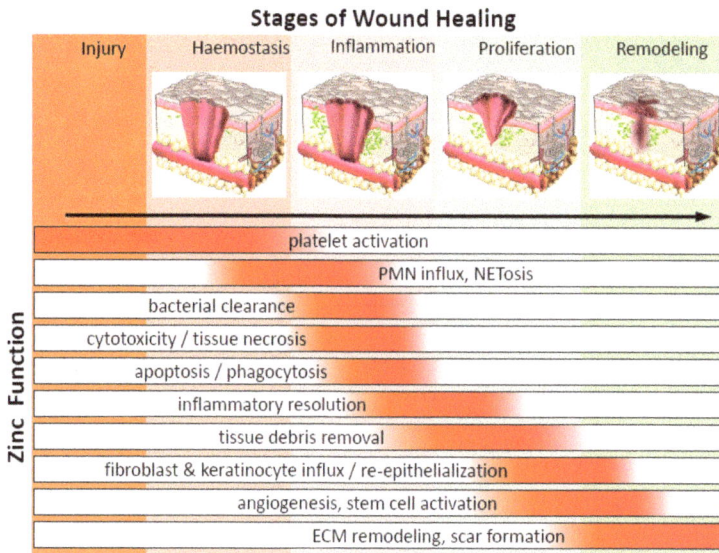

Figure 1. The function of zinc throughout the stages of wound healing. Zinc has a significant function in many cells over the entire process of wound repair. After injury wounded tissue must establish haemostasis via coagulation and clot formation. Injury is quickly followed by immune infiltration and inflammation as a means to clear the wound of damaged tissue and microbes, thus preventing infection and allowing room for granulation. Fibroblast, epithelial cells, keratinocytes and endothelial cells, will proliferate and migrate into wounds to deposit ECM and re-populate the injury site, facilitating wound closure. Finally, matrix deposition and clearance regulates the development of scar formation. PMN—polymorphonuclear leukocytes; NETosis—a novel form of programed neutrophil death that resulted in the formation of neutrophil extracellular traps (NETs); ECM—extracellular matrix.

2.1. Haemostasis and Platelets

Serious injury results in vasculature damage and it becomes imperative to stanch bleeding. The major mechanism by which haemostasis is accomplished is via activation and aggregation of platelet cells. Platelets are capable of responding to vascular damage by means of aggregating at the damage site to form an initial clot followed by fibrin deposition and polymerization to further strengthen the plug [45]. It has been understood for decades now that zinc is capable of enhancing platelet activity and aggregation [46,47]. Recently it was shown that the effect of zinc on platelets is mediated through Protein kinase C (PKC)-mediated tyrosine phosphorylation of platelet proteins [48,49]. Exogenous zinc treatment (at millimolar concentration range) induced zinc entry into the platelet cytosol and time-dependent (within 30 min) stimulation of tyrosine phosphorylation on certain high molecular weight proteins which could be blocked by PKC inhibitors. The intriguing role of zinc on pathophysiological thrombus formation during tissue injury is still largely unknown. Platelets are increasingly being recognized as immune cells capable of pathogen recognition and mediating an inflammatory response via cytokines and chemokines [50]. Platelets contain alpha-granules, which carry a plethora of proteins and factors, such as Chemokine (C-X-C motif) ligand 1 (CXCL1, GRO-α (growth regulated α protein), CXCL4, CXCL5 (ENA-78 ,epithelial-derived neutrophil-activating protein 78), CXCL7 (PPBP (Pro-Platelet basic protein), β-TG (Beta-Thromboglobulin), CTAP-III (connective tissue activating peptide III), NAP-2 (neutrophil-activating peptide-2)), CXCL8 (IL-8, interleukin-8), CXCL12 (SDF-1α, stromal cell-derived factor-1α), Chemokine (C-C motif) ligand 2 (CCL2, MCP-1 (monocyte chemoattractant protein-1)), CCL3 (MIP-1α, macrophage inflammatory protein 1-α) and CCL5 (RANTES, regulated upon activation normal T cell expressed and secreted); factors capable of recruiting and activating innate immune cells to the wound site [51]. It has been shown that zinc induces alpha-granule release [48]. These studies suggest that platelets and zinc play an important role in initiating the inflammatory phase of wound healing.

2.2. Inflammation and Immune Defence

During and after haemostasis, wounded tissue undergoes an inflammatory stage. This is an elaborate process involving coordination amongst a diversity of cell types. Innate immune cells migrate to and infiltrate injured tissue whereby they can rid the environment of cellular debris and infectious microbes. In experimental human studies of mild zinc deficiency, the affected elderly subjects (ages 55–85 years) had increased inflammatory cytokines and oxidative stress production [52]. Zinc supplementation in elderly subjects reduced plasma levels of oxidative stress markers, decreased ex vivo production of inflammatory cytokines like C-Reactive Protein (CRP) and IL-6, reduced chemokines such as monocyte chemoattractant protein-1 (MCP-1) and reduced secretary cell adhesion molecules (soluble vascular cell adhesion molecule-1 (sVCAM-1), soluble intercellular adhesion molecule-1 (sICAM-1) and s-E-selectin) which represent important biomarkers of cell damage-associated inflammation in endothelium and platelets [18,52,53]. Inflammation-associated vascular dysfunction could be due to peroxisome proliferator-activated receptors (PPAR) dysregulation during zinc deficiency [54].

Neutrophils are granular polymorphonuclear leukocytes (PMN), which often act as one of the first responders to tissue injury and bacterial infection. The migration of neutrophils and other leukocytes to infected/damaged sites is accomplished via increasing gradients of chemokines and cytokines, a process known as chemotaxis. In rhesus monkeys, zinc deficiency obstructs PMN chemotaxis while supplementation reverses the effects [55]. Upon arrival to wounds neutrophils are capable of secreting inflammatory cytokines and phagocytizing pathogens in order to prevent infection. In a study of zinc-deficient acquired immune deficiency syndrome (AIDS) patients, zinc supplementation was observed to enhance neutrophilic phagocytosis of opsonized zymosan particles, a Toll-like receptor-2 (TLR2) agonist [56].

Phagocytes, such as neutrophils, are able to destroy intracellular pathogens via ROS. Enzymes important for the generation of ROS precursors and bacterial clearance, are nicotinamide adenine dinucleotide phosphate (NADPH)-oxidases. Interestingly excess zinc, as well as zinc-deficiency, can both inhibit NADPH-oxidases and thereby hinder microbial elimination [57,58]. A unique mechanism by which neutrophils are able to eliminate pathogens is via the release of neutrophil extracellular traps (NETs). NETs are extracellular matrices consisting of granule proteins, chromatin and DNA; capable of trapping and killing microbes [59]. Absence of zinc, via chelators, compromises NETosis [60]. The contents of NETs include heterodimeric proteins known as calprotectin [61]. Calprotectin is able to bind and sequester zinc ions [62]. By sequestering zinc, calprotectin deprives bacteria of essential metals and hinders bacterial survival and expansion. This method of microbial control falls under a category known as "Nutritional Immunity", a process in which host cells sequester and limit the availability of essential trace elements thereby inhibiting pathogenic growth. Bacteria have developed their own response to combat strategies such as calprotectin. Some bacteria have evolved to express zinc uptake receptors with higher zinc-affinity than calprotectin, or even receptors that bind and repurpose calprotectin, thus allowing them to evade nutritional immunity [63,64].

Monocytes are pro-inflammatory innate immune cells. Monocytes respond to chemokines and migrate to affected tissue where they adhere to endothelial cells, infiltrate tissue and differentiate into macrophages capable of clearing pathogens/damaged tissue and propagating inflammation. It has been reported that zinc has conflicting roles on monocyte/endothelial adhesion. It has been shown that zinc-deficiency as well as zinc oxide treatment result in elevated monocyte adhesion [65,66]. Dierichs et al. recently reported that zinc could participate in modulation of monocyte differentiation into pro-inflammatory (M1) or immune-regulatory/wound healing (M2) macrophages [67]. M1 macrophages are important for early inflammation and microbial/debris clearance, while M2 macrophages are involved in immune suppression and later tissue remodelling/repair. Using the human monocyte cell line THP-1s (Tohoku Hospital Pediatrics-1), they discovered that both zinc deficiency and supplementation promote M1 phenotypes, while inhibiting M2 differentiation. Counterintuitively, they also report that zinc supplementation suppresses inducible nitric oxide synthases (iNOS) expression, an M1 hallmark associated with reactive nitrogen species production and pathogen clearance. Maintaining an appropriate balance between M1/M2 macrophage populations is complex and crucial during wound healing. Fully elucidating the effect of zinc on macrophage phenotypes and functions will aid in the advancement of wound healing treatments.

Macrophages eliminate inflammatory pathogens by phagocytosis, a process that microbes are taken up and trapped via membrane bound intracellular phagosomes. From there microbes can be killed by means of oxidation or lysosomal degradation. Phagosomes can fuse with lysosomes, whereby the protease-containing acidic environment can destroy bacteria. Many bacteria have developed strategies whereby they can live within intracellular phagosomes undetected and prevent lysosome fusion/degradation. Under these circumstances, similar to neutrophils, macrophages have developed their own forms of nutritional immunity. Through the use of zinc transporters, macrophages are able to shuttle zinc in or out of bacterial laden phagosomes. Depending on the microbes present, macrophages are able to deprive bacteria of zinc, essentially starving them, or alternatively poison bacteria with toxic levels of zinc and other heavy metals [68,69]. *M. tuberculosis* developed a defence to zinc toxicity however, via P-type ATPases, capable of exporting zinc and maintaining viable ion concentrations even within the toxic environment of phagosomes [70].

Macrophages and other immune cells, are major producers of cytokines. Many studies have shown that zinc modulation has an effect on cytokine production. Some of the major regulators of inflammatory cytokine production are T cell receptor (TLR) proteins. TLR proteins are capable of recognizing pathogen-specific molecular motifs and implement signalling cascades. Closely associated with TLRs is nuclear factor kappa-light-chain-enhancer of activated B cells (NF-κB) signalling. NF-κB is a potent transcriptional regulator involved in a plethora of cellular processes associated with wound healing including: inflammatory response, tissue remodelling, proliferation, apoptosis, cell adhesion, etc. [71]. Numerous reports have detailed the effects of zinc on TLR/NF-κB mediated inflammatory signalling, however studies have come to conflicting conclusions. Hasse et al. reported that lipopolysaccharide (LPS)/TLR4 mediated NF-κB signalling is dependent upon intracellular free zinc [72]. In their study sequestration of zinc via an intracellular membrane-permeable zinc ion chelator, TPEN (*N,N,N',N'*-tetrakis(2-pyridinylmethyl)-1,2-ethanediamine), completely abolishes NF-κB activation after LPS stimulus. In contrast, there is a growing body of evidence that zinc acts as an inhibitor of TLR/NF-κB signalling. Reports have shown that zinc is capable of negatively regulating NF-κB signalling via PPAR-α, A20, IκB kinase-β (IKKβ) and phosphodiesterase (PDE) [73–76].

Dynamic crosstalk exists between zinc homeostasis and inflammation. A negative feedback loop appears to exist within zinc/NF-κB signalling. It has been demonstrated that upon inflammatory stimulation NF-κB upregulates the zinc transporter ZIP8. ZIP8 translocates to the plasma membrane where it facilitates zinc uptake into the cell. Intracellular zinc is thereupon free to inhibit IKKβ and negatively regulate the inflammatory process [75]. In a similar negative feedback loop, IL-6 stimulus results in upregulation of ZIP14, which is also capable of attenuating inflammation in hepatocytes [77].

IL-1β and IL-18 are potent pro-inflammatory cytokines under the regulation of caspase 1 activation. Caspase-1 belongs to the pro-apoptotic endoprotease family of Caspases. Research has yielded conflicting results on the pro vs. anti-effects of zinc on apoptosis. While results have been ambiguous, zinc concentration appears to be an important factor [78]. Groups have shown that zinc has a direct inhibitory effect on the activity of caspases 3, 6, 7, 8 and 9 [79–81]. A similar study utilizing a zinc-containing compound, ziram, showed pro-caspase1, the inactive precursor of caspase1, degraded upon ziram treatment [82]. Degradation of the pro-inflammatory precursor (pro-caspase1) indicates a potential role for zinc in regulating caspase-mediated inflammation. This notion is supported by clinical studies showing higher levels of IL-1β expression in overweight patients with low dietary zinc intake, compared to patients with higher zinc intake [83].

As mentioned earlier, macrophages partake in the clearance of not only microbes but also damaged tissue. Lymphocytes and the adaptive immune system also play an important role in this element of wound healing. It has been shown that B-lymphocytes aid in wound clearance and repair [84,85]. Mature B-cells/plasma cells are capable of producing antibodies that detect injured tissue. These antibodies serve as signals by which macrophages recognize and phagocytize damaged cells. Zinc deficiency results in lowered populations of both precursor and mature B-cells and can reduce antibody production [86]. Diminishing B-cells populations and ergo circulating antibodies, would negatively affect phagocytosis causing hindered wound clearance and chronic wounds. In fact, it has been demonstrated in chronic diabetic skin lesions, that direct B-cell treatment accelerates wound healing [87].

2.3. Inflammatory Resolution and Tissue Growth (Proliferation) Stage

During wound healing, it is important to resolve inflammation and initiate re-epithelization, the process where epithelial cells proliferate and repopulate injured tissue for wound closure. M2 macrophages are one cell type that helps mitigate inflammation but there are numerous other immune cells that aid in this process. Zinc deficiency also has a significant impact on T lymphocyte populations [86,88]. Regulatory T lymphocytes (Tregs) regulate and suppress inflammation. Zinc supplementation is known to increase the number of Tregs in multiple circumstances: mixed lymphocyte cultures, in response to allergens and when combined with transforming growth factor-β (TGFβ) [89–91]. Cutaneous wound studies have shown that Tregs help resolve inflammation, promote re-epithelization and wound contraction [92]. It would be interesting to determine whether zinc supplementation is capable of upregulating a regulatory T-cell response in order to promote accelerated wound repair.

About two or three days after the wound occurs, fibroblasts begin to enter the wound site, marking the onset of the tissue proliferative phase. Fibroblast infiltration is associated with collagen/ECM deposition, which serves as a temporary scaffold for repair. Collagen serves as a bed enabling migration of epithelium, keratinocytes and microvasculature. One of the primary regulators of ECM deposition and fibrosis is TGFβ/SMAD (Mothers against decapentaplegic homolog protein) signalling. Zinc is a vital cofactor for SMAD signalling and thus plays a major role in formation of granulation tissue [91]. During re-epithelialization and wound closure, there is transient proliferation and migration of resident keratinocytes, fibroblasts, epithelial cells and endothelial cells with simultaneous activation and trans-differentiation of multiple epidermal stem cells populations [93]. The collaborative efforts of collagenases and plasminogen activators led to degradation of fibrin clots along with the zinc-dependent matrix metalloproteinase (MMP, discussed in more details below), which digest dermal basal membranes and ECM, allows room for cell growth, migration and angiogenesis.

Within the epidermis, apoptotic and necrotic cells stimulate epidermal cells proliferation and migration over granulation tissue in order to repair the epidermis. Topical zinc application enhanced re-epithelialization in porcine skin wound healing model [94]. Moreover, a study testing galvanic Cu/zinc (Zn) microparticles on wound closure reports ROS-mediated enhancement of human dermal fibroblast migration [95]. Similarly, zinc was shown to increase keratinocyte migration and participate in re-epithelialization of the epidermis [96]. Concurrent with re-epithelialization, endothelial cells migrate and proliferate into wound sites to establish new blood vessels in a process called neovascularization, or angiogenesis, thus supplying essential oxygen and nutrients for the growth of cells in the wound bed. Zinc has been shown effective for angiogenesis in vivo [97]. However, studies analysing the effect of micronutrient trace elements on vascular biology report contradictory findings in which zinc acts as an anti-angiogenic agent altering important genes and growth factors [98]. Further research and characterization is needed regarding zinc and this phase of tissue healing and regeneration.

2.4. Wound Resolution and Matrix Remodelling

ECM is composed of a complex mixture of insoluble molecules such as collagens, laminins, fibronectin, integrin and heparin sulphate proteoglycans and provide a solid supportive matrix scaffold for cells. The ECM network also serves as a reservoir of a plethora of cytokines, growth factors and molecular cues, both active and latent, to promote cellular migration, epithelialization, adhesion and wound contraction [99]. Among the many proteins essential for epidermal wound repair are the ECM-remodelling matrix metalloproteinase (MMPs) family proteins. MMPs are secreted by distinct cell types such as inflammatory cells, keratinocytes, endothelial cells and fibroblasts. MMPs are zinc-dependent endopeptidases which act to modulate growth factor activation, cleavage, degradation and composition of ECM, processing of cell-cell junctional adhesion molecules, cytokines and cell surface receptors and cell-matrix signalling during different stages of wound healing [100–103].

MMPs are synthesized as inactive zymogens (proMMPs) and their functions are modulated in four ways—namely gene expression, compartmentalization, proMMPs activation and MMPs enzymatic inactivation. The structures of MMPs are composed of four domains, the pro-peptide domain with a conserved cysteine switch motif PRCGXPD, the zinc-binding catalytic domain, a hinge region and the C-terminal hemopexin-like domain. Activation of MMPs is dependent on a "cysteine switch" mechanism [104]. The pro-peptide cysteine interacts with the catalytically important zinc ion in the active site to keep proMMPs in an enzymatic inactive state to prevent their interaction and cleavage of substrates. The C-terminal hemopexin-like domains determine substrate specificity and their interaction with MMP inhibitors, the tissue inhibitor of metalloproteinases (TIMPs). Many stimuli such as tissue injury [105], oxidative stress upon UV exposure [106], inflammatory cytokines such as TNFα or IL-1α [107] and certain growth factors like vascular endothelial growth factor (VEGF) trigger the activation of MMPs [108]. Secreted or cell surface localized TIMPs also play important roles in wound repair. TIMPs process a wide range of extracellular substrates such as ECM proteins, cytokines and their receptors through their regulations of metalloproteinase activities [109]. These intricate activation mechanisms keep MMPs activities under tight control and in dynamic homeostasis under different wound healing demands [110].

Coordinated MMP function is pivotal for ECM degradation, migration of keratinocytes over ECM (wound re-epithelialization) [111], neo-angiogenesis [112], cell proliferation, fibroblast activation/migration and collagen deposition and fibrous tissue (fibroplasia and scar) formation during tissue remodelling to restore epidermal tissue integrity [113]. Prolonged ECM deposition leads to tissue fibrosis, whereas MMPs dysfunction is linked to defective wound closure [100,114]. Zinc and calcium ions are required for optimal MMPs function in vitro [115], however, the molecular mechanism by how zinc regulates MMPs function in vivo is still not fully understood due to the complexity of their regulation and the numerous MMPs involved in wound healing.

3. Zinc Is an Antioxidant Micronutrient

Several studies have shown that zinc deficiency increases oxidative stress [22,116,117]. It is well accepted that oxidative damage is a major cause of tissue injury and redox regulation plays a prominent role in wound repair [118–120]. Superoxide radicals such as reactive oxygen species (ROS) and reactive nitrogen free radical species (RNS) are by-products of electron leakage during mitochondrial electron transfer and constitute various forms of oxidative stress [121,122]. Superoxide radicals can cause oxidative damage to biomolecules, such as DNA, protein and lipids, thus impairing their bioactivity.

In biology, zinc is redox-inert and opposes the absorption and activity of redox-active transition metals like copper and iron, which catalyse the production of highly reactive oxidative stress [123,124]. Metallothionein (MT) is a family of low molecular weight, cysteine-rich (cysteine constitutes 30% of MT amino acids) proteins capable of binding heavy metals through their sulfhydryl (-SH)-rich cysteine residues. A large percentage (nearly 20%) of intracellular zinc is bound to MTs and can be rapidly released according to physiological needs. MTs are redox-sensitive antioxidant proteins, crucial for zinc regulation and protection against heavy-metal toxicity and oxidative stress. Interestingly, synthesis of MTs is dependent on availability of the dietary zinc, copper and selenium [125]. Zinc exhibits acute antioxidant properties by means of binding to and thus protecting redox-sensitive sulfhydryl groups of MTs [124,125]. Zinc supplementation induces MT expression and has been shown to protect against UV immunosuppression [126]. Oxidative stress associated with long term zinc deficiencies can be attributed to a reduction in the synthesis of MTs and a decline in the antioxidant activity of zinc-containing Cu, Zn superoxide dismutase (SOD1) [127].

4. TRIM Proteins in Membrane Repair and Wound Healing

Tripartite motif family (TRIM) proteins are characterized by the presence of N-terminal Ring (Really Interesting New Gene)-finger domain, zinc-finger B-box domains and a coil-coil domain. There are over 80 identified human TRIM proteins which play important roles in regulating cellular processes such as protein degradation, innate immunity, cell survival/death, oncogenesis, development and intracellular signalling. TRIM proteins exhibit a wide breadth of diversity along their C-termini, resulting in 12 different subfamilies/classifications. Most TRIM proteins contain E3 ubiquitin ligase activity, a class of enzymes which catalyze the final step (E3 step) in the ubiquitination cascade to form an ubiquitin covalent bond with a substrate lysine. TRIM proteins have been widely studied and reviewed within the context of immunology, cell death/survival and cancer [128–131], however an emerging role in wound healing has developed.

Maintaining cell membrane integrity is vital to normal cell physiology and function [132–134]. Repair of damaged cellular membranes requires intracellular vesicle trafficking which leads to an accumulation of vesicles close to the plasma membrane [135]. Subsequent resealing of the cell membrane is imperative for the survival and long-term viability of cells. Disruption of membrane repair contributes to pathophysiological conditions such as dystrophic muscle [136], diabetes [137], poor wound healing, chronic ulcer and scarring [133,134].

We have previously identified a novel TRIM protein, Mitsugumin 53 (MG53) or TRIM72, as an essential component of the cell membrane repair machinery [138,139] and is highly expressed in muscle. MG53 is capable of sensing oxidative stress associated with cell membrane damage and responds by binding to phosphatidylserine containing intracellular vesicles and then shuttles pre-assembled sub-membrane/intracellular vesicles to patch plasma membrane disruptions caused by mechanical or chemical injury [138–140]. Furthermore, MG53 is capable of protecting against ROS-mediated cellular stress, as seen with ischemic reperfusion injuries and metabolic disorders and prevents cell death [141]. MG53 ablation in mice ($MG53^{-/-}$) results in defective membrane repair with progressive pathological consequences in skeletal and cardiac muscle and enhanced susceptibility to injuries in lungs, kidneys and skin [43,142–148]. The protective repair function of endogenous and recombinant human MG53 (rhMG53) protein have been reported in multiple tissue types ranging from skeletal muscle [136,144,149], heart [141,145,146,150], kidney [142], lung [143,151], skin [43,44] and brain [147].

The binding of zinc to TRIM family proteins is critical to their E3 ligase activities [152]. While membrane repair mechanisms can be context dependent, we have shown that zinc serves as a molecular switch linking oxidative stress and the membrane reseal function of MG53 [153]. MG53 consists of two zinc binding domains in the Ring-finger and B-box motifs [138,153]. Zinc binding appears to be essential for MG53-mediated membrane repair, as mutation of either zinc binding residue compromises the membrane resealing ability of MG53. Simultaneous disruption of both zinc binding motifs in double mutants further exacerbates this effect [153]. Moreover, defective MG53-mediated vesicular transport and membrane repair was observed in the absence of extracellular zinc via a biochemical zinc chelator. These results suggest that MG53 acts as an acceptor for zinc during cell membrane repair.

Current reports support the findings that TGFβ plays a central role throughout wound healing [154–156]. Excessive TGFβ signalling can lead to maladaptive repair conditions and tissue fibrosis [157]. Recently, we showed MG53 is a vital component of wound healing and topical application of rhMG53 protein promotes wound healing with reduced scar formation [43,44]. MG53 deficiency, in mice, leads to delayed wound healing with aberrant scar formation, while therapeutic treatment with rhMG53 accelerates healing and prevents scarring. In vitro assays revealed that rhMG53 induces fibroblast migration while simultaneously suppressing myofibroblast differentiation and production of fibrotic proteins. The underlying molecular mechanisms of MG53-mediated protection against dermal wounding involves membrane repair, modulation of cell migration and suppression of ECM protein synthesis via inhibition of TGFβ/SMAD signalling (Figure 2).

MG53 is a versatile molecule with function associated with various signalling pathways like reperfusion injury salvage kinase (RISK) [145], glycogen synthase kinase-3β (GSK3β) [136,145,158], cell survival kinase AKT, TGFβ [43] and modulation of inflammatory mediators [143]. These findings are promising with regards to MG53s translational potential in wound healing and tissue regeneration. However, how zinc impacts MG53 E3-ubiquitin ligase activity and the identities of the E3-ligase substrates involved in MG53-mediated wound healing remain elusive and requires further investigation.

Two other TRIM proteins have been identified that might play a role in wound healing. Beer et al. reported that TRIM16, also known as oestrogen-responsive B box protein (EBBP), is a regulator of keratinocyte differentiation. TRIM16 expression is downregulated in skin wounds and hyper-thickened epithelium [159]. Over expression of TRIM16 enhances early differentiation of keratinocytes and is believed to regulate the differentiation capacity of cells. TRIM16 has extensively been studied in the field of cancer but little attention as has been directed toward wound healing. Interestingly, a study on ovarian cancer metastasis showed that overexpression of TRIM16 inhibited expression of MMP2 and MMP9 [160]. It is possible that TRIM16 is downregulated during wound healing in order to allow for tissue granulation, re-epithelialization and remodelling.

Recently the function of TRIM28 in endothelium was investigated by Wang et al. They show that TRIM28 helps mediate not only inflammation but also angiogenesis in a VEGFR2 dependent manner. Scratch wound assay showed endothelial cell migration was significantly reduced, after TRIM28 siRNA treatment [161]. These findings have significant implications for inflammation and wound healing. While both TRIM16 and TRIM28 have promising potential for wound repair, they are yet to be directly applied to such a study. Additionally, characterizing the impact of zinc on these proteins' functions would be beneficial. Further research into zinc regulation of TRIM protein expression/function during wound healing would provide new and exciting insight on wound repair.

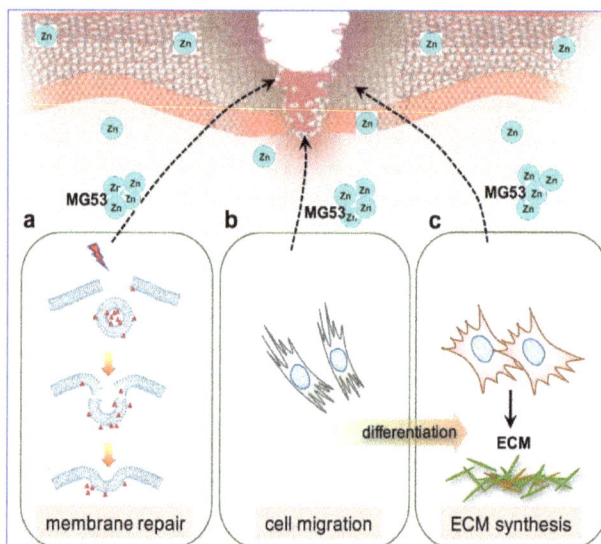

Figure 2. Proposed roles of zinc in MG53 mediated wound healing process. MG53 exists as intrinsic intracellular vesicles which could be secreted into blood circulation as a myokine to mediate wound healing. In response to dermal injury, MG53 could exert the following functions. (**a**) MG53-containing vesicles nucleate the cell membrane repair machinery and trafficking to damaged cell membrane to protect against acute membrane injury of keratinocytes and fibroblasts; (**b**) MG53 mediates cytoskeletal stress fibre remodelling to promote fibroblasts migration to the wound sites; and (**c**) MG53 regulates TGFβ signalling to modulate trans-differentiation of fibroblasts into myofibroblasts and suppresses deposition of ECM proteins during tissue remodelling stage of wound healing. Zinc is proposed to bind to MG53 on its two zinc-binding sites and modulates MG53-mediated wound healing process (Modified from JBC 290(40): 24592). MG53: Mitsugumin 53; ECM: extracellular matrix; TGFβ: transforming growth factor-β.

5. Zinc in Wound Healing—Clinical Perspectives

The role zinc plays in wound healing can be viewed from two perspectives: first, the impact of zinc deficiency and second, the effect of zinc supplementation (topical/local or systemic) on wound repair. The association between zinc deficiency and delayed wound healing has been described [32,35]. Treating zinc deficiency results in improved wound healing compared to those with zinc deficiency. For example, in patients considered to be at risk of refeeding syndrome, it may be appropriate to give a loading dose of 10–30 mg of Zn, followed by the daily maintenance dose of 2.5–5 mg [4]. However, the impact of zinc supplementation on wound healing in patients without zinc deficiency is less well known. There are very few well-done clinical studies on the topic and what little information currently available is inconsistent. For example, the Cochrane database reports 6 small studies on patients with arterial or venous ulcers and found that oral zinc supplementation did not improve wound healing [162]. Contrarily, another meta-analysis of topical zinc therapy with zinc oxide paste-medicated dressing containing zinc concentration between 6–15% for chronic venous leg ulcers showed improved healing, though the authors point out that the studies were small and of sub-optimal quality [163]. Cereda and co-authors performed a randomized, prospective trial in malnourished patients with chronic pressure ulcers [164]. They found a significant reduction in the size of the ulcers after 12 weeks of supplementation with a high calorie, high protein oral formula that was also supplemented with arginine, anti-oxidants and zinc (either orally or tube fed with 18–20 mg zinc daily). It is unknown how significant of a role the zinc supplementation played in this study. Attia and colleagues reported on 90 non-diabetic patients with uncomplicated wounds who were topically treated with one of two zinc-containing fluids (regular crystalline insulin or aqueous zinc chloride solutions at 0.2 mg/100 mL per 10 cm^2 wound) versus a control of 0.9% normal saline. The groups treated with the zinc-containing fluids had significantly improved healing [165]. On the other hand, a study of 42 patients with pressure ulcers treated with oral L-carnosine versus zinc containing polaprezinc (at 34 mg per day) showed no difference in healing [166]. It is clear that more studies utilizing more stringent controls will be necessary to fully understand the clinical potential of zinc supplementation.

Due to the loss of zinc during injury, zinc therapy has been used in wound care to enhance healing in zinc-deficient patients [32,167]. Topical zinc sulphate ($ZnSO_4$) application, usually at an optimal 3% concentration, has been widely used in wound healing for its antioxidant effect [30]. Other forms of application include 1% $ZnCl_2$ or the largely insoluble zinc oxide (ZnO). ZnO provides prolonged supply of zinc to wounds and enhance its healing ability. Additionally, ZnO increases collagen degradation in necrotic wounds [168]. It has been shown that topical zinc application induces mRNA expression of metallothionein, which could account for its anti-UV photoprotective effect [30,169]. A standard regimen for severe burn care includes regular daily dietary zinc supplementation equivalent or exceeding 22 mg [39,170]. Moreover, recent advances in drug delivery with zinc oxide nanoparticle (ZnO-NPs) technology has received considerable attention for the treatment of wounds due to their effective cell penetration, immunomodulation and antimicrobial capacity [171,172]. However, in-depth pharmacodynamics and toxicology studies are still needed prior to widespread applications [173].

6. Concluding Remarks and Future Perspectives

Zinc is a micronutrient that is essential to human health. Zinc plays a major role in regulating every phase of the wound healing process; ranging from membrane repair, oxidative stress, coagulation, inflammation and immune defence, tissue re-epithelialization, angiogenesis, to fibrosis/scar formation. With huge demands for improved wound care, we need a more thorough in-depth understanding of the molecular mechanisms in which zinc functions. A more thorough comprehension of the cellular cross-talks and MMP regulation would go a long way in progressing the field wound healing. The biological function and therapeutic potential of TRIM proteins, such as MG53, in wound repair is emerging. Understanding the precise mechanisms by which zinc regulates their activity remains unexplored, yet is crucial. Further inquiry into the mechanisms of zinc and the proteins for which it serves as a cofactor, will greatly advance the treatment and care of difficult-to-heal wounds.

Acknowledgments: Grant supports are provided to J.M. by the NIH (AR061385, AG056919, AR070752 and DK106394); to P.-H.L. by an OSU intramural Lockwood Research Fund.

Author Contributions: P.-H.L., M.S. and S.M.S. wrote manuscript. H.L., P.H.U.L. and J.M. contributed idea and edited manuscript.

Conflicts of Interest: J.M. is a founder of TRIM-edicine, Inc., a biotechnology company developing rhMG53 as a therapeutic protein. All other authors declare no competing financial interests.

Abbreviations

AE	Acrodermatitis enteropathica
CAM	Cell adhesion molecules
CXCL	Chemokine (C-X-C motif) ligand
CCL	Chemokine (C-C motif) ligand
CRP	C-reactive protein
ECM	Extracellular matrix
ILs	Interleukins
MCP-1	Monocyte chemoattractant protein-1
MMP	Matrix metalloproteinase
MG53	Mitsugumin 53

MT	Metallothioneins
NF-κB	Nuclear factor kappa-light-chain-enhancer of activated B cells
PPARα	Peroxisome proliferator activated receptors-a
PMN	Polymorphonuclear leukocytes
NET	Neutrophil extracellular traps
NADPH	Nicotinamide adenine dinucleotide phosphate
ROS	Reactive oxygen species
TIMP	Tissue inhibitor of metalloproteinases
TLR	Toll-like receptor
TRIM	Tripartite motif
TGFβ	Transforming Growth Factor-β
VEGF	Vascular endothelial growth factor
ZIPs	Zinc transporter proteins

References

1. Nussbaum, S.R.; Carter, M.J.; Fife, C.E.; da Vanzo, J.; Haught, R.; Nusgart, M.; Cartwright, D. An economic evaluation of the impact, cost, and medicare policy implications fo chronic nonhealing wounds. *Value Health* **2017**, in press. [CrossRef]

2. Roohani, N.; Hurrell, R.; Kelishadi, R.; Schulin, R. Zinc and its importance for human health: An integrative review. *J. Res. Med. Sci.* **2013**, *18*, 144–157. [PubMed]

3. Freeland-Graves, J.H.; Sanjeevi, N.; Lee, J.J. Global perspectives on trace element requirements. *J. Trace Elem. Med. Biol.* **2015**, *31*, 135–141. [CrossRef] [PubMed]

4. Livingstone, C. Zinc: Physiology, deficiency, and parenteral nutrition. *Nutr. Clin. Pract.* **2015**, *30*, 371–382. [CrossRef] [PubMed]

5. Zheng, J.; Lang, Y.; Zhang, Q.; Cui, D.; Sun, H.; Jiang, L.; Chen, Z.; Zhang, R.; Gao, Y.; Tian, W.; et al. Structure of human MDM2 complexed with RPL11 reveals the molecular basis of p53 activation. *Genes Dev.* **2015**, *29*, 1524–1534. [CrossRef] [PubMed]

6. Cho, J.G.; Park, S.; Lim, C.H.; Kim, H.S.; Song, S.Y.; Roh, T.Y.; Sung, J.H.; Suh, W.; Ham, S.J.; Lim, K.H.; et al. ZNF224, Kruppel like zinc finger protein, induces cell growth and apoptosis-resistance by down-regulation of p21 and p53 via miR-663a. *Oncotarget* **2016**, *7*, 31177–31190. [CrossRef] [PubMed]

7. Cronin, L.; Walton, P.H. Synthesis and structure of [Zn(OMe)(L)] × [Zn(OH)(L)] × 2(BPh4), L = cis,cis-1,3,5-tris[(E,E)-3-(2-furyl)acrylideneamino]cyclohexane: Structural models of carbonic anhydrase and liver alcohol dehydrogenase. *Chem. Commun. (Camb. Engl.)* **2003**, *13*, 1572–1573. [CrossRef]

8. Tomlinson, M.L.; Garcia-Morales, C.; Abu-Elmagd, M.; Wheeler, G.N. Three matrix metalloproteinases are required in vivo for macrophage migration during embryonic development. *Mechan. Dev.* **2008**, *125*, 1059–1070. [CrossRef] [PubMed]

9. Pawlak, K.; Mysliwiec, M.; Pawlak, D. The alteration in Cu/Zn superoxide dismutase and adhesion molecules concentrations in diabetic patients with chronic kidney disease: The effect of dialysis treatment. *Diabetes Res. Clin. Pract.* **2012**, *98*, 264–270. [CrossRef] [PubMed]

10. Choi, S.; Bird, A.J. Zinc'ing sensibly: Controlling zinc homeostasis at the transcriptional level. *Metallomics* **2014**, *6*, 1198–1215. [CrossRef] [PubMed]

11. Colvin, R.A.; Holmes, W.R.; Fontaine, C.P.; Maret, W. Cytosolic zinc buffering and muffling: Their role in intracellular zinc homeostasis. *Metallomics* **2010**, *2*, 306–317. [CrossRef] [PubMed]

12. Hojyo, S.; Fukada, T. Zinc transporters and signaling in physiology and pathogenesis. *Arch. Biochem. Biophys.* **2016**, *611*, 43–50. [CrossRef] [PubMed]

13. Kambe, T.; Tsuji, T.; Hashimoto, A.; Itsumura, N. The Physiological, Biochemical, and Molecular Roles of Zinc Transporters in Zinc Homeostasis and Metabolism. *Physiol. Rev.* **2015**, *95*, 749–784. [CrossRef] [PubMed]

14. Bozym, R.A.; Chimienti, F.; Giblin, L.J.; Gross, G.W.; Korichneva, I.; Li, Y.; Libert, S.; Maret, W.; Parviz, M.; Frederickson, C.J.; et al. Free zinc ions outside a narrow concentration range are toxic to a variety of cells in vitro. *Exp. Biol. Med.* **2010**, *235*, 741–750. [CrossRef] [PubMed]

15. Zhang, T.; Sui, D.; Hu, J. Structural insights of ZIP4 extracellular domain critical for optimal zinc transport. *Nat. Commun.* **2016**, *7*, 11979. [CrossRef] [PubMed]

16. Reilly-O'Donnell, B.; Robertson, G.B.; Karumbi, A.; McIntyre, C.; Bal, W.; Nishi, M.; Takeshima, H.; Stewart, A.J.; Pitt, S.J. Dysregulated Zn^{2+} homeostasis impairs cardiac type-2 ryanodine receptor and mitsugumin 23 functions, leading to sarcoplasmic reticulum Ca^{2+} leakage. *J. Biol. Chem.* **2017**, *292*, 13361–13373. [CrossRef] [PubMed]

17. Chappell, R.L.; Anastassov, I.; Lugo, P.; Ripps, H. Zinc-mediated feedback at the synaptic terminals of vertebrate photoreceptors. *Exp. Eye Res.* **2008**, *87*, 394–397. [CrossRef] [PubMed]

18. Prasad, A.S. Zinc is an Antioxidant and Anti-Inflammatory Agent: Its Role in Human Health. *Front. Nutr.* **2014**, *1*, 14. [CrossRef] [PubMed]

19. Moynahan, E.J. Letter: Acrodermatitis enteropathica: A lethal inherited human zinc-deficiency disorder. *Lancet* **1974**, *2*, 399–400. [CrossRef]

20. Tran, C.D.; Katsikeros, R.; Manton, N.; Krebs, N.F.; Hambidge, K.M.; Butler, R.N.; Davidson, G.P. Zinc homeostasis and gut function in children with celiac disease. *Am. J. Clin. Nutr.* **2011**, *94*, 1026–1032. [CrossRef] [PubMed]

21. Martinez, S.S.; Campa, A.; Li, Y.; Fleetwood, C.; Stewart, T.; Ramamoorthy, V.; Baum, M.K. Low Plasma Zinc Is Associated with Higher Mitochondrial Oxidative Stress and Faster Liver Fibrosis Development in the Miami Adult Studies in HIV Cohort. *J. Nutr.* **2017**, *147*, 556–562. [CrossRef] [PubMed]

22. Mariani, E.; Mangialasche, F.; Feliziani, F.T.; Cecchetti, R.; Malavolta, M.; Bastiani, P.; Baglioni, M.; Dedoussis, G.; Fulop, T.; Herbein, G.; et al. Effects of zinc supplementation on antioxidant enzyme activities in healthy old subjects. *Exp. Gerontol.* **2008**, *43*, 445–451. [CrossRef] [PubMed]

23. Gammoh, N.Z.; Rink, L. Zinc in Infection and Inflammation. *Nutrients* **2017**, *9*, 624. [CrossRef] [PubMed]

24. Mohammed, J.; Mehrotra, S.; Schulz, H.; Lim, R. Severe Infant Rash Resistant to Therapy Due to Zinc Deficiency. *Pediatr. Emerg. Care* **2017**, *33*, 582–584. [CrossRef] [PubMed]

25. Hagmeyer, S.; Haderspeck, J.C.; Grabrucker, A.M. Behavioral impairments in animal models for zinc deficiency. *Front. Behav. Neurosci.* **2014**, *8*, 443. [CrossRef] [PubMed]

26. Boycott, K.M.; Beaulieu, C.L.; Kernohan, K.D.; Gebril, O.H.; Mhanni, A.; Chudley, A.E.; Redl, D.; Qin, W.; Hampson, S.; Kury, S.; et al. Autosomal-Recessive Intellectual Disability with Cerebellar Atrophy Syndrome Caused by Mutation of the Manganese and Zinc Transporter Gene SLC39A8. *Am. J. Hum. Genet.* **2015**, *97*, 886–893. [CrossRef] [PubMed]

27. Rotter, I.; Kosik-Bogacka, D.I.; Dolegowska, B.; Safranow, K.; Kuczynska, M.; Laszczynska, M. Analysis of the relationship between the blood concentration of several metals, macro- and micronutrients and endocrine disorders associated with male aging. *Environ. Geochem. Health* **2016**, *38*, 749–761. [CrossRef] [PubMed]

28. Zorrilla, P.; Gomez, L.A.; Salido, J.A.; Silva, A.; Lopez-Alonso, A. Low serum zinc level as a predictive factor of delayed wound healing in total hip replacement. *Wound Repair Regen.* **2006**, *14*, 119–122. [CrossRef] [PubMed]

29. Henzel, J.H.; DeWeese, M.S.; Lichti, E.L. Zinc concentrations within healing wounds. Significance of postoperative zincuria on availability and requirements during tissue repair. *Arch. Surg.* **1970**, *100*, 349–357. [CrossRef] [PubMed]

30. Rostan, E.F.; DeBuys, H.V.; Madey, D.L.; Pinnell, S.R. Evidence supporting zinc as an important antioxidant for skin. *Int. J. Dermatol.* **2002**, *41*, 606–611. [CrossRef] [PubMed]

31. Gupta, M.; Mahajan, V.K.; Mehta, K.S.; Chauhan, P.S. Zinc therapy in dermatology: A review. *Dermatol. Res. Pract.* **2014**, *2014*, 709152. [CrossRef] [PubMed]

32. Lansdown, A.B.; Mirastschijski, U.; Stubbs, N.; Scanlon, E.; Agren, M.S. Zinc in wound healing: Theoretical, experimental, and clinical aspects. *Wound Repair Regen.* **2007**, *15*, 2–16. [CrossRef] [PubMed]

33. Wang, K.; Zhou, B.; Kuo, Y.M.; Zemansky, J.; Gitschier, J. A novel member of a zinc transporter family is defective in acrodermatitis enteropathica. *Am. J. Hum. Genet.* **2002**, *71*, 66–73. [CrossRef] [PubMed]

34. Perafan-Riveros, C.; Franca, L.F.; Alves, A.C.; Sanches, J.A., Jr. Acrodermatitis enteropathica: Case report and review of the literature. *Pediatr. Dermatol.* **2002**, *19*, 426–431. [CrossRef] [PubMed]

35. Kogan, S.; Sood, A.; Garnick, M.S. Zinc and Wound Healing: A Review of Zinc Physiology and Clinical Applications. *Wounds Compend. Clin. Res. Pract.* **2017**, *29*, 102–106.

36. Besecker, B.Y.; Exline, M.C.; Hollyfield, J.; Phillips, G.; Disilvestro, R.A.; Wewers, M.D.; Knoell, D.L. A comparison of zinc metabolism, inflammation, and disease severity in critically ill infected and noninfected adults early after intensive care unit admission. *Am. J. Clin. Nutr.* **2011**, *93*, 1356–1364. [CrossRef] [PubMed]

37. Rech, M.; To, L.; Tovbin, A.; Smoot, T.; Mlynarek, M. Heavy metal in the intensive care unit: A review of current literature on trace element supplementation in critically ill patients. *Nutr. Clin. Pract.* **2014**, *29*, 78–89. [CrossRef] [PubMed]

38. Kurmis, R.; Greenwood, J.; Aromataris, E. Trace Element Supplementation Following Severe Burn Injury: A Systematic Review and Meta-Analysis. *J. Burn Care Res.* **2016**, *37*, 143–159. [CrossRef] [PubMed]

39. Adjepong, M.; Agbenorku, P.; Brown, P.; Oduro, I. The role of antioxidant micronutrients in the rate of recovery of burn patients: A systematic review. *Burns Trauma* **2016**, *4*, 18. [CrossRef] [PubMed]

40. Mirastschijski, U.; Martin, A.; Jorgensen, L.N.; Sampson, B.; Agren, M.S. Zinc, copper, and selenium tissue levels and their relation to subcutaneous abscess, minor surgery, and wound healing in humans. *Biol. Trace Elem. Res.* **2013**, *153*, 76–83. [CrossRef] [PubMed]

41. Posthauer, M.E. Nutrition: Fuel for pressure ulcer prevention and healing. *Nursing* **2014**, *44*, 67–69. [CrossRef] [PubMed]

42. Sernekos, L.A. Nutritional treatment of pressure ulcers: What is the evidence? *J. Am. Assoc. Nurse Pract.* **2013**, *25*, 281–288. [CrossRef] [PubMed]

43. Li, H.; Duann, P.; Lin, P.H.; Zhao, L.; Fan, Z.; Tan, T.; Zhou, X.; Sun, M.; Fu, M.; Orange, M.; et al. Modulation of wound healing and scar formation by MG53 protein-mediated cell membrane repair. *J. Biol. Chem.* **2015**, *290*, 24592–24603. [CrossRef] [PubMed]

44. Li, M.; Li, H.; Li, X.; Zhu, H.; Xu, Z.; Liu, L.; Ma, J.; Zhang, M. A Bioinspired Alginate-Gum Arabic Hydrogel with Micro-/Nanoscale Structures for Controlled Drug Release in Chronic Wound Healing. *ACS Appl. Mater. Interfaces* **2017**, *9*, 22160–22175. [CrossRef] [PubMed]

45. Didar, U.; Sekhon, S.; Gupta, A.S. Platelets and Platelet-Inspired Biomaterials Technologies in Wound Healing Applications. *ACS Biomater. Sci. Eng.* **2017**. [CrossRef]

46. Heyns Adu, P.; Eldor, A.; Yarom, R.; Marx, G. Zinc-induced platelet aggregation is mediated by the fibrinogen receptor and is not accompanied by release or by thromboxane synthesis. *Blood* **1985**, *66*, 213–219. [PubMed]

47. Marx, G.; Krugliak, J.; Shaklai, M. Nutritional zinc increases platelet reactivity. *Am. J. Hematol.* **1991**, *38*, 161–165. [CrossRef] [PubMed]

48. Taylor, K.A.; Pugh, N. The contribution of zinc to platelet behaviour during haemostasis and thrombosis. *Metallomics Integr. Biomet. Sci.* **2016**, *8*, 144–155. [CrossRef] [PubMed]

49. Watson, B.R.; White, N.A.; Taylor, K.A.; Howes, J.M.; Malcor, J.D.; Bihan, D.; Sage, S.O.; Farndale, R.W.; Pugh, N. Zinc is a transmembrane agonist that induces platelet activation in a tyrosine phosphorylation- dependent manner. *Metallomics Integr. Biomet. Sci.* **2016**, *8*, 91–100. [CrossRef] [PubMed]

50. Morrell, C.N.; Aggrey, A.A.; Chapman, L.M.; Modjeski, K.L. Emerging roles for platelets as immune and inflammatory cells. *Blood* **2014**, *123*, 2759–2767. [CrossRef] [PubMed]

51. Blair, P.; Flaumenhaft, R. Platelet alpha-granules: Basic biology and clinical correlates. *Blood Rev.* **2009**, *23*, 177–189. [CrossRef] [PubMed]

52. Bao, B.; Prasad, A.S.; Beck, F.W.; Fitzgerald, J.T.; Snell, D.; Bao, G.W.; Singh, T.; Cardozo, L.J. Zinc decreases C-reactive protein, lipid peroxidation, and inflammatory cytokines in elderly subjects: A potential implication of zinc as an atheroprotective agent. *Am. J. Clin. Nutr.* **2010**, *91*, 1634–1641. [CrossRef] [PubMed]

53. Prasad, A.S. Zinc: An antioxidant and anti-inflammatory agent: Role of zinc in degenerative disorders of aging. *J. Trace Elem. Med. Biol.* **2014**, *28*, 364–371. [CrossRef] [PubMed]

54. Shen, H.; Oesterling, E.; Stromberg, A.; Toborek, M.; MacDonald, R.; Hennig, B. Zinc deficiency induces vascular pro-inflammatory parameters associated with NF-kappaB and PPAR signaling. *J. Am. Coll. Nutr.* **2008**, *27*, 577–587. [CrossRef] [PubMed]

55. Vruwink, K.G.; Fletcher, M.P.; Keen, C.L.; Golub, M.S.; Hendrickx, A.G.; Gershwin, M.E. Moderate zinc deficiency in rhesus monkeys. An intrinsic defect of neutrophil chemotaxis corrected by zinc repletion. *J. Immunol.* **1991**, *146*, 244–249. [PubMed]

56. Zazzo, J.F.; Rouveix, B.; Rajagopalon, P.; Levacher, M.; Girard, P.M. Effect of zinc on the immune status of zinc-depleted AIDS related complex patients. *Clin. Nutr.* **1989**, *8*, 259–261. [CrossRef]

57. DeCoursey, T.E.; Morgan, D.; Cherny, V.V. The voltage dependence of NADPH oxidase reveals why phagocytes need proton channels. *Nature* **2003**, *422*, 531–534. [CrossRef] [PubMed]

58. Hasegawa, H.; Suzuki, K.; Suzuki, K.; Nakaji, S.; Sugawara, K. Effects of zinc on the reactive oxygen species generating capacity of human neutrophils and on the serum opsonic activity in vitro. *Lumin. J. Biol. Chem. Lumin.* **2000**, *15*, 321–327. [CrossRef]

59. Brinkmann, V.; Reichard, U.; Goosmann, C.; Fauler, B.; Uhlemann, Y.; Weiss, D.S.; Weinrauch, Y.; Zychlinsky, A. Neutrophil extracellular traps kill bacteria. *Science* **2004**, *303*, 1532–1535. [CrossRef] [PubMed]
60. Hasan, R.; Rink, L.; Haase, H. Zinc signals in neutrophil granulocytes are required for the formation of neutrophil extracellular traps. *Innate Immun.* **2013**, *19*, 253–264. [CrossRef] [PubMed]
61. Li, A.; Lu, G.; Qi, J.; Wu, L.; Tian, K.; Luo, T.; Shi, Y.; Yan, J.; Gao, G.F. Structural basis of nectin-1 recognition by pseudorabies virus glycoprotein D. *PLoS Pathog.* **2017**, *13*, e1006314. [CrossRef] [PubMed]
62. Sohnle, P.G.; Collins-Lech, C.; Wiessner, J.H. The zinc-reversible antimicrobial activity of neutrophil lysates and abscess fluid supernatants. *J. Infect. Dis.* **1991**, *164*, 137–142. [CrossRef] [PubMed]
63. Lappann, M.; Danhof, S.; Guenther, F.; Olivares-Florez, S.; Mordhorst, I.L.; Vogel, U. In vitro resistance mechanisms of Neisseria meningitidis against neutrophil extracellular traps. *Mol. Microbiol.* **2013**, *89*, 433–449. [CrossRef] [PubMed]
64. Stork, M.; Grijpstra, J.; Bos, M.P.; Manas Torres, C.; Devos, N.; Poolman, J.T.; Chazin, W.J.; Tommassen, J. Zinc piracy as a mechanism of Neisseria meningitidis for evasion of nutritional immunity. *PLoS Pathog.* **2013**, *9*, e1003733. [CrossRef] [PubMed]
65. Lee, S.; Eskin, S.G.; Shah, A.K.; Schildmeyer, L.A.; McIntire, L.V. Effect of zinc and nitric oxide on monocyte adhesion to endothelial cells under shear stress. *Ann. Biomed. Eng.* **2012**, *40*, 697–706. [CrossRef] [PubMed]
66. Suzuki, Y.; Tada-Oikawa, S.; Ichihara, G.; Yabata, M.; Izuoka, K.; Suzuki, M.; Sakai, K.; Ichihara, S. Zinc oxide nanoparticles induce migration and adhesion of monocytes to endothelial cells and accelerate foam cell formation. *Toxicol. Appl. Pharmacol.* **2014**, *278*, 16–25. [CrossRef] [PubMed]
67. Dierichs, L.; Kloubert, V.; Rink, L. Cellular zinc homeostasis modulates polarization of THP-1-derived macrophages. *Eur. J. Nutr.* **2017**. [CrossRef] [PubMed]
68. Subramanian Vignesh, K.; Landero Figueroa, J.A.; Porollo, A.; Caruso, J.A.; Deepe, G.S., Jr. Granulocyte macrophage-colony stimulating factor induced Zn sequestration enhances macrophage superoxide and limits intracellular pathogen survival. *Immunity* **2013**, *39*, 697–710. [CrossRef] [PubMed]
69. Botella, H.; Stadthagen, G.; Lugo-Villarino, G.; de Chastellier, C.; Neyrolles, O. Metallobiology of host-pathogen interactions: An intoxicating new insight. *Trends Microbiol.* **2012**, *20*, 106–112. [CrossRef] [PubMed]
70. Botella, H.; Peyron, P.; Levillain, F.; Poincloux, R.; Poquet, Y.; Brandli, I.; Wang, C.; Tailleux, L.; Tilleul, S.; Charriere, G.M.; et al. Mycobacterial p(1)-type ATPases mediate resistance to zinc poisoning in human macrophages. *Cell Host Microbe* **2011**, *10*, 248–259. [CrossRef] [PubMed]
71. Tabruyn, S.P.; Griffioen, A.W. A new role for NF-kappaB in angiogenesis inhibition. *Cell Death Differ.* **2007**, *14*, 1393–1397. [CrossRef] [PubMed]
72. Haase, H.; Ober-Blobaum, J.L.; Engelhardt, G.; Hebel, S.; Heit, A.; Heine, H.; Rink, L. Zinc signals are essential for lipopolysaccharide-induced signal transduction in monocytes. *J. Immunol.* **2008**, *181*, 6491–6502. [CrossRef] [PubMed]
73. Reiterer, G.; Toborek, M.; Hennig, B. Peroxisome proliferator activated receptors alpha and gamma require zinc for their anti-inflammatory properties in porcine vascular endothelial cells. *J. Nutr.* **2004**, *134*, 1711–1715. [PubMed]
74. Prasad, A.S.; Bao, B.; Beck, F.W.; Kucuk, O.; Sarkar, F.H. Antioxidant effect of zinc in humans. *Free Radic. Biol. Med.* **2004**, *37*, 1182–1190. [CrossRef] [PubMed]
75. Liu, M.J.; Bao, S.; Galvez-Peralta, M.; Pyle, C.J.; Rudawsky, A.C.; Pavlovicz, R.E.; Killilea, D.W.; Li, C.; Nebert, D.W.; Wewers, M.D.; et al. ZIP8 regulates host defense through zinc-mediated inhibition of NF-kappaB. *Cell Rep.* **2013**, *3*, 386–400. [CrossRef] [PubMed]
76. Von Bulow, V.; Dubben, S.; Engelhardt, G.; Hebel, S.; Plumakers, B.; Heine, H.; Rink, L.; Haase, H. Zinc-dependent suppression of TNF-alpha production is mediated by protein kinase A-induced inhibition of Raf-1, I kappa B kinase beta, and NF-kappa B. *J. Immunol.* **2007**, *179*, 4180–4186. [CrossRef] [PubMed]
77. Aydemir, T.B.; Chang, S.M.; Guthrie, G.J.; Maki, A.B.; Ryu, M.S.; Karabiyik, A.; Cousins, R.J. Zinc transporter ZIP14 functions in hepatic zinc, iron and glucose homeostasis during the innate immune response (endotoxemia). *PLoS ONE* **2012**, *7*, e48679.
78. Cummings, J.E.; Kovacic, J.P. The ubiquitous role of zinc in health and disease. *J. Vet. Emerg. Crit. Care* **2009**, *19*, 215–240. [CrossRef] [PubMed]
79. Stennicke, H.R.; Salvesen, G.S. Biochemical characteristics of caspases-3, -6, -7, and -8. *J. Biol. Chem.* **1997**, *272*, 25719–25723. [CrossRef] [PubMed]

80. Huber, K.L.; Hardy, J.A. Mechanism of zinc-mediated inhibition of caspase-9. *Protein Sci. Publ. Protein Soc.* **2012**, *21*, 1056–1065. [CrossRef] [PubMed]

81. Velazquez-Delgado, E.M.; Hardy, J.A. Zinc-mediated allosteric inhibition of caspase-6. *J. Biol. Chem.* **2012**, *287*, 36000–36011. [CrossRef] [PubMed]

82. Muroi, M.; Tanamoto, K. Zinc- and oxidative property-dependent degradation of pro-caspase-1 and NLRP3 by ziram in mouse macrophages. *Toxicol. Lett.* **2015**, *235*, 199–205. [CrossRef] [PubMed]

83. Costarelli, L.; Muti, E.; Malavolta, M.; Cipriano, C.; Giacconi, R.; Tesei, S.; Piacenza, F.; Pierpaoli, S.; Gasparini, N.; Faloia, E.; et al. Distinctive modulation of inflammatory and metabolic parameters in relation to zinc nutritional status in adult overweight/obese subjects. *J. Nutr. Biochem.* **2010**, *21*, 432–437. [CrossRef] [PubMed]

84. Nishio, N.; Ito, S.; Suzuki, H.; Isobe, K. Antibodies to wounded tissue enhance cutaneous wound healing. *Immunology* **2009**, *128*, 369–380. [CrossRef] [PubMed]

85. Iwata, Y.; Yoshizaki, A.; Komura, K.; Shimizu, K.; Ogawa, F.; Hara, T.; Muroi, E.; Bae, S.; Takenaka, M.; Yukami, T.; et al. CD19, a response regulator of B lymphocytes, regulates wound healing through hyaluronan-induced TLR4 signaling. *Am. J. Pathol.* **2009**, *175*, 649–660. [CrossRef] [PubMed]

86. Fraker, P.J.; King, L.E. Reprogramming of the immune system during zinc deficiency. *Ann. Rev. Nutr.* **2004**, *24*, 277–298. [CrossRef] [PubMed]

87. Sirbulescu, R.F.; Boehm, C.K.; Soon, E.; Wilks, M.Q.; Ilies, I.; Yuan, H.; Maxner, B.; Chronos, N.; Kaittanis, C.; Normandin, M.D.; et al. Mature B cells accelerate wound healing after acute and chronic diabetic skin lesions. *Wound Repair Regen.* **2017**. [CrossRef] [PubMed]

88. King, L.E.; Frentzel, J.W.; Mann, J.J.; Fraker, P.J. Chronic zinc deficiency in mice disrupted T cell lymphopoiesis and erythropoiesis while B cell lymphopoiesis and myelopoiesis were maintained. *J. Am. Coll. Nutr.* **2005**, *24*, 494–502. [CrossRef] [PubMed]

89. Rosenkranz, E.; Metz, C.H.; Maywald, M.; Hilgers, R.D.; Wessels, I.; Senff, T.; Haase, H.; Jager, M.; Ott, M.; Aspinall, R.; et al. Zinc supplementation induces regulatory T cells by inhibition of Sirt-1 deacetylase in mixed lymphocyte cultures. *Mol. Nutr. Food Res.* **2016**, *60*, 661–671. [CrossRef] [PubMed]

90. Rosenkranz, E.; Hilgers, R.D.; Uciechowski, P.; Petersen, A.; Plumakers, B.; Rink, L. Zinc enhances the number of regulatory T cells in allergen-stimulated cells from atopic subjects. *Eur. J. Nutr.* **2017**, *56*, 557–567. [CrossRef] [PubMed]

91. Maywald, M.; Meurer, S.K.; Weiskirchen, R.; Rink, L. Zinc supplementation augments TGF-beta1-dependent regulatory T cell induction. *Mol. Nutr. Food Res.* **2017**, *61*, 3. [CrossRef] [PubMed]

92. Nosbaum, A.; Prevel, N.; Truong, H.A.; Mehta, P.; Ettinger, M.; Scharschmidt, T.C.; Ali, N.H.; Pauli, M.L.; Abbas, A.K.; Rosenblum, M.D. Cutting Edge: Regulatory T Cells Facilitate Cutaneous Wound Healing. *J. Immunol.* **2016**, *196*, 2010–2014. [CrossRef] [PubMed]

93. Arwert, E.N.; Hoste, E.; Watt, F.M. Epithelial stem cells, wound healing and cancer. *Nat. Rev. Cancer* **2012**, *12*, 170–180. [CrossRef] [PubMed]

94. Agren, M.S.; Chvapil, M.; Franzen, L. Enhancement of re-epithelialization with topical zinc oxide in porcine partial-thickness wounds. *J. Surg. Res.* **1991**, *50*, 101–105. [CrossRef]

95. Tandon, N.; Cimetta, E.; Villasante, A.; Kupferstein, N.; Southall, M.D.; Fassih, A.; Xie, J.; Sun, Y.; Vunjak-Novakovic, G. Galvanic microparticles increase migration of human dermal fibroblasts in a wound-healing model via reactive oxygen species pathway. *Exp. Cell Res.* **2014**, *320*, 79–91. [CrossRef] [PubMed]

96. Tenaud, I.; Leroy, S.; Chebassier, N.; Dreno, B. Zinc, copper and manganese enhanced keratinocyte migration through a functional modulation of keratinocyte integrins. *Exp. Dermatol.* **2000**, *9*, 407–416. [CrossRef] [PubMed]

97. Li, H.; Chang, J. Bioactive silicate materials stimulate angiogenesis in fibroblast and endothelial cell co-culture system through paracrine effect. *Acta Biomater.* **2013**, *9*, 6981–6991. [CrossRef] [PubMed]

98. Saghiri, M.A.; Asatourian, A.; Orangi, J.; Sorenson, C.M.; Sheibani, N. Functional role of inorganic trace elements in angiogenesis-Part II: Cr, Si, Zn, Cu, and S. *Crit. Rev. Oncol. Hematol.* **2015**, *96*, 143–155. [CrossRef] [PubMed]

99. Tracy, L.E.; Minasian, R.A.; Caterson, E.J. Extracellular Matrix and Dermal Fibroblast Function in the Healing Wound. *Adv. Wound Care* **2016**, *5*, 119–136. [CrossRef] [PubMed]

100. McCarty, S.M.; Cochrane, C.A.; Clegg, P.D.; Percival, S.L. The role of endogenous and exogenous enzymes in chronic wounds: A focus on the implications of aberrant levels of both host and bacterial proteases in wound healing. *Wound Repair Regen.* **2012**, *20*, 125–136. [CrossRef] [PubMed]

101. Martins, V.L.; Caley, M.; O'Toole, E.A. Matrix metalloproteinases and epidermal wound repair. *Cell Tissue Res.* **2013**, *351*, 255–268. [CrossRef] [PubMed]

102. Caley, M.P.; Martins, V.L.; O'Toole, E.A. Metalloproteinases and Wound Healing. *Adv. Wound Care* **2015**, *4*, 225–234. [CrossRef] [PubMed]

103. Xue, M.; Le, N.T.; Jackson, C.J. Targeting matrix metalloproteases to improve cutaneous wound healing. *Expert Opin. Ther. Targets* **2006**, *10*, 143–155. [CrossRef] [PubMed]

104. Van Wart, H.E.; Birkedal-Hansen, H. The cysteine switch: A principle of regulation of metalloproteinase activity with potential applicability to the entire matrix metalloproteinase gene family. *Proc. Natl. Acad. Sci. USA* **1990**, *87*, 5578–5582. [CrossRef] [PubMed]

105. Jansen, P.L.; Rosch, R.; Jansen, M.; Binnebosel, M.; Junge, K.; Alfonso-Jaume, A.; Klinge, U.; Lovett, D.H.; Mertens, P.R. Regulation of MMP-2 gene transcription in dermal wounds. *J. Investig. Dermatol.* **2007**, *127*, 1762–1767. [CrossRef] [PubMed]

106. Venditti, E.; Bruge, F.; Astolfi, P.; Kochevar, I.; Damiani, E. Nitroxides and a nitroxide-based UV filter have the potential to photoprotect UVA-irradiated human skin fibroblasts against oxidative damage. *J. Dermatol. Sci.* **2011**, *63*, 55–61. [CrossRef] [PubMed]

107. Zhou, L.; Yan, C.; Gieling, R.G.; Kida, Y.; Garner, W.; Li, W.; Han, Y.P. Tumor necrosis factor-alpha induced expression of matrix metalloproteinase-9 through p21-activated kinase-1. *BMC Immunol.* **2009**, *10*, 15. [CrossRef] [PubMed]

108. Kim, C.H.; Lee, J.H.; Won, J.H.; Cho, M.K. Mesenchymal stem cells improve wound healing in vivo via early activation of matrix metalloproteinase-9 and vascular endothelial growth factor. *J. Korean Med. Sci.* **2011**, *26*, 726–733. [CrossRef] [PubMed]

109. Gill, S.E.; Parks, W.C. Metalloproteinases and their inhibitors: Regulators of wound healing. *Int. J. Biochem. Cell Biol.* **2008**, *40*, 1334–1347. [CrossRef] [PubMed]

110. Chen, Q.; Jin, M.; Yang, F.; Zhu, J.; Xiao, Q.; Zhang, L. Matrix metalloproteinases: Inflammatory regulators of cell behaviors in vascular formation and remodeling. *Mediat. Inflamm.* **2013**, *2013*, 928315. [CrossRef] [PubMed]

111. Kyriakides, T.R.; Wulsin, D.; Skokos, E.A.; Fleckman, P.; Pirrone, A.; Shipley, J.M.; Senior, R.M.; Bornstein, P. Mice that lack matrix metalloproteinase-9 display delayed wound healing associated with delayed reepithelization and disordered collagen fibrillogenesis. *Matrix Biol. J. Int. Soc. Matrix Biol.* **2009**, *28*, 65–73. [CrossRef] [PubMed]

112. Zigrino, P.; Ayachi, O.; Schild, A.; Kaltenberg, J.; Zamek, J.; Nischt, R.; Koch, M.; Mauch, C. Loss of epidermal MMP-14 expression interferes with angiogenesis but not with re-epithelialization. *Eur. J. Cell Biol.* **2012**, *91*, 748–756. [CrossRef] [PubMed]

113. Gawronska-Kozak, B. Scarless skin wound healing in FOXN1 deficient (nude) mice is associated with distinctive matrix metalloproteinase expression. *Matrix Biol. J. Int. Soc. Matrix Biol.* **2011**, *30*, 290–300. [CrossRef] [PubMed]

114. Binnebosel, M.; Junge, K.; Schwab, R.; Antony, A.; Schumpelick, V.; Klinge, U. Delayed wound healing in sacrococcygeal pilonidal sinus coincides with an altered collagen composition. *World J. Surg.* **2009**, *33*, 130–136. [CrossRef] [PubMed]

115. Tezvergil-Mutluay, A.; Agee, K.A.; Hoshika, T.; Carrilho, M.; Breschi, L.; Tjaderhane, L.; Nishitani, Y.; Carvalho, R.M.; Looney, S.; Tay, F.R.; et al. The requirement of zinc and calcium ions for functional MMP activity in demineralized dentin matrices. *Dent. Mater.* **2010**, *26*, 1059–1067. [CrossRef] [PubMed]

116. Sun, Q.; Zhong, W.; Zhang, W.; Zhou, Z. Defect of mitochondrial respiratory chain is a mechanism of ROS overproduction in a rat model of alcoholic liver disease: Role of zinc deficiency. *Am. J. Physiol. Gastrointest. Liver Physiol.* **2016**, *310*, G205–G214. [CrossRef] [PubMed]

117. Slepchenko, K.G.; Lu, Q.; Li, Y.V. Cross talk between increased intracellular zinc (Zn^{2+}) and accumulation of reactive oxygen species in chemical ischemia. *Am. J. Physiol. Cell Physiol.* **2017**, *313*, C448–C459. [CrossRef] [PubMed]

118. Sen, C.K. The general case for redox control of wound repair. *Wound Repair Regen.* **2003**, *11*, 431–438. [CrossRef] [PubMed]

119. Sen, C.K.; Khanna, S.; Gordillo, G.; Bagchi, D.; Bagchi, M.; Roy, S. Oxygen, oxidants, and antioxidants in wound healing: An emerging paradigm. *Ann. N. Y. Acad. Sci.* **2002**, *957*, 239–249. [CrossRef] [PubMed]

120. Kivisaari, J.; Vihersaari, T.; Renvall, S.; Niinikoski, J. Energy metabolism of experimental wounds at various oxygen environments. *Ann. Surg.* **1975**, *181*, 823–828. [CrossRef] [PubMed]

121. Drose, S.; Brandt, U. Molecular mechanisms of superoxide production by the mitochondrial respiratory chain. *Adv. Exp. Med. Biol.* **2012**, *748*, 145–169. [PubMed]

122. Henderson, J.R.; Swalwell, H.; Boulton, S.; Manning, P.; McNeil, C.J.; Birch-Machin, M.A. Direct, real-time monitoring of superoxide generation in isolated mitochondria. *Free Radic. Res.* **2009**, *43*, 796–802. [CrossRef] [PubMed]

123. Kloubert, V.; Rink, L. Zinc as a micronutrient and its preventive role of oxidative damage in cells. *Food Funct.* **2015**, *6*, 3195–3204. [CrossRef] [PubMed]

124. Valko, M.; Jomova, K.; Rhodes, C.J.; Kuca, K.; Musilek, K. Redox- and non-redox-metal-induced formation of free radicals and their role in human disease. *Arch. Toxicol.* **2016**, *90*, 1–37. [CrossRef] [PubMed]

125. Ruttkay-Nedecky, B.; Nejdl, L.; Gumulec, J.; Zitka, O.; Masarik, M.; Eckschlager, T.; Stiborova, M.; Adam, V.; Kizek, R. The role of metallothionein in oxidative stress. *Int. J. Mol. Sci.* **2013**, *14*, 6044–6066. [CrossRef] [PubMed]

126. Hanada, K.; Sawamura, D.; Hashimoto, I.; Kida, K.; Naganuma, A. Epidermal proliferation of the skin in metallothionein-null mice. *J. Investig. Dermatol.* **1998**, *110*, 259–262. [CrossRef] [PubMed]

127. Penkowa, M.; Giralt, M.; Thomsen, P.S.; Carrasco, J.; Hidalgo, J. Zinc or copper deficiency-induced impaired inflammatory response to brain trauma may be caused by the concomitant metallothionein changes. *J. Neurotrauma* **2001**, *18*, 447–463. [CrossRef] [PubMed]

128. Hatakeyama, S. TRIM Family Proteins: Roles in Autophagy, Immunity, and Carcinogenesis. *Trends Biochem. Sci.* **2017**, *42*, 297–311. [CrossRef] [PubMed]

129. Ozato, K.; Shin, D.M.; Chang, T.H.; Morse, H.C., 3rd. TRIM family proteins and their emerging roles in innate immunity. *Nat. Rev. Immunol.* **2008**, *8*, 849–860. [CrossRef] [PubMed]

130. Rajsbaum, R.; Garcia-Sastre, A.; Versteeg, G.A. TRIMmunity: The roles of the TRIM E3-ubiquitin ligase family in innate antiviral immunity. *J. Mol. Biol.* **2014**, *426*, 1265–1284. [CrossRef] [PubMed]

131. Versteeg, G.A.; Benke, S.; Garcia-Sastre, A.; Rajsbaum, R. InTRIMsic immunity: Positive and negative regulation of immune signaling by tripartite motif proteins. *Cytokine Growth Factor Rev.* **2014**, *25*, 563–576. [CrossRef] [PubMed]

132. Cooper, S.T.; McNeil, P.L. Membrane Repair: Mechanisms and Pathophysiology. *Physiol. Rev.* **2015**, *95*, 1205–1240. [CrossRef] [PubMed]

133. Demonbreun, A.R.; McNally, E.M. Plasma Membrane Repair in Health and Disease. *Curr. Top. Membr.* **2016**, *77*, 67–96. [PubMed]

134. Tan, T.; Ko, Y.G.; Ma, J. Dual function of MG53 in membrane repair and insulin signaling. *BMB Rep.* **2016**, *49*, 414–423. [CrossRef] [PubMed]

135. McNeil, P.L.; Kirchhausen, T. An emergency response team for membrane repair. *Nat. Rev. Mol. Cell Biol.* **2005**, *6*, 499–505. [CrossRef] [PubMed]

136. He, B.; Tang, R.H.; Weisleder, N.; Xiao, B.; Yuan, Z.; Cai, C.; Zhu, H.; Lin, P.; Qiao, C.; Li, J.; et al. Enhancing muscle membrane repair by gene delivery of MG53 ameliorates muscular dystrophy and heart failure in delta-Sarcoglycan-deficient hamsters. *Mol. Ther.* **2012**, *20*, 727–735. [CrossRef] [PubMed]

137. Howard, A.C.; McNeil, A.K.; Xiong, F.; Xiong, W.C.; McNeil, P.L. A novel cellular defect in diabetes: Membrane repair failure. *Diabetes* **2011**, *60*, 3034–3043. [CrossRef] [PubMed]

138. Cai, C.; Masumiya, H.; Weisleder, N.; Matsuda, N.; Nishi, M.; Hwang, M.; Ko, J.K.; Lin, P.; Thornton, A.; Zhao, X.; et al. MG53 nucleates assembly of cell membrane repair machinery. *Nat. Cell Biol.* **2009**, *11*, 56–64. [CrossRef] [PubMed]

139. Cai, C.; Weisleder, N.; Ko, J.K.; Komazaki, S.; Sunada, Y.; Nishi, M.; Takeshima, H.; Ma, J. Membrane repair defects in muscular dystrophy are linked to altered interaction between MG53, caveolin-3, and dysferlin. *J. Biol. Chem.* **2009**, *284*, 15894–15902.

140. Demonbreun, A.R.; Quattrocelli, M.; Barefield, D.Y.; Allen, M.V.; Swanson, K.E.; McNally, E.M. An actin-dependent annexin complex mediates plasma membrane repair in muscle. *J. Cell Biol.* **2016**, *213*, 705–718. [CrossRef] [PubMed]

141. Cao, C.M.; Zhang, Y.; Weisleder, N.; Ferrante, C.; Wang, X.; Lv, F.; Song, R.; Hwang, M.; Jin, L.; Guo, J.; et al. MG53 constitutes a primary determinant of cardiac ischemic preconditioning. *Circulation* **2010**, *121*, 2565–2574. [CrossRef] [PubMed]

142. Duann, P.; Li, H.; Lin, P.; Tan, T.; Wang, Z.; Chen, K.; Zhou, X.; Gumpper, K.; Zhu, H.; Ludwig, T.; et al. MG53-mediated cell membrane repair protects against acute kidney injury. *Sci. Transl. Med.* **2015**, *7*, 279ra236. [CrossRef] [PubMed]

143. Jia, Y.; Chen, K.; Lin, P.; Lieber, G.; Nishi, M.; Yan, R.; Wang, Z.; Yao, Y.; Li, Y.; Whitson, B.A.; et al. Treatment of acute lung injury by targeting MG53-mediated cell membrane repair. *Nat. Commun.* **2014**, *5*, 4387. [CrossRef] [PubMed]

144. Weisleder, N.; Takizawa, N.; Lin, P.; Wang, X.; Cao, C.; Zhang, Y.; Tan, T.; Ferrante, C.; Zhu, H.; Chen, P.J.; et al. Recombinant MG53 protein modulates therapeutic cell membrane repair in treatment of muscular dystrophy. *Sci. Transl. Med.* **2012**, *4*, 139ra185. [CrossRef] [PubMed]

145. Zhang, Y.; Lv, F.; Jin, L.; Peng, W.; Song, R.; Ma, J.; Cao, C.M.; Xiao, R.P. MG53 participates in ischaemic postconditioning through the RISK signalling pathway. *Cardiovasc. Res.* **2011**, *91*, 108–115. [CrossRef] [PubMed]

146. Liu, J.; Zhu, H.; Zheng, Y.; Xu, Z.; Li, L.; Tan, T.; Park, K.H.; Hou, J.; Zhang, C.; Li, D.; et al. Cardioprotection of recombinant human MG53 protein in a porcine model of ischemia and reperfusion injury. *J. Mol. Cell. Cardiol.* **2015**, *80*, 10–19. [CrossRef] [PubMed]

147. Yao, Y.; Zhang, B.; Zhu, H.; Li, H.; Han, Y.; Chen, K.; Wang, Z.; Zeng, J.; Liu, Y.; Wang, X.; et al. MG53 permeates through blood-brain barrier to protect ischemic brain injury. *Oncotarget* **2016**, *7*, 22474–22485. [CrossRef] [PubMed]

148. Wang, C.; Wang, H.; Wu, D.; Hu, J.; Wu, W.; Zhang, Y.; Peng, X. A novel perspective for burn-induced myopathy: Membrane repair defect. *Sci. Rep.* **2016**, *6*, 31409. [CrossRef] [PubMed]

149. Gushchina, L.V.; Bhattacharya, S.; McElhanon, K.E.; Choi, J.H.; Manring, H.; Beck, E.X.; Alloush, J.; Weisleder, N. Treatment with Recombinant Human MG53 Protein Increases Membrane Integrity in a Mouse Model of Limb Girdle Muscular Dystrophy 2B. *Mol. Ther. J. Am. Soc. Gene Ther.* **2017**, *25*, 2360–2371. [CrossRef] [PubMed]

150. Zhang, C.; Chen, B.; Wang, Y.; Guo, A.; Tang, Y.; Khataei, T.; Shi, Y.; Kutschke, W.J.; Zimmerman, K.; Weiss, R.M.; et al. MG53 is dispensable for T-tubule maturation but critical for maintaining T-tubule integrity following cardiac stress. *J. Mol. Cell. Cardiol.* **2017**, *112*, 123–130. [CrossRef] [PubMed]

151. Nagre, N.; Wang, S.; Kellett, T.; Kanagasabai, R.; Deng, J.; Nishi, M.; Shilo, K.; Oeckler, R.A.; Yalowich, J.C.; Takeshima, H.; et al. TRIM72 modulates caveolar endocytosis in repair of lung cells. *Am. J. Physiol. Lung Cell. Mol. Physiol.* **2016**, *310*, L452–L464. [CrossRef] [PubMed]

152. Lipkowitz, S.; Weissman, A.M. RINGs of good and evil: RING finger ubiquitin ligases at the crossroads of tumour suppression and oncogenesis. *Nat. Rev. Cancer* **2011**, *11*, 629–643. [CrossRef] [PubMed]

153. Cai, C.; Lin, P.; Zhu, H.; Ko, J.K.; Hwang, M.; Tan, T.; Pan, Z.; Korichneva, I.; Ma, J. Zinc Binding to MG53 Protein Facilitates Repair of Injury to Cell Membranes. *J. Biol. Chem.* **2015**, *290*, 13830–13839. [CrossRef] [PubMed]

154. Pakyari, M.; Farrokhi, A.; Maharlooei, M.K.; Ghahary, A. Critical Role of Transforming Growth Factor Beta in Different Phases of Wound Healing. *Adv. Wound Care* **2013**, *2*, 215–224. [CrossRef] [PubMed]

155. Hameedaldeen, A.; Liu, J.; Batres, A.; Graves, G.S.; Graves, D.T. FOXO1, TGF-beta regulation and wound healing. *Int. J. Mol. Sci.* **2014**, *15*, 16257–16269. [CrossRef] [PubMed]

156. Morikawa, M.; Derynck, R.; Miyazono, K. TGF-beta and the TGF-beta Family: Context-Dependent Roles in Cell and Tissue Physiology. *Cold Spring Harb. Perspect. Biol.* **2016**, *8*, a021873. [CrossRef] [PubMed]

157. Boo, S.; Dagnino, L. Integrins as Modulators of Transforming Growth Factor Beta Signaling in Dermal Fibroblasts During Skin Regeneration After Injury. *Adv. Wound Care* **2013**, *2*, 238–246. [CrossRef] [PubMed]

158. Ma, H.; Liu, J.; Bian, Z.; Cui, Y.; Zhou, X.; Zhang, B.; Adesanya, T.M.; Yi, F.; Park, K.H.; Tan, T.; et al. Effect of metabolic syndrome on mitsugumin 53 expression and function. *PLoS ONE* **2015**, *10*, e0124128. [CrossRef] [PubMed]

159. Beer, H.D.; Munding, C.; Dubois, N.; Mamie, C.; Hohl, D.; Werner, S. The estrogen-responsive B box protein: A novel regulator of keratinocyte differentiation. *J. Biol. Chem.* **2002**, *277*, 20740–20749. [CrossRef] [PubMed]

160. Tan, H.; Qi, J.; Chu, G.; Liu, Z. Tripartite Motif 16 Inhibits the Migration and Invasion in Ovarian Cancer Cells. *Oncol. Res.* **2017**, *25*, 551–558. [CrossRef] [PubMed]

161. Wang, Y.; Li, J.; Huang, Y.; Dai, X.; Liu, Y.; Liu, Z.; Wang, Y.; Wang, N.; Zhang, P. Tripartite motif-containing 28 bridges endothelial inflammation and angiogenic activity by retaining expression of TNFR-1 and -2 and VEGFR2 in endothelial cells. *FASEB J.* **2017**, *31*, 2026–2036. [CrossRef] [PubMed]

162. Wilkinson, E.A. Oral zinc for arterial and venous leg ulcers. *Cochrane Database Syst. Rev.* **2012**, *8*, CD001273.

163. O'Connor, S.; Murphy, S. Chronic venous leg ulcers: Is topical zinc the answer? A review of the literature. *Adv. Skin Wound Care* **2014**, *27*, 35–44. [CrossRef] [PubMed]

164. Cereda, E.; Gini, A.; Pedrolli, C.; Vanotti, A. Disease-specific, versus standard, nutritional support for the treatment of pressure ulcers in institutionalized older adults: A randomized controlled trial. *J. Am. Geriatr. Soc.* **2009**, *57*, 1395–1402. [CrossRef] [PubMed]

165. Attia, E.A.; Belal, D.M.; El Samahy, M.H.; El Hamamsy, M.H. A pilot trial using topical regular crystalline insulin vs. aqueous zinc solution for uncomplicated cutaneous wound healing: Impact on quality of life. *Wound Repair Regen.* **2014**, *22*, 52–57. [CrossRef] [PubMed]

166. Sakae, K.; Agata, T.; Kamide, R.; Yanagisawa, H. Effects of L-carnosine and its zinc complex (Polaprezinc) on pressure ulcer healing. *Nutr. Clin. Pract.* **2013**, *28*, 609–616. [CrossRef] [PubMed]

167. Lansdown, A.B. Zinc in the healing wound. *Lancet* **1996**, *347*, 706–707. [CrossRef]

168. Agren, M.S. Zinc oxide increases degradation of collagen in necrotic wound tissue. *Br. J. Dermatol.* **1993**, *129*, 221. [CrossRef] [PubMed]

169. Pinnell, S.R. Cutaneous photodamage, oxidative stress, and topical antioxidant protection. *J. Am. Acad. Dermatol.* **2003**, *48*, 1–19. [CrossRef] [PubMed]

170. Berger, M.M.; Baines, M.; Raffoul, W.; Benathan, M.; Chiolero, R.L.; Reeves, C.; Revelly, J.P.; Cayeux, M.C.; Senechaud, I.; Shenkin, A. Trace element supplementation after major burns modulates antioxidant status and clinical course by way of increased tissue trace element concentrations. *Am. J. Clin. Nutr.* **2007**, *85*, 1293–1300. [PubMed]

171. Xiong, H.M. ZnO nanoparticles applied to bioimaging and drug delivery. *Adv. Mater.* **2013**, *25*, 5329–5335. [CrossRef] [PubMed]

172. Oyarzun-Ampuero, F.; Vidal, A.; Concha, M.; Morales, J.; Orellana, S.; Moreno-Villoslada, I. Nanoparticles for the Treatment of Wounds. *Curr. Pharm. Des.* **2015**, *21*, 4329–4341. [CrossRef] [PubMed]

173. Pati, R.; Das, I.; Mehta, R.K.; Sahu, R.; Sonawane, A. Zinc-Oxide Nanoparticles Exhibit Genotoxic, Clastogenic, Cytotoxic and Actin Depolymerization Effects by Inducing Oxidative Stress Responses in Macrophages and Adult Mice. *Toxicol. Sci.* **2016**, *150*, 454–472. [CrossRef] [PubMed]

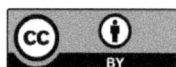

![nutrients logo]

Article

Prospective Study of Dietary Zinc Intake and Risk of Cardiovascular Disease in Women

Abul Hasnat Milton *, Khanrin P. Vashum, Mark McEvoy, Sumaira Hussain, Patrick McElduff, Julie Byles and John Attia

Centre for Clinical Epidemiology and Biostatistics (CCEB), School of Medicine and Public Health, Faculty of Health and Medicine, The University of Newcastle, University Drive, Callaghan, NSW 2308, Australia; khanrin.vashum@newcastle.edu.au (K.P.V.); mark.mcevoy@newcatle.edu.au (M.M.); sumaira.87@gmail.com (S.H.); patrick.mcelduff@newcastle.edu.au (P.M.); julie.byles@newcastle.edu.au (J.B.); john.attia@newcastle.edu.au (J.A.)
* Correspondence: milton.hasnat@newcastle.edu.au; Tel.: +61-2-4042-0525

Received: 28 November 2017; Accepted: 15 December 2017; Published: 4 January 2018

Abstract: Several animal and human studies have shown that zinc is associated with cellular damage and cardiac dysfunction. This study aims to investigate dietary zinc and the zinc-iron ratio, as predictors of incident cardiovascular disease (CVD) in a large longitudinal study of mid-age Australian women (aged 50–61 years). Data was self-reported and validated food frequency questionnaires were used to assess dietary intake. Energy-adjusted zinc was ranked using quintiles and predictors of incident CVD were examined using stepwise logistic regression. After six years of follow-up, 320 incident CVD cases were established. A positive association between dietary zinc intake, zinc-iron ratio and risk of CVD was observed even after adjusting for potential dietary and non-dietary confounders. Compared to those with the lowest quintile of zinc, those in the highest quintile (Odds Ratio (OR) = 1.67, 95% Confidence Interval (CI) = 1.08–2.62) and zinc-iron ratio (OR = 1.72, 95% CI = 1.05–2.81) had almost twice the odds of developing CVD (p trend = 0.007). This study shows that high dietary zinc intake and zinc-iron ratio is associated with a greater incidence of CVD in women. Further studies are required detailing the source of zinc and iron in diet and their precise roles when compared to other essential nutrients.

Keywords: diet; cohort; Australia; zinc; women; cardiovascular disease

---

1. Introduction

The prevalence of chronic diseases has been increasing in the past few decades. Cardiovascular diseases (CVDs) are the number one cause of death globally: more people die annually from CVDs than from any other cause [1]. CVD has a strong genetic basis and it is modified by environmental factors. To date, the most accessible method of preventing or lowering occurrence of CVD is through modification of lifestyle factors, especially diet and exercise. A review in 1996 by Houtman about trace elements and CVD obtained from epidemiological, biochemical and cell biological studies concluded that zinc has the potential to counteract the development of cardiovascular disease [2]; however, the strength of this effect on public health is difficult to measure. Recently, there has been growing interest in the relation of dietary intake, especially micronutrients present in the diet, and risk of CVDs [3–6]. Zinc is one of those micronutrients present in our diet whose deficiency may play an important role in the appearance of diseases and has three major biological roles, as catalyst, structural, and regulatory ion [4]. Zinc has been reported to have antioxidant and anti-atherosclerotic effects [4,5,7]. Zinc deficiency leads to cellular damage and atherosclerosis [5] and is known to cause sensitivity to oxidative damage, leading to an increased release of interleukin 1 and tumour necrosis factor-α, which causes increased endothelial cell apoptosis [7].

Experimental studies have shown that zinc administration during reperfusion improves myocardial recovery to almost 100%, protects against cardiac mechanical and/or electrical dysfunction, decreases the incidence of arrhythmias and improves post-ischemic myocardial recovery [8]. Another recent experimental study demonstrated that decreased level of zinc in the diet could induce hypertension and cardiac dysfunction [9]. Inadequate intake of zinc in humans was persistently observed in patients with heart disease [10] and trace element analysis of hair showed that CVD patients had lower concentrations of zinc [11]. Similarly, decreased serum zinc level was observed in ischemic stroke patients when compared to control patients [12].

Trials have explored the contribution of zinc supplementation in different conditions. In stroke patients, zinc supplementation has been shown to decrease the risk of mortality (Lixian trial) [13] and enhance neurological recovery [14]. However, according to a systematic review on the effect of zinc supplements in humans, besides the observed adverse effect on plasma high-density lipoprotein cholesterol (HDL-C) concentrations, the effect of zinc supplementation on heart disease risk remains unclear [15]. A more recent review of prospective cohort studies on zinc status and CVDs revealed no association between zinc intake and CVD events [6]. To the best of the authors' knowledge, apart from the inconclusive findings in the aforementioned reviews [6,15], no prospective study has been carried out to investigate the association between dietary zinc intake and risk of incident CVD in women. Consequently, the objective of this study was to investigate whether dietary zinc was associated with incident cardiovascular disease in a large cohort of Australian women. A secondary aim was to examine the association of dietary zinc-iron ratio with CVD because minerals with similar physical or chemical properties such as iron and zinc may compete with each other biologically [16] and previous studies in humans have shown that iron interferes with the absorption of zinc [17].

2. Methods

2.1. The Australian Longitudinal Study on Women's Health (ALSWH)

The Australian Longitudinal Study on Women's Health (ALSWH) is a national cohort study examining the health and wellbeing of women of different ages. This paper uses data from the 1946–1951 cohort, who were 45–50 years of age during Survey 1 in 1996. Ethical approval was obtained by the Human Research Ethics Committees of the University of Newcastle (H-076-0795) prior to baseline data collection in 1996, with written informed consent provided by participants. Ethical clearance for ALSWH was obtained from the University of Newcastle and University of Queensland. Details of ALSWH's methods and recruitment have been previously published [18,19]. Briefly, women were randomly selected from Medicare, the National Health Insurance Database, which includes all permanent residents of Australia. ALSWH collects self-reported data using mailed and online surveys at roughly 3-year intervals and has linked the study data with administrative records after the women gave their consent to participate in the study. The surveys include questions about: health conditions, symptoms, and diagnoses; use of health services; health-related quality of life; social circumstances, including work and time use; demographic factors; and health behaviors.

The response rate for the 1946–1951 cohort at Survey 3 in 2001 (then aged 50–55 years) was 83% of those who had completed Survey 1 (1996) and had not died ($n = 115$) or become too ill to complete further surveys ($n = 21$). Complete food frequency questionnaire (FFQ) data were available for 11,196 women aged 50–55 years (Survey 3, 2001) and 9264 of these women had data available for analysis when they were 56–61 years (Survey 5 in 2007).

2.2. Dietary Assessment

ALSWH uses the Dietary Questionnaire for Epidemiological Studies (DQES) Version 2 FFQ. Both the development of the questionnaire [20] and its validation in young Australian women has been previously reported [21]. This questionnaire asks respondents to report their usual consumption of 74 foods and six alcoholic beverages over the preceding 12 months using a 10-point frequency scale. Additional questions are asked about the number of serves or type of fruit, vegetables, bread, dairy products, eggs, fat spreads and sugar and further details are provided in Hodge et al. [21]. Nutrient intakes were computed from NUTTAB 1995, a national government food composition database of Australian foods NUTTAB 95 [22], using software developed by the Cancer Council of Victoria. The validation of the FFQ against a 7-day weighted food record showed Pearson correlation coefficient = 0.40 for dietary zinc and 0.44 for dietary iron. The FFQ validation study deemed the correlation coefficient acceptable as it is of similar magnitude to those previously reported [21].

2.3. Ascertainment of Cardiovascular Disease

History of CVD was collected at both baseline and follow-up. Participants were classified as having CVD if they had been diagnosed/treated by a doctor for heart attack and/or stoke which was self-reported. In this paper, incident cases of CVD at follow-up were classified as individuals with a diagnosis/treatment of heart attack and/or stroke, after excluding the prevalent cases; that is, those who self-reported a diagnosis/treatment of the condition at Survey 1, 2, or Survey 3.

2.4. Measurement of Non-Dietary Factors

Social and behavioral characteristics were based on information collected at Survey 3 in 2001. Participants were asked to report frequency of engaging in vigorous (e.g., aerobics, jogging) and less vigorous (e.g., walking and swimming) exercise lasting for <20 min in a normal week. Responses were scored using approximate weekly frequencies of exercise. The resulting physical activity scores ranged from 0 to 80 and were categorized as "nil/sedentary (<5)", "low (5 to 15)", "moderate (16 to 25)", or "high (>25)". A score of 15 is commensurate with the current recommendation of moderate intensity activity on most days of the week. This measure is described in more detail elsewhere [23] and has previously been shown to have acceptable test-retest reliability [24]. Standard questions were used to categorize respondents as never-smoker, ex-smoker, or current smoker; body mass index (BMI) was calculated as self-reported weight in kilograms, divided by height in meter squared. Medical history of hypertension and diabetes as diagnosed by a physician along with use of hormone replacement therapy (HRT) (coded as either yes or no) were all self-reported. The participants were also asked to report the number of supplements being used and categorized as taking multivitamin & mineral supplements (yes or no). Alcohol intake was quantified and classified according to Australian National Health & Medical Research (NHMRC, CBR, Australia) guidelines [25]. Annual household income and level of education was sub-classified into different categories.

2.5. Statistical Analysis

Zinc and iron were adjusted for total energy intake using the residual method [26]. The macronutrient variables are adjusted for total energy intake by calculating their component of total energy (as a %). The micronutrients are adjusted for total energy by regressing (using linear regression) the natural log of the micronutrient on the natural log of total energy and extracting the standardized residuals.

Associations between baseline characteristics and quintiles of energy-adjusted zinc were tested using chi-square for categorical variables and analysis of variance (ANOVA) for continuous variables. Quintiles of energy-adjusted zinc were obtained using the *xtile* command in Stata. Predictors of 6-year incidence of CVD were examined using forward stepwise multivariable logistic regression in stepped approach, with the main predictor being energy adjusted zinc and zinc-iron ratio measured at Survey 3 used to predict incidence of CVD by Survey 5.

The multivariable analysis controlled for dietary factors (energy adjusted fiber, fat and iron), non-dietary factors (BMI, smoking status, education, marital status, HRT, exercise group, history (yes/no) of hypertension and diabetes) along with alcohol intake and use of multivitamins/minerals. *p*-values for trends were conducted by treating quintile of energy-adjusted zinc as a continuous variable.

Statistical significance was considered when 2-sided $p < 0.05$. STATA software version 11 was used for all statistical analyses.

3. Results

The baseline characteristics at Survey 3 of the participants by quintile of energy-adjusted dietary zinc (quintile 1 = lowest intake; quintile 5 = highest intake) are shown in Table 1. The dietary zinc intakes of the lowest and highest quintiles were 5.94 mg/day (95% Confidence Interval (CI) = 5.90, 5.99) and 17.35 mg/day (95% CI = 17.12, 17.59) respectively, with a mean intake of 10.66 mg/day. At baseline, (Table 1) non-dietary factors found to be significantly different across quintiles included: smoking status, exercise, education, household income, BMI, HRT, hypertension and age. Energy-adjusted dietary factors found both macronutrients and micronutrient to be significantly different across quintiles. Women in the highest quintile of zinc intake were more likely to be a current smoker and also have a higher level of alcohol intake. Interestingly, women with a higher intake of zinc also had a higher BMI whereas women in the lower quintiles were found to have a more sedentary lifestyle with little or no exercise. Mean age was similar across all the quintiles.

Table 1. Characteristics of subjects at baseline (Survey 3) by quintile of energy-adjusted zinc intake.

Characteristic	Sub-Group/Mean (SD)	Quintile of Energy-Adjusted Zinc Intake			*p*-Value
		Q1 Lowest (*n* = 2125)	Q3 Middle (*n* = 2125)	Q5 Highest (*n* = 2124)	
Smoking status	Never a smoker	948 (* 53%)	1033 (58%)	922 (52%)	<0.001
	Former smoker	568 (32%)	531 (30%)	569 (32%)	
	Current smoker	261 (15%)	215 (12%)	287 (16%)	
Alcohol Intake	Abstainer/rarely drinks	960 (49.84%)	762 (39.08%)	748 (37.72%)	<0.001
	Low risk/moderate drinker	902 (46.83%)	1088 (55.79%)	1049 (52.90%)	
	Binge/risky drinker	53 (2.75%)	93 (4.77%)	156 (7.87%)	
	Chronic/High risk drinker	11 (0.57%)	7 (0.36%)	30 (1.51%)	
Exercise group	Nil/sedentary	321 (19%)	271 (16%)	323 (19%)	0.003
	Low	621 (37%)	683 (40%)	622 (36%)	
	Moderate	318 (19%)	355 (21%)	338 (20%)	
	High	437 (26%)	408 (24%)	433 (25%)	
Education	No formal qualification	417 (19.80%)	300 (14.23%)	365 (17.29%)	<0.001
	School/intermediate certificate	597 (28.35%)	658 (31.21%)	764 (36.19%)	
	Secondary schooling completed	343 (16.29%)	372 (17.65%)	342 (16.20%)	
	Trade qualification/TAFE	415 (19.71)	435 (20.64%)	397 (18.81%)	
	University/other tertiary study	334 (15.86%)	343 (16.27%)	243 (11.51%)	
Annual household income	$1–$15,999	127 (9.25%)	82 (5.27%)	86 (5.66%)	<0.001
	$16,000–$36,999	415 (30.23%)	398 (25.56%)	428 (28.18%)	
	$37,000–$77,999	472 (34.38%)	589 (37.83%)	545 (35.88%)	
	$78,000 or more	189 (13.77%)	276 (17.73%)	253 (16.66%)	
	Don't know or missing	170 (12.38%)	212 (13.62%)	2017 (13.63%)	
Hormone Replacement Therapy (HRT)	No	1250 (70%)	1193 (67%)	1160 (65%)	0.020
	Yes	535 (30%)	591 (33%)	624 (35%)	
Hypertension	No	1498 (85%)	1495 (85%)	1449 (82%)	0.038
	Yes	271 (15%)	274 (15%)	316 (18%)	
Diabetes	No	1724 (99.60%)	1790 (99.50%)	1719 (99.42%)	0.659
	Yes	7 (0.40%)	9 (0.50%)	10 (0.58%)	
Use of multivitamins/minerals	No	957 (45.38%)	918 (43.47%)	989 (46.78%)	0.260
	Yes	1152 (54.62%)	1194 (56.53%)	1125 (53.22%)	
Age	mean (SD)	52.6 (1.4)	52.6 (1.5)	52.4 (1.5)	0.004
Body Mass Index	mean (SD)	26.0 (5.4)	26.5 (5.1)	27.2 (5.4)	<0.001
Total energy intake (KJ/day)	mean (SD)	6676 (2415)	6604 (2275)	6687 (2790)	0.508
Carbohydrates (% of energy)	mean (SD)	48.2 (5.8)	45.6 (5.8)	41.0 (7.5)	<0.001
Dietary fibre (% of energy)	mean (SD)	2.4 (0.7)	2.5 (0.6)	2.5 (0.8)	<0.001
Total protein (% of energy)	mean (SD)	17.1 (2.1)	20.8 (1.7)	25.1 (2.8)	<0.001
Total fat (% of energy)	mean (SD)	35.5 (5.5)	34.3 (5.9)	34.5 (6.6)	<0.001
Saturated fat (energy adjusted)	mean (SD)	14.0 (3.8)	13.5 (3.4)	13.9 (3.3)	<0.001
Polyunsaturated fat (% of energy)	mean (SD)	6.3 (2.3)	5.5 (1.9)	4.7 (1.5)	<0.001

Table 1. *Cont.*

| Characteristic | Sub-Group/Mean (SD) | Quintile of Energy-Adjusted Zinc Intake | | | *p*-Value |
		Q1 Lowest (*n* = 2125)	Q3 Middle (*n* = 2125)	Q5 Highest (*n* = 2124)	
Monounsaturated fat (% of energy)	mean (SD)	12.1 (2.2)	12.1 (2.4)	12.6 (2.8)	<0.001
Iron mg/day (energy adjusted)	mean (SD)	−0.605 (0.984)	0.022 (0.905)	0.543 (0.897)	<0.001
Cholesterol mg/day (energy adjusted)	mean (SD)	−0.584 (1.170)	−0.043 (0.827)	0.607 (0.855)	<0.001
Retinol ug/day (energy adjusted)	mean (SD)	0.451 (0.947)	0.030 (0.932)	−0.525 (0.993)	<0.001
Vitamin C mg/day (energy adjusted)	mean (SD)	−0.092 (1.198)	0.024 (0.957)	0.028 (0.895)	0.001
Vitamin E mg/day (energy adjusted)	mean (SD)	0.346 (1.094)	0.035 (0.923)	−0.407 (0.939)	<0.001
Calcium mg/day (energy adjusted)	mean (SD)	−0.374 (0.901)	0.126 (0.940)	0.089 (1.166)	<0.001
Magnesium mg/day (energy adjusted)	mean (SD)	−0.453 (1.001)	0.064 (0.901)	0.268 (1.069)	<0.001
Sodium mg/day (energy adjusted)	mean (SD)	−0.432 (1.030)	0.026 (0.930)	0.345 (0.999)	<0.001
Potassium mg/day (energy adjusted)	mean (SD)	−0.594 (1.072)	0.067 (0.891)	0.454 (0.915)	<0.001

* The percentage (%) for each characteristic in the quintile columns is % of the total. *p*-Values are for trends.

Tables 2 and 3 show the output of the stepwise approach that examined energy adjusted zinc intake and zinc-iron ratio as independent predictors of incident CVD respectively. At the end of the six years follow-up, 320 (3.6%) incident cases of CVD were identified out of 9264 participants.

In an age adjusted analysis there was no significant association across quintiles 2, 3 and 4 but quintile 5 showed a significant association (OR = 1.43, 95% CI = 1.01–2.04) between energy-adjusted zinc and risk of CVD (Table 2). After adjustment for non-dietary factors including age, the findings did not change and quintile 5 remained statistically significant with *p* = 0.029 (OR = 1.44, 95% CI = 1.01–2.10). Further adjustment for dietary factors lead to an overall increase in odds of developing CVD and strengthened the association (*p* = 0.011). Additional adjustment for alcohol intake and use of supplements (multivitamins/minerals) also showed a statistically significant increase in the odds of developing CVD across quintiles (P_{trend} = 0.007). Compared with the lowest quintile of energy-adjusted zinc those in the highest quintile had almost twice the odds of developing CVD (OR = 1.67, 95% CI = 1.08–0.77).

The association between the energy-adjusted zinc–iron ratio and odds of developing CVD (Table 3) was significant (*p* = 0.002) after adjusting for age with a consistent increase in the odds of developing CVD across the quintiles. A borderline statistically significant association was observed (P_{trend} = 0.057) after adjusting for age and non-dietary factors. A statistically significant increase in the odds of developing CVD across quintiles of energy-adjusted zinc–iron ratio was observed with further adjustment for energy-adjusted dietary factors (*p* = 0.015) and alcohol intake and use of supplements (*p* = 0.007). Those in quintile 4 (OR = 1.78, 95% CI =1.13–2.79) and 5 (OR = 1.72, 95% CI = 1.05–2.81) had almost twice the odds of developing CVD compared with the lowest quintile of energy-adjusted zinc-iron ratio.

Table 2. Stepwise multivariable logistic regression to examine energy-adjusted zinc intake as an independent predictor of a new diagnosis of cardiovascular disease.

| | Quintile of Energy-Adjusted Zinc Intake | | | | | |
	Q1	Q2	Q3	Q4	Q5	*p
Energy-adjusted zinc (median (min, max))	−1.25 (−4.8, −0.79)	−0.48 (−0.79, −0.23)	0.01 (−0.23, 0.26)	0.50 (0.26, 0.79)	1.24 (0.79, 4.45)	
Number of cardiovascular disease	54	55	62	72	77	
Odds ratio						
Age adjusted	1.00	0.99 (0.68 to 1.46)	1.10 (0.76 to 1.60)	1.28 (0.90 to 1.84)	1.43 (1.01 to 2.04)	0.015
Age & non-dietary [†] factors adjusted	1.00	0.92 (0.63 to 1.48)	1.19 (0.84 to 1.88)	1.16 (0.82 to 1.83)	1.44 (1.01 to 2.10)	0.029
Age, non-dietary [†] and dietary [‡] factors adjusted	1.00	0.96 (0.62 to 1.47)	1.26 (0.84 to 1.90)	1.25 (0.82 to 1.90)	1.63 (1.07 to 1.90)	0.011
Age, non-dietary [†] and dietary [‡] factors adjusted plus alcohol intake and use of supplements	1.00	0.94 (0.60 to 1.48)	1.18 (0.76 to 1.82)	1.36 (0.84 to 2.00)	1.67 (1.08 to 2.62)	0.007

[†] Non-dietary factors were BMI; smoking status; HRT; exercise group; education level and history of diabetes and hypertension; [‡] Dietary factors were energy-adjusted fiber, iron and fat. Adjustment for family income in the models resulted in a loss of 1300 observations but education was adjusted for. * *p*-Value for trends.

Table 3. Stepwise multivariable logistic regression to examine zinc–iron ratio as an independent predictor of a new diagnosis of cardiovascular disease.

| | Quintile of Zinc-Iron Ratio | | | | | |
	Q1	Q2	Q3	Q4	Q5	*p
Zinc-iron ratio (median(min, max))	0.69 (0.28, 0.77)	0.84 (0.77, 0.90)	0.95 (0.90, 1.00)	1.06 (1.00, 1.12)	1.21 (1.12, 1.75)	
Number of cardiovascular disease	51	52	69	74	74	
Odds ratio						
Age adjusted	1	1.02 (0.69 to 1.51)	1.38 (0.96 to 1.99)	1.51 (1.05 to 2.17)	1.55 (1.08 to 2.23)	0.002
Age & non-dietary [†] factors adjusted	1	0.95 (0.61 to 1.47)	1.38 (0.92 to 2.06)	1.47 (0.99 to 2.09)	1.40 (0.93 to 2.09)	0.057
Age, non-dietary [†] and dietary [‡] factors adjusted	1	1.03 (0.66 to 1.59)	1.45 (0.95 to 2.20)	1.57 (1.02 to 2.42)	1.54 (0.97 to 2.45)	0.015
Age, non-dietary [†] and dietary [‡] factors adjusted plus alcohol intake and use of supplements	1	1.15 (0.73 to 1.83)	1.52 (0.97 to 2.36)	1.78 (1.13 to 2.79)	1.72 (1.05 to 2.81)	0.007

[†] Non-dietary factors were BMI; smoking status; HRT; exercise group; education level and history of diabetes and hypertension. [‡] Dietary factors were energy-adjusted fiber and fat. * *p*-Value for trends.

Nutrients **2018**, *10*, 38

4. Discussion

Findings from this longitudinal study showed that dietary zinc intake was associated with a higher incidence of CVD in women aged 50 years and older, even after adjusting for potential dietary and non-dietary confounders. The same association was also observed between zinc-iron ratio and risk of CVD. To our knowledge, this is the only longitudinal study that has looked at the relationship between dietary zinc and zinc-iron ratio with incident CVD in an adult women population.

The association between dietary zinc and CVD suggests that high dietary zinc might increase the risk of CVD. The only other prospective study that looked at dietary intake of zinc and iron and CVD was the Iowa women's health study [27]. The study found that dietary zinc and iron were not associated with risk of CVD mortality but the study might have lacked power. Furthermore, the end point of the study was CVD mortality and CVD incidence data was not measured; consequently, cases of CVD with a different cause of death may have been missed. A key observation noted was that the benefit of higher zinc intake in CVD mortality occurred only in the presence of a trigger such as alcohol ($\geq$10 g/day) that could disturb iron homeostasis. Contrastingly, another study reported that alcohol consumption (>40 mL/day) was negatively linked to serum zinc [28]. Lee et al. 2005 also observed that women with higher dietary zinc intake were less likely to smoke and engaged in more physical activity [27], which differs from the characteristics observed in our study. It is widely known that smoking and BMI are modifiable risk factors for CVD and could be a possible explanation for the observed benefit of higher zinc intake in CVD mortality despite the presence of alcohol intake ($\geq$10 g/day). The study also does not appear to have controlled for type 2 diabetes though it has considered other dietary and non-dietary factors as independent variables.

The relationship between type 2 diabetes and CVD is established: CVD events related to type 2 diabetes and the high incidence of other macrovascular complications are a major cause of chronic disease burden [29]. It has been shown that the age-adjusted prevalence of coronary heart disease is twice as high among those with type 2 diabetes than among those without diabetes [30,31]. Hence, zinc status in patients with type 2 diabetes and CVD events was assessed [32,33], which showed low serum zinc and high concentration of urinary zinc excretion in patients with diabetes mellitus and all CVD events [32,33]. Zinc intake was also assessed in an older population of men and women in Australia [34] and in the same cohort of women with type 2 diabetes [35]. These studies showed that a high zinc intake was inversely associated with risk of insulin resistance and type 2 diabetes.

In contrast to the observed association between type 2 diabetes and dietary zinc intake in the same cohort, the finding from this study indicates that dietary zinc intake after a certain level increases the risk of CVD and that those in the highest quintiles are above the threshold and was zinc replete. A possible explanation for this could be the fact that the participants are residents in Australia, a mainly affluent Western society, with reasonably good nutrition and were zinc replete. Of particular interest in this study, it was observed that those in the highest quintile of zinc also had the highest quintile of dietary iron intake. The most commonly recorded dietary source of zinc and iron was meat as the highest contributor, which could explain the increase in iron as zinc intake increases, though fish, poultry, cereals and dairy products were other substantial source. We cannot be sure whether the zinc intake is directly increasing the incidence of CVD, as zinc intake tends to increase as other micronutrients intakes increase (for example, iron in this study), or diet quality more generally. However, recent studies have shown that high intake of red meat in multivariable analyses including age, smoking, and other risk factors [36] and specifically, zinc and heme iron from red meat and not other sources [3] was associated with increased risk of CVD. Findings from these studies lend support to the association observed in our study, as the main source of zinc and iron in the majority of the cohort was most likely to be meat based on the Australian diet.

The secondary aim of this study was also to look at dietary zinc-iron ratio as part of the analysis because iron is known to interact with the absorption of zinc [16]. Zinc causes dose-dependent inhibition of iron binding to phospholipids and competition of zinc for iron binding sites is particularly relevant as zinc deficiency promotes intracellular iron accumulation [37]. We observed that risk of CVD was positively associated with higher quintiles of zinc-iron ratio. This suggests that the proportion of zinc intake in relation to iron is a relevant determinant of CVD risk. The association of zinc-iron ratio has also been observed in diabetes [35] in the same cohort even though the direction of association was different.

The main strengths of this study are the prospective design, where dietary assessment preceded the outcome, and the generalizability, this being a population-based cohort rather than a clinic sample. The main advantage of the prospective design is that it reduces selection bias and potential recall bias. It is also the only prospective study so far that looks at incident CVD with both dietary zinc and zinc-iron ratio. The large sample size also means that it is possible to obtain reasonably stable parameter estimates.

Despite the good generalizability of this study there are some limitations. Use of FFQ to collect dietary information (especially micronutrients) has limitations due to the lack of homogeneity in food composition tables [38] and over or under reporting of certain foods/food groups. However, the use of FFQs to collect dietary information in large population-based samples is the most cost-effective and feasible method available. In this study the use of an FFQ to estimate dietary zinc intake will have underestimated the amount of zinc consumed by study participants and biased the effect size towards the null [39]. A further limitation is that dietary assessment was carried out at one time only. However, instead of excluding participants who developed comorbidities during the follow-up period, we controlled for these in the analysis so as to account for any change in dietary habit that may have occurred following the development of comorbid conditions. Adjustments were made for all known major confounders but residual confounding cannot be entirely excluded. Also despite controlling for type 2 diabetes and alcohol intake, stratifying analysis by alcohol status to duplicate findings by Lee et al. 2005 [27] will be worthwhile in the future.

This study also considered the use of supplementary multivitamins/minerals and analysis showed that the proportion of people taking supplements were not significantly different between quintiles of zinc intake. Although multiple dietary assessments are useful to reduce random measurement error, given that single dietary assessment is likely to bias results toward the null, the fact that we still observed a significant association is an indication that the association is likely to be robust and even stronger than that observed in this study.

In conclusion, this prospective study showed that higher total dietary zinc intake and zinc–iron ratio is associated with a higher incidence of CVD in women aged 50 and above. This study finding is preliminary and needs to be investigated further. Future research is necessary to confirm this association in both men and women across different age groups. A positive finding should prompt further research to investigate the association of zinc and iron from meat and other major sources because these dietary aspects would encourage change in dietary guidelines recommended for reducing CVD burden.

Acknowledgments: The authors wish to sincerely thank all affiliates, together with the numerous academics and university staff that made valuable contributions to this project. We are also truly grateful to the women participants of the Australian Longitudinal Study on Women's Health (ALSWH) who provided and gave permission for information about their health to be used for research purposes. The authors thank Graham Giles of the Cancer Epidemiology Centre of Cancer Council Victoria, for permission to use the Dietary Questionnaire for Epidemiological Studies (Version 2), Melbourne: Cancer Council Victoria, 1996. We are grateful to the Australian Government Department of Health and Ageing for funding. The funding source had no role in the concept formation, study design and writing of the study manuscript.

Author Contributions: K.P.V., A.H.M., M.M. and J.A. conceived and designed the study. J.B. contributed in study design and in data collection. K.P.V. and P.M. carried out the data analysis and data interpretation was carried out along with M.M. All authors contributed substantially to the development of manuscript.

Conflicts of Interest: The authors declare no conflict of interest. The founding sponsor had no role in the design of the study; in the collection, analyses, or interpretation of data; in the writing of the manuscript, and in the decision to publish the results.

References

1. Alwan, A. *Global Status Report on Noncommunicable Diseases 2010*; World Health Organization: Geneva, Switzerland, 2011.
2. Houtman, J.P.W. Trace elements and cardiovascular diseases. *J. Cardiovasc. Risk* **1996**, *3*, 18–24. [CrossRef] [PubMed]
3. De Oliveira Otto, M.C.; Alonso, A.; Lee, D.H.; Delclos, G.L.; Bertoni, A.G.; Jiang, R.; Lima, J.A.; Symanski, E.; Jacobs, D.R., Jr.; Nettleton, J.A. Dietary intakes of zinc and heme iron from red meat, but not from other sources, are associated with greater risk of metabolic syndrome and cardiovascular disease. *J. Nutr.* **2012**, *142*, 526–533. [CrossRef] [PubMed]
4. Chasapis, C.T.; Loutsidou, A.C.; Spiliopoulou, C.A.; Stefanidou, M.E. Zinc and human health: An update. *Arch. Toxicol.* **2012**, *86*, 521–534. [CrossRef] [PubMed]
5. Little, P.J.; Bhattacharya, R.; Moreyra, A.E.; Korichneva, I.L. Zinc and cardiovascular disease. *Nutrition* **2010**, *26*, 1050–1057. [CrossRef] [PubMed]
6. Chu, A.; Foster, M.; Samman, S. Zinc Status and Risk of Cardiovascular Diseases and Type 2 Diabetes Mellitus—A Systematic Review of Prospective Cohort Studies. *Nutrients* **2016**, *8*, 707. [CrossRef] [PubMed]
7. Giannoglou, G.D.; Konstantinou, D.M.; Kovatsi, L.; Chatzizisis, Y.S.; Mikhailidis, D.P. Association of reduced zinc status with angiographically severe coronary atherosclerosis: A pilot study. *Angiology* **2010**, *61*, 449–455. [CrossRef] [PubMed]
8. Karagulova, G.; Yue, Y.; Moreyra, A.; Boutjdir, M.; Korichneva, I. Protective role of intracellular zinc in myocardial ischemia/reperfusion is associated with preservation of protein kinase C isoforms. *J. Pharmacol. Sci. Exp. Ther.* **2007**, *321*, 517–525. [CrossRef] [PubMed]
9. Suzuki, Y.; Mitsushima, S.; Kato, A.; Yamaguchi, T.; Ichihara, S. High-phosphorus/zinc-free diet aggravates hypertension and cardiac dysfunction in a rat model of the metabolic syndrome. *Cardiovasc. Pathol.* **2014**, *23*, 43–49. [CrossRef] [PubMed]
10. Lourenço, B.H.; Vieira, L.P.; Macedo, A.; Nakasato, M.; Marucci, M.F.; Bocchi, E.A. Nutritional status and adequacy of energy and nutrient intakes among heart failure patients. *Arq. Bras. Cardiol.* **2009**, *93*, 541–548. [PubMed]
11. Tan, C.; Chen, H.; Xia, C. The prediction of cardiovascular disease based on trace element contents in hair and a classifier of boosting decision stumps. *Biol. Trace Elem. Res.* **2009**, *129*, 9–19. [CrossRef] [PubMed]
12. Munshi, A.; Babu, S.; Kaul, S.; Shafi, G.; Rajeshwar, K.; Alladi, S.; Jyothy, A. Depletion of serum zinc in ischemic stroke patients. *Methods Find. Exp. Clin. Pharmacol.* **2009**, *32*, 433–436.
13. Mark, S.D.; Wang, W.; Fraumeni, J.F.; Li, J.Y.; Taylor, P.R.; Wang, G.Q.; Dawsey, S.M.; Li, B.; Blot, W.J. Do nutritional supplements lower the risk of stroke or hypertension? *Epidemiology* **1998**, *9*, 9–15. [CrossRef] [PubMed]
14. Aquilani, R.; Baiardi, P.; Scocchi, M.; Iadarola, P.; Verri, M.; Sessarego, P.; Boschi, F.; Pasini, E.; Pastoris, O.; Viglio, S. Normalization of zinc intake enhances neurological retrieval of patients suffering from ischemic strokes. *Nutr. Neurosci.* **2009**, *12*, 219–225. [CrossRef] [PubMed]
15. Hughes, S.; Samman, S. The effect of zinc supplementation in humans on plasma lipids, antioxidant status and thrombogenesis. *J. Am. Coll. Nutr.* **2006**, *25*, 285–291. [CrossRef] [PubMed]
16. Whittaker, P. Iron and zinc interactions in humans. *Am. J. Clin. Nutr.* **1998**, *68*, 442S–446S. [PubMed]
17. Lönnerdal, B. Dietary factors influencing zinc absorption. *J. Nutr.* **2000**, *130*, 1378S–1383S. [PubMed]
18. Lee, C.; Dobson, A.J.; Brown, W.J.; Bryson, L.; Byles, J.; Warner-Smith, P.; Young, A.F. Cohort profile: The Australian longitudinal study on women's health. *Int. J. Epidemiol.* **2005**, *34*, 987–991. [CrossRef] [PubMed]
19. Brown, W.J.; Byles, J.E.; Dobson, A.J.; Lee, C.; Mishra, G.; Schofield, M. Women's Health Australia: Recruitment for a national longitudinal cohort study. *Women Health* **1999**, *28*, 23–40. [CrossRef]
20. Ireland, P.; Jolley, D.; Giles, G.; O'Dea, K.; Powles, J.; Rutishauser, I.; Wahlqvist, M.L.; Williams, J. Development of the Melbourne FFQ: A food frequency questionnaire for use in an Australian prospective study involving an ethnically diverse cohort. *Asia Pac. J. Clin. Nutr.* **1994**, *3*, 19–31. [PubMed]
21. Hodge, A.; Patterson, A.J.; Brown, W.J.; Ireland, P.; Giles, G. The Anti Cancer Council of Victoria FFQ: Relative validity of nutrient intakes compared with weighed food records in young to middle aged women in a study of iron supplementation. *Aust. N. Z. J. Public Health Policy* **2000**, *24*, 576–583. [CrossRef]

22. Lewis, J.; Milligan, G.; Hunt, A. *NUTTAB95: Nutrient Data Table for Use in Australia*; Australian Government Publishing Service: Canberra, CBR, Australia, 1995.
23. Brown, W.J.; Mishra, G.; Lee, C.; Bauman, A. Leisure time physical activity in Australian women: Relationship with well being and symptoms. *Res. Q. Exerc. Sport* **2000**, *71*, 206–216. [CrossRef] [PubMed]
24. Booth, M.L.; Owen, N.; Bauman, A.E.; Gore, C.J. Retest reliability of recall measures of leisure-time physical activity in Australian adults. *Int. J. Epidemiol.* **1996**, *25*, 153–159. [CrossRef] [PubMed]
25. National Health and Medical Research Council (NHMRC). *Australian Guidelines to Reduce Health Risks from Drinking Alcohol*; Commonwealth of Australia: Canberra, CBR, Australia, 2009.
26. Willett, W. *Nutritional Epidemiology*, 2nd ed.; Oxford University Press: New York, NY, USA, 1998.
27. Lee, D.-H.; Folsom, A.R.; Jacobs, D.R. Iron, zinc, and alcohol consumption and mortality from cardiovascular diseases: The Iowa Women's Health Study. *Am. Clin. Nutr.* **2005**, *81*, 787–791.
28. Leone, N.; Dominique, C.; Pierre, D.; Mahmoud, Z. Zinc, copper, and magnesium and risks for all-cause, cancer, and cardiovascular mortality. *Epidemiology* **2006**, *17*, 308–314. [CrossRef] [PubMed]
29. Gæde, P.; Vedel, P.; Larsen, N.; Jensen, G.V.H.; Parving, H.H.; Pedersen, O. Multifactorial intervention and cardiovascular disease in patients with type 2 diabetes. *N. Engl. J. Med.* **2003**, *348*, 383–393. [CrossRef] [PubMed]
30. Wingard, D.L.; Barrett-Connor, E. Heart disease and diabetes. *Diabetes Am.* **1995**, *2*, 429–448.
31. Gu, K.; Cowie, C.C.; Harris, M.I. Diabetes and decline in heart disease mortality in US adults. *JAMA* **1999**, *281*, 1291–1297. [CrossRef] [PubMed]
32. Shokrzadeh, M.; Ghaemian, A.; Salehifar, E.; Aliakbari, S.; Saravi, S.S.S.; Ebrahimi, P. Serum zinc and copper levels in ischemic cardiomyopathy. *Biol. Trace Elem. Res.* **2009**, *127*, 116–123. [CrossRef] [PubMed]
33. Soinio, M.; Marniemi, J.; Laakso, M.; Pyörälä, K.; Lehto, S.; Rönnemaa, T. Serum zinc level and coronary heart disease events in patients with type 2 diabetes. *Diabetes Care* **2007**, *30*, 523–528. [CrossRef] [PubMed]
34. Vashum, K.P.; McEvoy, M.; Milton, A.H.; Islam, M.R.; Hancock, S.; Attia, J. Is serum zinc associated with pancreatic beta cell function and insulin sensitivity in pre-diabetic and normal individuals? Findings from the Hunter Community Study. *PLoS ONE* **2014**, *9*. [CrossRef] [PubMed]
35. Vashum, K.P.; McEvoy, M.; Shi, Z.; Milton, A.H.; Islam, M.R.; Sibbritt, D.; Patterson, A.; Byles, J.; Loxton, D.; Attia, J. Is dietary zinc protective for type 2 diabetes? Results from the Australian longitudinal study on women's health. *BMC Endocr. Disord.* **2013**, *13*, 40. [CrossRef] [PubMed]
36. Bernstein, A.M.; Sun, Q.; Hu, F.B.; Stampfer, M.J.; Manson, J.E.; Willett, W.C. Major dietary protein sources and risk of coronary heart disease in women. *Circulation* **2010**, *122*, 876–883. [CrossRef] [PubMed]
37. Zago, M.P.; Oteiza, P.I. The antioxidant properties of zinc: Interactions with iron and antioxidants. *Free Radic. Biol. Med.* **2001**, *31*, 266–274. [CrossRef]
38. Liu, L.; Wang, P.P.; Roebothan, B.; Ryan, A.; Tucker, C.S.; Colbourne, J.; Baker, N.; Cotterchio, M.; Yi, Y.; Sun, G. Assessing the validity of a self-administered food-frequency questionnaire (FFQ) in the adult population of Newfoundland and Labrador, Canada. *Nutr. J.* **2013**, *12*, 49. [CrossRef] [PubMed]
39. Smith, W.; Mitchell, P.; Reay, E.M.; Webb, K.; Harvey, P.W. Validity and reproducibility of a self-administered food frequency questionnaire in older people. *Aust. N. Z. J. Public Health* **1998**, *22*, 456–463. [CrossRef] [PubMed]

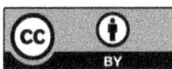

nutrients

MDPI

Review

Associations between Zinc Deficiency and Metabolic Abnormalities in Patients with Chronic Liver Disease

Takashi Himoto [1,*] and Tsutomu Masaki [2]

[1] Department of Medical Technology, Kagawa Prefectural University of Health Sciences, 281-1, Hara, Mure-Cho, Takamatsu, Kagawa 761-0123, Japan
[2] Department of Gastroenterology and Neurology, Kagawa University School of Medicine, Kagawa 761-0123, Japan; tmasaki@med.kagawa-u.ac.jp
* Correspondence: himoto@chs.pref.kagawa.jp; Tel.: +81-87-870-1240

Received: 14 December 2017; Accepted: 5 January 2018; Published: 14 January 2018

Abstract: Zinc (Zn) is an essential trace element which has favorable antioxidant, anti-inflammatory, and apoptotic effects. The liver mainly plays a crucial role in maintaining systemic Zn homeostasis. Therefore, the occurrence of chronic liver diseases, such as chronic hepatitis, liver cirrhosis, or fatty liver, results in the impairment of Zn metabolism, and subsequently Zn deficiency. Zn deficiency causes plenty of metabolic abnormalities, including insulin resistance, hepatic steatosis and hepatic encephalopathy. Inversely, metabolic abnormalities like hypoalbuminemia in patients with liver cirrhosis often result in Zn deficiency. Recent studies have revealed the putative mechanisms by which Zn deficiency evokes a variety of metabolic abnormalities in chronic liver disease. Zn supplementation has shown beneficial effects on such metabolic abnormalities in experimental models and actual patients with chronic liver disease. This review summarizes the pathogenesis of metabolic abnormalities deriving from Zn deficiency and the favorable effects of Zn administration in patients with chronic liver disease. In addition, we also highlight the interactions between Zn and other trace elements, vitamins, amino acids, or hormones in such patients.

Keywords: zinc deficiency; HCV-related chronic liver disease; nonalcoholic steatohepatitis; liver cirrhosis; insulin resistance; hepatic steatosis; hepatic encephalopathy; iron overload; lipid peroxidation; insulin-like growth factor-1

1. Introduction

Zinc (Zn) is an essential trace element that plays pivotal roles in cellular integrity and biological functions related to cell division, growth and development [1,2]. Zn acts as a cofactor for many enzymes and proteins involved in anti-oxidant, anti-inflammatory and apoptotic effects [3]. Zinc-binding proteins represent approximately 10% of human proteomes, with more than 300 enzymes having zinc ions within their catalytic domains [4]. Two types of Zn transporters that maintain Zn homeostasis are identified: ZnTs (zinc transporters) and ZIPs (Zrt-, Irt-like proteins) [5]. ZnTs lower cytoplasmic Zn by transporting Zn through cell-surface membranes and intracellular organelles, while ZIPs increase cytoplasmic Zn.

Zn homeostasis is primarily regulated in the liver. Therefore, chronic liver damage results in the impairment of zinc homeostasis, and eventually zinc deficiency [6–11]. Zn deficiency consequently initiates a variety of metabolic abnormalities, including insulin resistance, hepatic steatosis, iron overload and hepatic encephalopathy (HE) in patients with chronic liver disease. By contrast, a decrease in albumin synthesis leads to Zn deficiency in patients with liver cirrhosis [12]. Recent studies have revealed the putative mechanisms by which Zn deficiency evokes a variety of metabolic abnormalities in patients with fatty liver, chronic hepatitis, or liver cirrhosis. The interactions between Zn deficiency and these metabolic abnormalities are summarized in Table 1.

Table 1. Metabolic abnormalities causing zinc deficiency and metabolic abnormalities deriving from zinc deficiency.

Disease	Cause of Zinc Deficiency	Outcomes of Zinc Deficiency	References
Liver cirrhosis	Decrease in albumin synthesis and relative increase in α2-macroglobulin		[13,14]
	Decrease in Zn absorption from the small intestine		[15]
Hepatic encephalopathy	Liver cirrhosis	Decrease in ornithine transcarbamylase activity	[16]
Insulin resistance	Oxidative stress	Iron overload	[17]
		Decrease in free IGF-1 level	[18]
Hepatic steatosis	Oxidative stress	Enhancement of lipid peroxidation	[17]

IGF-1, insulin-like growth factor.

Here, we mainly focus on the metabolic abnormalities deriving from Zn deficiency in patients with chronic liver disease and the beneficial effects resulting from zinc administration in such patients. Finally, the interactions between Zn deficiency and levels of other trace elements, vitamins, amino acids, or hormones are described.

2. Association between Zn Metabolism and Its Metabolic Abnormality

2.1. Zn Deficiency and Liver Cirrhosis

Liver cirrhosis is considered the most advanced stage of chronic liver disease. An unfavorable hepatic reserve results in numerous metabolic disorders, such as hypoalbuminemia. Consequently, a relative increase in α2 macroglobulin, which more strongly binds to Zn [13], caused a substantial increase in the urinary excretion of Zn [14]. Moreover, Zn absorption from the small intestine was often impaired in patients with liver cirrhosis [15,19]. Such mechanisms result in severe Zn deficiency in patients with liver cirrhosis.

2.2. Zn Deficiency and Hepatic Encephalopathy

Hepatic encephalopathy (HE) is one of the most common neuropsychiatric complications in patients with liver cirrhosis. The pathogenesis of HE has not been completely understood, although ammonia is considered to play a key role. Approximately 90% of patients with liver cirrhosis and HE have elevated ammonia levels in the plasma [9]. HE in liver cirrhosis patients was associated with a high prevalence of Zn deficiency [20]. Poor Zn status resulted in the impairment of nitrogen metabolism by reducing the activity of urea cycle enzyme, ornithine transcarbamylase, in the liver [16,21] and of glutamine synthetase in the muscle [22]. Indeed, serum Zn levels were inversely correlated with blood ammonia levels in patients with liver cirrhosis [23].

2.3. Zn Deficiency and Hepatocellular Carcinoma

Hepatocellular carcinoma (HCC) is the fifth most common form of cancer worldwide [24]. Liver cirrhosis appears to be a decisive risk factor leading to the progression to HCC.

The roles of trace elements underlying hepatocarcinogenesis have not been fully understood yet, although previous studies have identified a number of signal transduction pathways that are involved in this process. Elevated serum copper (Cu) levels were associated with the development of HCC [25–28]. Hepatic Cu content was significantly higher in the HCC tissue than that in the surrounding liver parenchyma [29,30]. By contrast, Zn concentrations in HCC tissues were lower than those in the surrounding hepatic parenchyma [29,30]. Zn may be involved in the regulation of apoptosis in HCC cells [31]. Zn also has a possibility to downregulate hypoxia-inducible factor-1α (HIF-1α) in the malignant cells [32]. Therefore, Zn deficiency may account for the proliferation of HCC cells. However, no significant difference in serum Zn levels was apparent between HCC and liver cirrhosis patients [33,34].

Based on the observations of intracellular Zn concentrations in different carcinomas, it has been postulated that these changes in Zn levels may contribute to the development of tumors by affecting a wide variety of molecular structures, such as receptors, kinases, caspases, phosphatases and transcriptional factors [35].

The decisive role of Zn in malignant transformation may derive from change in the expression of Zn transporters such as Zip4, Zip6, Zip7 and Zip10, as shown by the previous studies on certain types of carcinomas [36–38]. Notably, the expression of Zip14 was decreased during the development of HCC, coupled with a reduction in intracellular Zn levels [39]. Zip14 localizes to the cell membrane of normal hepatocytes and is a functional transmembrane transporter involved in the uptake of zinc into the cell. Therefore, its downregulation may explain the decreased Zn levels in HCC cells. On the other hand, the expression of Zip 4 gene, which is associated with acrodermatitis enteropathica [40], was upregulated in human and mouse HCC tissues, compared with surrounding non-cancerous tissues [41]. Zip4 influenced the expression of matrix metalloproteinase (MMP)-2 and MMP-9, which are directly involved in angiogenesis and the degradation of basement membrane collagen, in the HCC cell lines [42]. MMP-2 and MMP-9 are in the family of zinc-containing enzymes [43]. Therefore, Zip4 may regulate the expression of MMP-2 and MMP-9 by influencing Zn concentration in the HCC tissues.

Serum Zn status may be recognized as a prognostic serological hallmark after initial hepatectomy in HCV-related HCC patients. Imai and colleagues elucidated that HCC patients with lower serum Zn levels at the preoperative stage had significantly lower overall survival than those with a normal range of Zn levels [44].

2.4. Zn Deficiency and HCV Infection

Hepatitis C virus (HCV) is known to induce a spectrum of chronic liver diseases from chronic hepatitis to liver cirrhosis, and ultimately to HCC. More than 184 million people worldwide are estimated to be infected with HCV worldwide at present [45]. Persistent HCV infection often evokes mitochondrial oxidative stress [46], and a variety of resulting metabolic abnormalities, including insulin resistance, dyslipidemia, iron overload and hepatic steatosis [47,48]. Zn has potential cytoprotective effects against oxidative stress, apoptosis and inflammation [49].

Zn deficiency may trigger oxidative stress in patients with HCV-related chronic hepatitis and liver cirrhosis, termed HCV-related chronic liver disease (CLD) [50]. A decrease in serum Zn levels was observed in patients with asymptomatic HCV-carrier as well as those with HCV-related CLD, compared with serum Zn levels in normal healthy controls [51]. However, no significant correlation was found between serum Zn levels and loads of HCV RNA in patients infected with HCV. These data may imply that HCV infection probably affects Zn metabolism, although HCV itself has no direct effect on serum Zn levels in those patients.

Previously, NS3 proteinase, which is involved in the process of HCV replication, proved to be a zinc-containing enzyme [52]. In addition, NS5A protein was considered a Zn metalloprotein [53]. These findings suggest that Zn may have inhibitory effects in the proliferation and replication of HCV.

2.5. Zn Deficiency in Nonalcoholic Steatohepatitis

Nonalcoholic fatty liver disease (NAFLD) is currently the most prevalent liver disease worldwide, characterized by the accumulation of triglycerides in the liver, and the absence of excessive alcohol consumption. NAFLD covers a spectrum of liver diseases that range from simple steatosis called nonalcoholic fatty liver (NAFL) through nonalcoholic steatohepatitis (NASH), which is associated with hepatic inflammation and fibrosis in addition to simple steatosis [54].

Previous studies elucidated that dietary habits are likely to affect Zn metabolism in patients with NAFLD. Lower oral intake of Zn was observed in patients with NAFLD than in normal healthy controls [55]. NASH patients had significantly lower oral intake of Zn than NAFL patients [56]. Zn deficiency in such patients may be due to this lower Zn intake. Zn deficiency results in mitochondrial oxidative stress and subsequently iron over load, insulin resistance, and hepatic steatosis in patients with NASH.

Zn and zinc transporters play crucial roles in the attenuation of endoplasmic reticulum (ER) stress-related signaling and the unfolded protein response (UPR) [57]. Therefore, Zn deficiency may potentially induce or exacerbate ER stress and apoptosis. Kim and colleagues recently elucidated that consumption of a zinc-deficient diet exacerbated ER-stress-induced apoptosis and hepatic steatosis in experimental mice models [58]. The authors proposed that Zip14 mediated Zn transport into hepatocytes to inhibit protein-tyrosine phosphatase 1B, which suppressed apoptosis and steatosis associated with ER stress [59].

2.6. Zn Deficiency and Insulin Resistance in Patients with HCV-Related CLD

Zn plays a pivotal role in the secretion and activation of insulin. Specifically, Zn participates as a potent physiological regulator of insulin signal transduction through its inhibitory effect on protein tyrosine phosphatase 1b, the key phosphatase that dephosphorylates the insulin receptor [60]. Therefore, it has been well known that Zn is absolutely indispensable for the regulation of glucose homeostasis. Zn deficiency seems to be associated with the pathogenesis of type 2 diabetes mellitus (DM), supporting the notion that Zn deficiency may result in the exacerbation of insulin resistance. Zn deficiency may derive from hyperzincuria in patients with type 2 DM [61].

Insulin resistance and/or concurrent type 2 DM are often associated with the occurrence of HCV-related CLD [62]. Previously, we elucidated that Zn deficiency caused the exacerbation of insulin resistance in patients with HCV-related CLD [17,63]. Zn deficiency may contribute to higher serum ferritin levels and lower IGF-1/IGFBP-3 ratios, surrogate measures for circulating free IGF-1 levels [64], and thus substantially exacerbate the insulin resistance in such patients [18].

Depressed serum Zn levels were found in some patients with NAFLD (unpublished data). Zn deficiency is likely to evoke insulin resistance in such patients by way of almost the same mechanism as chronic HCV infection, including hyperferritinemia and/or lower circulating free IGF-1 levels [65].

Zn deficiency is also observed in patients with primary biliary cholangitis (PBC), an autoimmune liver disease characterized by progressive destruction of the intrahepatic bile ducts, leading to cholestasis [66]. Serum Zn levels are gradually decreased as the hepatic fibrosis develops in those patients. Advanced-stage PBC patients also have higher insulin resistance, suggesting that Zn deficiency may exacerbate insulin resistance in such patients [67].

2.7. Zn Deficiency and Iron Overload in Patients with HCV-Related CLD

Persistent HCV infection and nonalcoholic fatty liver disease (NAFLD) are well recognized cofactors affecting body iron storage [48]. A patient's serum ferritin level is ordinarily used as an indicator of iron storage in the liver. We previously showed an inverse correlation between serum Zn and ferritin levels in patients with HCV-related CLD, implying that Zn deficiency might result in iron overload in those patients [17,63].

It has been well established that Zn and iron may compete for access to transporters. Formigari and colleagues suggested that divalent metal transporter 1 (DMT1) is a possible candidate zinc-iron transporter [68]. It is of interest that Zn competed with iron uptake in cells overexpressing Zip14, implicating Zip14 as another possible candidate for transport of both Zn and iron in the liver [69].

2.8. Iron Overload and Insulin Resistance

Iron often influences glucose metabolism. The amount of iron storage in the body was found to be significantly associated with the development of glucose intolerance or type 2 DM in a general population [70].

In addition, iron overload reciprocally seems to affect insulin action. Iron storage interferes with the production of glucose by the liver. Hepatic extraction of insulin and the body's metabolism of insulin is reduced with increasing iron storage, leading to peripheral hyperinsulinemia.

This status is called "iron overload-related insulin resistance" [71]. Iron overload-related insulin resistance was observed in CLD-C and NAFLD patients with hyperferritinemia, who are frequently associated with hepatic steatosis and/or fibrosis [48,72].

2.9. Decrease in Circulating Free IGF-1 Levels and Insulin Resistance in Patients with HCV-Related CLD

Insulin-like growth factor-1 (IGF-1), a liver-derived humoral growth factor, has crucial anabolic and metabolic actions. It is secreted from hepatocytes and has a negative feedback control on growth hormone release from the pituitary gland. The biological activity of IGF-1 is primarily dependent on IGF-binding proteins (IGFBPs). The binding of IGFBP-3 to IGF-1 has been shown to inhibit the bioavailability of IGF-1 [73]. Therefore, free IGF-1 is considered the bioactive form of IGF-1 (Figure 1). However, free IGF-1 levels are difficult to determine directly. The ratio of IGF-1/IGFBP-3 is usually used as a surrogate estimate of free IGF-1 [64].

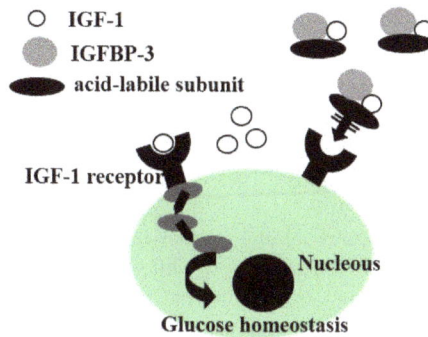

Figure 1. Putative mechanisms by which a decrease in free IGF-1 levels cause insulin resistance in patients with HCV-related CLD. IGF-1, insulin-like growth factor; IGFBP, IGF-binding protein; HCV, Hepatitis C virus; CLD, chronic liver disease.

Zn is likely to participate in the stabilization of IGF-1 transcripts [74]. Thus, the IGF-1/IGFBP-3 ratio, a surrogate measure for circulating free IGF-1 level, had a positive correlation with serum Zn levels in patients with HCV-related CLD [18]. It is of interest that the IGF-1/IGFBP-3 ratio was inversely associated with the values of homeostasis model for assessment of insulin resistance (HOMA-IR), an indicator for insulin resistance, suggesting that a lower circulating free IGF-1 concentration might result in the exacerbation of insulin resistance in such patients.

2.10. Zn Deficiency and Hepatic Steatosis in Patients with HCV-Related CLD

A previous study demonstrated that Zn deficiency was linked to hepatic steatosis in an experimental animal model of fatty liver induced by tetracycline [75]. We confirmed that serum Zn levels were decreased as the degrees of hepatic steatosis developed in patients with HCV-related CLD [17]. Moreover, serum Zn levels were decreased in inverse proportion to the intensity of 4-hydroxy-2'-nonenal (4-HNE), an indicator for lipid peroxidation, in the liver of those patients [17].

Zn has been considered to participate in the enhancement of peroxisome proliferator-activated receptor-α (PPAR-α), a regulator of lipid homeostasis [76]. Zn is necessary for the DNA-binding activity of PPAR-α. Therefore, Zn deficiency may result in a decline of DNA-binding activity, and thereby facilitate lipid peroxidation, ultimately exacerbating hepatic steatosis.

We also revealed that a lower IGF-1/IGFBP-3 ratio might cause more advanced hepatic steatosis in patients with HCV-related CLD [18]. A significant correlation was confirmed between insulin resistance and the severity of hepatic steatosis in those patients. Higher insulin resistance may result in a lower ratio of IGF-1/IGFBP-3 in HCV-related CLD patients with severe steatosis (Figure 2). The lower ratio of IGF-1/IGFBP-3 was also observed in patients with NAFLD [77], suggesting that a decrease in circulating free IGF-1 levels may account for exacerbation of insulin resistance and advanced hepatic steatosis.

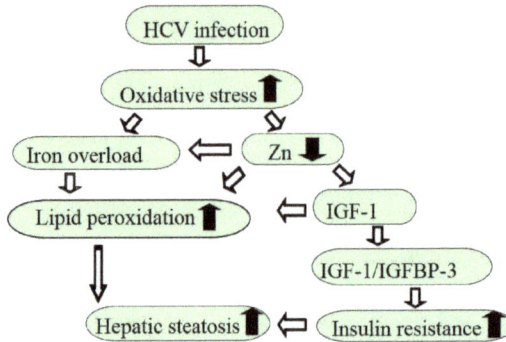

Figure 2. Putative mechanisms by which chronic HCV infection evokes insulin resistance and hepatic steatosis.

Iron overload is also believed to cause lipid peroxidation, and subsequently to lead to hepatic steatosis in patients with HCV-related CLD [72]. We confirmed a significant correlation between the intensity of hepatic 4-HNE expression and serum ferritin levels in such patients [17].

2.11. Zn Metabolism and Wilson's Disease

Wilson's disease is an autosomal recessive, hereditary disorder of Cu metabolism due to defective Cu-transporting ATPase activity, leading to the accumulation of Cu in the liver and basal ganglia of the brain [78]. The accumulation of Cu may affect the metabolisms of other trace elements, including Zn and iron. However, few studies have focused on imbalances of trace elements in patients with Wilson's disease. Ferenci and colleagues previously documented that slightly increased hepatic accumulation of Zn and iron were observed in such patients [79].

2.12. Zn Metabolism and Hemochromatosis

Patients with hereditary hemochromatosis, characterized by HFE point mutations [80], are more susceptible to iron overload when factors such as alcohol, HCV infection, and abnormal porphyrin metabolism are present [48]. Even in the absence of hereditary hemochromatosis, there are several conditions associated with secondary iron overload. A few studies have focused on the relationships between iron overload and other trace element statuses either in experimental models of hemochromatosis or in patients with hemochromatosis. Unfortunately, Zn status in patients with hemochromatosis remains controversial. Vayenas and colleagues elucidated that hepatic Zn content was increased in iron-overload Wister rats [81]. Adams and colleagues also revealed that hepatic zinc content was significantly higher in the livers of patients with hemochromatosis than that in normal livers [82]. The increase in hepatic Zn content might substantially derive from increased intestinal absorption of Zn and hepatic sequestration. To the contrary, Beckett and colleagues recently documented that iron overload did not have a significant effect on Zn status [83].

3. Therapeutic Effects of Zn Administration

Zinc administration has shown favorable effects on metabolic abnormalities in patients with chronic liver disease. The effects of zinc supplementation and possible mechanisms of these effects are summarized in Table 2, and described in detail below.

Table 2. Beneficial effects of zinc administration in patients with chronic liver disease.

Disease	Type of Zn Compound	Effect of Zinc Supplementation	Putative Mechanism	Reference
Hepatic encephalopathy	Zinc sulfate	Reduced ammonia levels	Recovery of OTC activity	[84]
	Zinc-hydrogen-asparate or zinc-histidine	Reduced ammonia levels	Recovery of OTC activity	[85]
	Zinc acetate	Reduced ammonia levels	Recovery of OTC activity	[86,87]
	Polaprezinc	Reduced ammonia levels	Recovery of OTC activity	[88]
Diabetes mellitus	Zinc sulfate	Reduced glucose levels	Improvement of insulin resistance	[89]
Chronic hepatitis	Polaprezinc	Reduced ALT levels	Improvement of iron overload	[90]
	Polaprezinc + IFN-based treatment	Higher rate of HCV eradication		[91]
	Polaprezinc + IFN-based treatment	Lower ALT levels		[92]
Wilson's disease	Zinc acetate	Inhibition of Cu absorption	Increase in MT synthesis	[93]
HCC	Polaprezinc	Lower incidence of HCC development	Maintenance of hepatic reserve	[94]

OTC, ornithine transcarbamylase; HCV, hepatitis C virus; IFN, interferon; ALT, alanine aminotransferase; MT, metallothioneine; HCC, hepatocellular carcinoma.

3.1. Attenuation of Hepatic Inflammation

Zn has beneficial effects on hepatic inflammation in patients with HCV-related CLD. We previously documented that the administration of polaprezinc, a complex of Zn and L-carnosine, showed anti-inflammatory effects in the liver by attenuating hepatic iron storage in such patients [90]. However, the administration of zinc did not directly affect HCV viremia in our study, although Takagi and colleagues revealed that the combination therapy of zinc with interferon (IFN)-α was more effective against HCV eradication than IFN treatment alone [91]. Likewise, Zn administration also prevented an increase in serum alanine aminotransferase (ALT) levels of patients with chronic hepatitis C during IFN-based treatment [92].

3.2. Improvement of Insulin Resistance

Zn supplementation is likely to have favorable effects on impaired glucose tolerance. Yoshikawa and colleagues demonstrated that oral administration of Zn (II)-dithiocarbamate complex improved hyperglycemia, glucose intolerance and insulin resistance in an experimental animal model of type 2 DM [95]. It is of interest that an increase in adiponectin synthesis by the administration of Zn complexes resulted in the improvement of insulin resistance in those experimental animal models.

Oral Zn administrations, using zinc sulfate or zinc acetate, have been prescribed in patients with T2DM. A systemic review by Jayawardena documented that Zn supplementation had beneficial effects on glycemic control in such patients [96]. The authors speculated that the effect of Zn might be mediated by increasing IGF-1. Surprisingly, the authors revealed that Zn administration also improved dyslipidemia in T2DM patients. However, all these studies included dietary supplementation with other antioxidant vitamins and minerals together with Zn. Hence, it is difficult to conclude that the beneficial effects were due to Zn alone.

It is of interest that long-term Zn treatment improved impaired glucose tolerance in patients with advanced liver cirrhosis [89]. Further examinations will be required to clarify the efficacy of Zn administration in HCV-related CLD or NAFLD patients accompanied by insulin resistance.

3.3. Attenuation of Hepatic Steatosis

Sugino and colleagues investigated the effect of Zn (polaprezinc) in a mouse model of NASH. Zn supplementation did not affect the steatosis, but visibly attenuated fibrosis in the liver [97]. Another study documented that treatment with zinc sulfate reversed alcohol-induced steatosis in male mice via reactivation of hepatocyte nuclear factor-4α (HNF-4α) and PPAR-α [98].

Unfortunately, the effects of Zn administration on hepatic steatosis in patients with CLD-C or NAFLD has not been fully verified yet. Hence, Zn supplementation should be evaluated as an optional treatment for such patients [99].

3.4. Improvement of Hepatic Encephalopathy

Long-term Zn supplementation significantly improved the grade of HE and blood ammonia levels in patients with liver cirrhosis [84–88]. Zn administration in patients with liver cirrhosis and HE potentially resulted in the recovery of urea synthesis in the liver and glutamine synthesis in the muscle. Supplementation with branched-chain amino acids (BCAAs) enhances detoxification of ammonia from the skeletal muscles by the amidation process for glutamine synthesis [100]. Interestingly, it was found that a combination treatment with BCAAs and Zn decreased blood ammonia levels more than a treatment with BCAAs alone in patients with liver cirrhosis [101].

3.5. Inhibitory Effect on the Development of HCC

Zn administration appears to have a preventive effect on the development of HCC. Matsumura and colleagues documented that chronic hepatitis C patients treated with polaprezinc, a complex of zinc and L-carnosine, had a significantly lower incidence of HCC than those without administration of polaprezinc [94]. Maintenance of favorable hepatic reserve by Zn supplementation may account for the lower incidence of HCC.

Insulin resistance seems to be one of the risk factors for the development of HCC [102]. Zn supplementation may result in an improvement of insulin resistance in patients with HCV-related CLD or NASH. Accordingly, a treatment with Zn should be considered as a therapeutic strategy in such patients [103].

3.6. Reduced Cu Absorption from the Small Intestine

It has been widely established that oral Zn administration often provides Wilson's disease patients with favorable effects. Zn administration induced the synthesis of metallothionein (MT), a copper-binding protein [104], in the small intestine and the liver. MT binds to newly absorbed Cu and prevents it from passing from the small intestine into the circulation. Some studies, using experimental animal models for Wilson's disease, have also revealed an increase in hepatic MT synthesis, and sequestration of excess hepatic Cu content by the administration of Zn [105]. A significant correlation was found between MT and Zn concentrations in the duodenal mucosa of 15 patients with Wilson's disease by the treatment with zinc sulfate or penicillamine [106]. Accordingly, Zn acetate has been approved for the treatment of Wilson's disease, especially in early stage patients [93].

4. Interactions between Zinc and Other Trace Elements or Vitamins

It has been widely recognized that some trace elements, including Cu and iron, compete with Zn, while selenium and vitamin A are positively associated with Zn status. Table 3 shows interactions between Zn and other trace elements, vitamins, amino acids, or hormones status.

Table 3. Interactions between zinc and other trace elements, vitamins, amino acids, or hormones in chronic liver disease.

Other Trace Elements, Vitamins, Amino Acids, or Hormones	Disease or Condition	Correlation	Reference
Copper	Liver cirrhosis	Increase in Cu/Zn ratio	[33]
	Liver cirrhosis	Increase in Cu/Zn ratio	[34]
	HCC	Increase in Cu/Zn ratio	[33]
	HCC	Increase in Cu/Zn ratio	[34]
	HCC	Increase in Cu/Zn ratio	[107]
	High dose of Zn prescription	Cu deficiency	[108]
Iron	HCV-related CLD	Inverse correlation	[17]
	HCV-related CLD with NAFLD	Inverse correlation	[109]
Selenium	Alcoholic liver disease, PBC, liver cirrhosis and autoimmune hepatitis	Positive correlation	[110]
	HCV-related CLD	Positive correlation	[111]
Vitamin A	Liver cirrhosis	Positive correlation	[112]
Retinol-Binding Protein	Liver cirrhosis	Positive correlation	
Vitamin D	Primary ovarian insufficiency	Positive correlation	[113]
	HCV-related CLD	No significant correlation	[114]
Branched-chain amino acids	HCV-related CLD	No significant correlation	[51]
Tyrosine	HCV-related CLD	Inverse correlation	[51]
IGF-1	HCV-related CLD	Positive correlation	[18]
Testosterone	Infertile males	Positive correlation	[115]

Cu, copper; Zn, zinc; HCC, hepatocellular carcinoma; HCV, hepatitis C virus; CLD, chronic liver disease; NAFLD, nonalcoholic fatty liver disease, PBC, primary biliary cholangitis; IGF-1, insulin-like growth factor-1.

4.1. Zn and Cu

It is well known that Zn competes with Cu [8]. The risk of Cu deficiency in patients with continuously high dose of Zn prescription has been warranted [108,116]. High-dose Zn supplementation causes enterocytes to produce MT which binds to Zn. Whereas, Cu binds more avidly to MT than Zn, eventually leading to Cu deficiency [117]. We previously performed the additional treatment with polaprezinc (51mg/day of Zn for 6 months) in 14 patients with HCV-related CLD. However, none of the HCV-related CLD patients on this regimen suffered from Cu deficiency [90]. To the contrary, a lower intake of Zn was more effective than a moderately higher intake of Zn in inducing changes associated with a decreased Cu status in postmenopausal women [118].

The ratio of serum Cu to Zn levels has been utilized as a clinical assessment in certain diseases [119]. Among chronic liver diseases, elevated Cu/Zn ratios have been observed in patients with liver cirrhosis or HCC [33,34]. Therefore, the ratio of Cu/Zn can be monitored for estimating the severity of liver damage. However, the ratio cannot discriminate HCC patients from liver cirrhosis patients. It is of interest that elevation of the Cu/Zn ratio was observed in HCC patients alone among hepatobiliary cancer patients [107].

4.2. Zn and Iron

Zn also competes with iron. We previously showed a weakly inverse correlation between serum zinc and ferritin levels in patients with HCV-related chronic liver disease [17]. The inverse correlation between serum Zn and ferritin was also found in HCV-related CLD patients associated with NAFLD [109]. The putative mechanism is explained in the paragraph regarding "zinc deficiency and iron overload" in this review.

Interestingly, Zn supplementation caused an increased iron concentration in the duodenal mucosa of patients with Wilson's disease, although the mechanism of this change remains unclear [106]. Further examinations will be required to clarify this phenomenon in such patients.

4.3. Zn and Selenium

We previously revealed that serum selenium levels were positively associated with serum Zn levels in patients with HCV-related CLD [111]. We also confirmed a positive correlation between serum selenium and albumin levels in such patients. Therefore, selenium deficiency might result in hypoalbuminemia, and subsequently cause Zn deficiency in those patients. Likewise, Thuluvath and Triger found a positive correlation between serum zinc and selenium levels among patients with various chronic liver diseases, including alcoholic liver disease, primary biliary cholangitis, cryptogenic cirrhosis, chronic active autoimmune hepatitis [110].

It is of interest that the administration of selenium modulated serum Zn levels in diabetic rats fed a zinc-deficient diet [120].

4.4. Zn and Vitamin A

A previous study elucidated that significant correlations between serum Zn and vitamin A or retinol-binding protein (RBP) levels were found in patients with liver cirrhosis [112]. Zn deficiency seems to impair the synthesis of RBP [7,121,122]. Therefore, the authors speculated that Zn deficiency might result in portosystemic shunting, and subsequent vitamin A deficiency by decreasing the release of RBP in such patients [112].

4.5. Zn and Vitamin D

Serum 25-hydroxy vitamin D (25-OH vitamin D) levels are also decreased in proportion to the severity of hepatic fibrosis as well as serum Zn levels in patients with HCV-related CLD [123]. Surprisingly, no significant correlation was found between serum 25-OH vitamin D and Zn levels in such patients [114], although serum Zn levels were significantly associated with serum 25-OH vitamin D levels among women with primary ovarian insufficiency [113].

4.6. Zinc and Amino Acids

Moriyama and colleagues documented that there was not a significant correlation between serum Zn and BCAA levels in patients with HCV-related CLD, but that an inverse correlation between serum Zn and tyrosine levels did exist [51]. Therefore, an inverse correlation was found between serum zinc levels and the ratio of BCAA to tyrosine (BTR) in such patients.

Surprisingly, oral administration of BCAA granules caused a decrease in serum Zn levels of patients with liver cirrhosis [124]. The authors speculated that the protein synthesis was facilitated by the administration of BCAAs resulting in consumption of Zn, because Zn acts at multiple steps in amino acid- and insulin-regulated intracellular signaling pathways, including mTOR. It is of interest that the amount of urinary Zn secretion was related to the infusion of amino acid in patients who received parenteral nutrition [125]. Surprisingly, Zn bound to amino acids such as aspartate, cysteine and histidine showed the highest absorption concentration, followed by zinc chloride, sulfate and acetate, while zinc oxide showed the lowest bioavailability [116].

4.7. Zn and Hormones

It has been well established that Zn plays a fundamental role in the stability of IGF-1 transcripts [74]. Therefore, Zn deficiency eventually caused a decrease in the synthesis of IGF-1 in patients with HCV-related CLD [18]. Zn supplementation may increase the production of IGF-1 in the livers of patients with liver cirrhosis.

Zn seems to participate in modulating serum testosterone levels in normal men. Therefore, hypogonadism has been linked to Zn deficiency [126]. In contrast, Fuse and colleagues found a significant correlation between serum Zn and testosterone levels among infertile male patients [115]. Indeed, Zn supplementation facilitated the synthesis of testosterone in elderly men with marginal Zn deficiency [9].

5. Conclusions

This review complied overwhelming evidence that Zn deficiency is common in patients with chronic liver diseases such as chronic hepatitis and NASH, as well as liver cirrhosis. In such patients, Zn deficiency causes various types of metabolic abnormalities, including insulin resistance, hepatic steatosis, iron overload and hepatic encephalopathy. As expected, these metabolic abnormalities may be recovered by Zn supplementation. Further trials will be required to verify the beneficial effects of Zn administration on theses metabolic abnormalities especially in NASH patients.

Author Contributions: T.H. wrote the manuscript. T.M. made critical revision.

Conflicts of Interest: The authors have no conflicts of interest to declare.

References

1. Wessels, I.; Maywald, M.; Rink, L. Zinc as a gatekeeper of immune function. *Nutrients* **2017**, *9*, 1286. [CrossRef] [PubMed]
2. Vallee, B.L.; Falchuk, K.H. The biochemical basis of zinc physiology. *Physiol. Rev.* **1993**, *73*, 79–118. [CrossRef] [PubMed]
3. Powell, S.R. The antioxidant properties of zinc. *J. Nutr.* **2000**, *130*, S1447–S1454.
4. Leoni, G.; Rosato, A.; Perozzi, G. Zinc proteome interaction network as a model to identify nutrient-affected pathways in human pathologies. *Genes. Nutr.* **2014**, *9*, 436. [CrossRef] [PubMed]
5. Liuzzi, J.P.; Cousins, R.J. Mammalian zinc transporters. *Annu. Rev. Nutr.* **2004**, *24*, 151–172. [CrossRef] [PubMed]
6. Prasad, A.S. The role of zinc in gastrointestinal and liver disease. *Clin. Gastroenterol.* **1983**, *12*, 713–741. [PubMed]
7. Ritland, S.; Aaseth, J. Trace elements and liver. *J. Hepatol.* **1987**, *5*, 118–122. [CrossRef]
8. McClain, C.J.; Marsano, L.; Burk, R.F.; Bacon, B. Trace metals in liver disease. *Semin. Liver Dis.* **1991**, *11*, 321–339. [CrossRef] [PubMed]
9. Grüngreiff, K. Zinc in liver disease. *J. Trace Elem. Exp. Med.* **2002**, *15*, 67–78. [CrossRef]
10. Mohammad, M.K.; Zhou, Z.; Cave, M.; Barve, A.; McClain, C.J. Nutrition in clinical practice. *Nutr. Clin. Pract.* **2012**, *27*, 8–20. [CrossRef] [PubMed]
11. Grüngreiff, K.; Reinhold, D.; Wedemeyer, H. The role of zinc in liver cirrhosis. *Ann. Hepatol.* **2016**, *15*, 7–16. [CrossRef] [PubMed]
12. Goode, H.F.; Kelleher, J.; Walker, B.E. Relation between zinc status and hepatic functional reserve in patients with liver disease. *Gut* **1990**, *41*, 694–697. [CrossRef]
13. Schechter, P.J.; Giroux, E.L.; Schlienger, J.L.; Hoenig, V.; Sjoerdsma, A. Distribution of serum zinc between albumin and α^2 -macroglobulin in patients with decompensated hepatic cirrhosis. *Eur. J. Clin. Investig.* **1976**, *31*, 147–150. [CrossRef]
14. Kiilerich, S.; Christiansen, C. Distribution of serum zinc between albumin and α^2-macroglobulin in patients with different zinc metabolic disorders. *Clin. Chim. Acta* **1986**, *154*, 1–6. [CrossRef]
15. Karayalcin, S.; Arcasoy, A.; Uzunalimoglu, O. Zinc plasma levels after zinc tolerance test in nonalcoholic cirrhosis. *Dig. Dis. Sci.* **1988**, *33*, 1096–1102. [CrossRef] [PubMed]
16. McClain, C.J.; Antonow, D.R.; Cohen, D.A.; Shedlofsky, S.I. Zinc metabolism in alcoholic liver disease. *Alcohol. Clin. Exp. Res.* **1986**, *10*, 582–589. [CrossRef]
17. Grüngreiff, K.; Franke, D.; Lössner, B.; Abicht, K.; Kleine, F.D. Zinc deficiency-A factor in the pathogenesis of hepatic encephalopathy. *Z. Gastroenterol.* **1991**, *29*, 101–106.
18. Rabbani, P.; Prasad, A.S. Plasma ammonia and liver ornithine carbamyltransferase activity in deficient rats. *Am. J. Physiol.* **1978**, *235*, E203–E206. [PubMed]
19. Riggio, O.; Merli, M.; Capocaccia, L.; Cashera, M.; Zullo, A.; Pinto, G.; Gaudio, E.; Franchitto, A.; Spagnoli, R.; D'Aquilino, E.; et al. Zinc supplementation reduces blood ammonia and increases liver transcarbamylase activity in experimental cirrhosis. *Hepatology* **1992**, *16*, 785–789. [CrossRef] [PubMed]

20. Yoshida, Y.; Higashi, T.; Nouso, K.; Nakatsukasa, H.; Nakamura, S.I.; Watanabe, A. Effects of zinc deficiency/zinc supplementation on ammonia metabolism in patients with decompensated liver cirrhosis. *Acta Med. Okayama* **2001**, *55*, 349–355. [PubMed]

21. Grüngreiff, K.; Presser, H.J.; Franke, D.; Lössner, B.; Kleine, F.D. Correlations between zinc, amino acids and ammonia in liver cirrhosis. *Z. Gastroenteriol.* **1989**, *27*, 731–735.

22. El-Serag, H.B. Hepatocellular carcinoma. *N. Engl. J. Med.* **2011**, *365*, 1118–1127. [CrossRef] [PubMed]

23. Miatto, O.; Casaril, M.; Gabrielli, B.G.; et al. Diagnostic and prognostic value of serum copper and plasma fibrinogen in hepatic carcinoma. *Cancer* **1985**, *55*, 774–778. [CrossRef]

24. Pramoolsinsap, C.; Promvanit, N.; Komindr, S.; Lerdverasirikul, P.; Srianujata, S. Serum trace metals in chronic viral hepatitis and hepatocellular carcinoma in Thailand. *J. Gastroenterol.* **1994**, *29*, 610–615. [CrossRef] [PubMed]

25. Grussamy, K. Trace element concentration in primary liver cancers-a systematic review. *Biol. Trace Elem. Res.* **2007**, *118*, 191–206. [CrossRef] [PubMed]

26. Himoto, T.; Fujita, K.; Nomura, T.; Tani, J.; Miyoshi, H.; Morishita, A.; Yoneyaka, H.; Kubota, S.; Haba, R.; Suzuki, Y.; Masaki, T. Roles of hepatocarcinogenesis via the activation of hypoxia-inducible factor-1. *Biol. Trace Elem. Res.* **2016**, *174*, 58–64. [CrossRef] [PubMed]

27. Ebara, M.; Fukuda, H.; Hatano, R.; Saisho, H.; Nagato, Y.; Suzuki, K.; Nakajima, K.; Yukawa, M.; Kondo, F.; Nakayama, A.; Sakurai, H. Relationship between copper, zinc and metallothionein in hepatocellular carcinoma and its surrounding liver parenchyma. *J. Hepatol.* **2000**, *33*, 415–422. [CrossRef]

28. Maeda, T.; Shimada, M.; Harimoto, N.; Tsujita, E.; Maehara, S.; Rikimaru, T.; Tanaka, S.; Shirabe, K.; Maehara, Y. Role of tissue trace elements in liver cancers and non-cancerous liver parenchyma. *Hepatogastroenterology* **2005**, *52*, 187–190. [PubMed]

29. Franklin, R.B.; Costello, L.C. The important role of the apoptitic effects of zinc in the development of cancers. *J. Cell Biochem.* **2009**, *106*, 750–757. [CrossRef] [PubMed]

30. Nardinocci, L.; Pantisano, V.; Puca, R.; Porru, M.; Aiello, A.; Graselli, A.; Leonetti, C.; Safran, M.; Rechavi, G.; Givol, D.; et al. Zinc downregulates HIF-1 and inhibits its activity in tumor cells in vitro and in vivo. *PLoS ONE* **2010**, *13*, e15048.

31. Poo, J.L.; Rosas-Romero, R.; Montemayor, A.C.; Isoard, F.; Uribe, M. Diagnostic value of the copper/zinc ratio in hepatocellular carcinoma: A case control study. *J. Gastroenterol.* **2003**, *38*, 45–51. [CrossRef] [PubMed]

32. Lin, C.C.; Huang, J.F.; Tsai, L.Y.; Huang, Y.L. Selenium, iron, copper, and zinc levels and copper-to-zinc ratios in xserum of patients at different stages of viral hepatic diseases. *Biol. Trace Elem. Res.* **2006**, *109*, 15–23. [CrossRef]

33. Overbeck, S.; Rink, L.; Haase, H. Modulating the immune response by oral zinc supplemrentation: A single approach for multiple diseases. *Arch. Immunol. Ther. Exp.* **2008**, *56*, 15–30. [CrossRef] [PubMed]

34. Zhang, Y.; Chen, C.; Yao, Q.; Li, M. ZIP4 upregulates the expression of neuropilin-1, vascular endothelial growth factor, and matrix metalloproteases in pancreatic cancer cell lines and xenografts. *Cancer Biol. Ther.* **2010**, *9*, 234–242. [CrossRef]

35. Hogstrand, C.; Kille, P.; Nicholson, R.I.; Taylor, K.M. Zinc transporters and cancer: A potential role for ZIP7 as a hub for tyrosine kinase activation. *Trends Mol. Med.* **2009**, *15*, 101–111. [CrossRef] [PubMed]

36. Kagara, N.; Tanaka, N.; Noguchi, S.; Hirano, T. Zinc and its regulator ZIP10 are involved in invasive behavior of breast cancer cells. *Cancer Sci.* **2007**, *98*, 692–697. [CrossRef] [PubMed]

37. Franklin, R.B.; Levy, B.A.; Zou, J.; Hanna, N.; Desouki, M.M.; Bagasra, O.; Johnson, L.A.; Costello, L.C. ZIP14 zinc transporter downregulation and zinc depletion in the development and progression of hepatocellular cancer. *J. Gastroenterol. Cancer* **2012**, *43*, 249–257. [CrossRef] [PubMed]

38. Wang, F.D.; Kim, B.E.; Dufner-Beattie, J.; Petris, M.J.; Andrews, G.; Eide, D.J. Acrodermatitis enteropathica mutations affect transport activity, localization and zinc-responsiveness trafficking of the mouse ZIP4 zinc transporter. *Hum. Mol. Genet.* **2004**, *13*, 563–571. [CrossRef] [PubMed]

39. Weaver, B.P.; Zhang, Y.; Hiscox, S.; Guo, G.L.; Apte, U.; Taylor, K.M.; Sheline, C.T.; Wang, L.; Andrews, G.K. Zip4 (Slc39a4) expression is activated in hepatocellular carcinomas and functions to repress apoptosis, enhance cell cycle and increase migration. *PLoS ONE* **2010**, *5*, e13158. [CrossRef] [PubMed]

40. Xu, X.; Guo, H.J.; Xie, H.Y.; Li, J.; Zhung, R.Z.; Ling, Q.; Zhou, L.; Wei, X.Y.; Liu, Z.K.; Ding, S.M.; et al. ZIP4, a novel determinant of tumor invasion in hepatocellular carcinoma, contributes to tumor recurrence after liver transplantation. *Int. J. Biol. Sci.* **2014**, *10*, 235–256. [CrossRef] [PubMed]

41. Consolo, M.; Amoroso, A.; Spandidos, D.A.; Mazzarino, M.C. Matrix metalloproteinases and their inhibitors as markers of inflammation and fibrosis in chronic liver disease (Review). *Int. J. Mol. Med.* **2009**, *24*, 143–152. [PubMed]

42. Imai, K.; Beppu, T.; Yamao, T.; Okabe, H.; Hayashi, H.; Nitta, H.; Hashimoto, D.; Mima, K.; Nakagawa, S.; Sakamoto, K.; et al. Clinicopathological and prognostic significance of preoperative serum zinc status in patients with hepatocellular carcinoma after initial hepatectomy. *Ann. Surg. Oncol.* **2014**, *21*, 3817–3826. [CrossRef] [PubMed]

43. Thrift, A.P.; El-Serag, H.B.; Kanwal, F. Global epidemiology and burden of HCV infection and HCV-related disease. *Nat. Rev. Gastroenterol. Hepatol.* **2017**, *14*, 122–132. [CrossRef] [PubMed]

44. Okuda, M.; Li, K.; Beard, M.R.; Showalter, L.A.; Scholle, F.; Lemon, S.M.; Weinman, S.A. Mitochondrial injury, oxidative stress, and antioxidant gene expression are induced by hepatitis C virus core protein. *Gastroenterology* **2002**, *122*, 366–375. [CrossRef] [PubMed]

45. Negro, F.; Sanyal, A.J. Hepatitis C virus, steatosis and lipid abnormalities: Clinical and pathologic data. *Liver Int.* **2009**, *29*, 26–37. [CrossRef] [PubMed]

46. Kohgo, Y.; Ikuta, K.; Ohtake, T.; Torimoto, Y.; Kato, J. Iron overload and cofactors with special reference to alcohol, hepatitis C virus infection and steatosis/insulin resistance. *World J. Gastroenterol.* **2007**, *13*, 4699–4706. [CrossRef] [PubMed]

47. Prasad, A.S.; Boa, B.; Beck, F.W.; Kucuk, O.; Sarkar, F.H. Antioxidant effects of zinc in human. *Free Radic. Biol. Med.* **2004**, *37*, 1182–1190. [CrossRef] [PubMed]

48. Ko, W.S.; Guo, C.H.; Yeh, M.S.; Lin, L.Y.; Hsu, G.S.; Chen, P.C.; Luo, M.C.; Lin, C.Y. Blood micronutrient, oxidative stress, and viral load in patients with chronic hepatitis C. *World J. Gastroenterol.* **2005**, *11*, 4697–4702. [CrossRef] [PubMed]

49. Moriyama, M.; Matsumura, H.; Fukushima, A.; Ohkido, K.; Arakawa, Y.; Nirei, K.; Aoki, H.; Yamagami, H.; Kaneko, M.; Tanaka, N.; Arakawa, Y. Clinical significance of evaluation of serum zinc concentrations in C-virus chronic liver disease. *Dig. Dis. Sci.* **2006**, *51*, 1967–1977. [CrossRef] [PubMed]

50. Stempniak, M.; Hostomska, Z.; Nodes, B.R.; Hostomsky, Z. The NS3 proteinase domain of hepatitis C virus is a zinc-containing enzyme. *J. Virol.* **1997**, *71*, 2881–2886. [PubMed]

51. Tellinghuisen, T.L.; Marcotrigiano, J.; Gorbalenya, A.E.; Rice, C.M. The NS5A protein of hepatitis C virus is a zinc metalloprotein. *J. Biol. Chem.* **2004**, *279*, 48576–48587. [CrossRef] [PubMed]

52. Chalasani, N.; Younossi, Z.; Lavine, J.E.; Diehl, A.M.; Brunt, E.M.; Cusi, K.; Charlton, M.; Sanyal, A.J. The diagnosis and management of non-alcoholic fatty liver disease: Practice guideline by the American association for the study of liver diseases, American College of Gastroenterology, and the American Gastroenterological Association. *Hepatology* **2012**, *55*, 2005–2023. [CrossRef] [PubMed]

53. Zolfaghari, H.; Askari, G.; Siassi, F.; Feizi, A.; Sotoudeh, G. Intake of nutrients, fiber, and sugar in patients with nonalcoholic fatty liver disease in comparison to healthy individuals. *Int. J. Prev. Med.* **2016**, *7*, 98. [PubMed]

54. Toshimitsu, K.; Matsuura, B.; Ohkubo, I.; Niiya, T.; Furukawa, S.; Hiasa, Y.; Kawamura, M.; Ebihara, K.; Onji, M. Dietary habits and nutrient intake in non-alcoholic steatohepatitis. *Nutrition* **2007**, *23*, 46–52. [CrossRef] [PubMed]

55. Malhi, H.; Kaufman, R.J. Endoplasmic reticulum stress in liver disease. *J. Hepatol.* **2011**, *54*, 795–809. [CrossRef] [PubMed]

56. Kim, M.H.; Aydemir, T.B.; Cousins, R.J. Dietary zinc regulates apoptosis through the phosphorylated eukaryotic initiation factor 2α/activating transcription factor-4/C/EBP-homologous protein pathway during pharmacologically induced endoplasmic reticulum stress in livers of mice. *J. Nutr.* **2016**, *146*, 2180–2186. [CrossRef] [PubMed]

57. Kim, M.H.; Aydemir, T.B.; Kim, J.; Cousins, R.J. Hepatic ZIP14-mediated zinc transport is required for adaptation to endoplasmic reticulum stress. *Proc. Natl. Acad. Sci. USA* **2017**, *114*, E5805–E5814. [CrossRef] [PubMed]

58. Sakurai, H.; Adachi, Y. The pharmacology of the insulinomimetic effect of zinc complexes. *Biometals* **2005**, *18*, 319–323. [CrossRef] [PubMed]

59. Walter, R.M., Jr.; Uriu-Hare, J.Y.; Olin, K.L.; Oster, M.H.; Anawalt, B.D.; Critchfield, J.W.; Keen, K.L. Copper, zinc, manganese, and magnesium status and complications of diabetes mellitus. *Diabetes Care* **1991**, *14*, 1050–1056. [CrossRef] [PubMed]

60. Allison, M.E.; Wreghitt, T.; Palmer, C.R.; Alexander, G.J. Evidence for a link between hepatitis C virus infection and diabetes mellitus in a cirrhotic population. *J. Hepatol.* **1994**, *21*, 1135–1139. [CrossRef]

61. Himoto, T.; Yoneyama, H.; Deguchi, A.; Kurokohchi, K.; Inukai, M.; Masugata, H.; Goda, F.; Senda, S.; Haba, R.; Watanabe, S.; Kubota, S.; Kuriyama, S.; Masaki, T. Insulin resistance derived from zinc deficiency in non-diabetic patients with chronic hepatitis C. *Exp. Ther. Med.* **2010**, *1*, 707–711. [CrossRef] [PubMed]

62. Himoto, T.; Nomura, T.; Tani, J.; Miyoshi, H.; Morishita, A.; Yoneyama, H.; Haba, R.; Masugata, H.; Masaki, T. Exacerbation of insulin resistance and hepatic steatosis deriving from zinc deficiency in patients with HCV-related chronic liver disease. *Biol. Trace. Elem. Res.* **2015**, *163*, 81–88. [CrossRef] [PubMed]

63. Rajaram, S.; Baylink, D.J.; Mohan, S. Insulin-like growth factor-binding proteins in serum and other biological fluids: Regulation and functions. *Endocr. Rev.* **1997**, *18*, 801–831. [CrossRef] [PubMed]

64. Himoto, T.; Tani, J.; Miyoshi, H.; Yoneyama, H.; Mori, H.; Inukai, M.; Masugata, H.; Goda, F.; Senda, S.; Haba, R.; Masaki, T. The ratio of insulin-like growth factor-I/insulin-like growth factor-binding protein-3 in sera of patients with chronic hepatitis C virus-related chronic liver disease as a predictive marker of insulin resistance. *Nutr. Res.* **2013**, *33*, 27–33. [CrossRef] [PubMed]

65. Ichikawa, T.; Nakao, K.; Hamasaki, K.; Furukawa, R.; Tsuruta, S.; Ueda, Y.; Taura, N.; Shibata, H.; fujimoto, M.; Toriyama, K.; Eguchi, K. Role of growth hormone, insulin-like growth factor 1 and insulin-like growth factor-binding protein 3 in development of non-alcoholic fatty liver disease. *Hepatol. Int.* **2007**, *1*, 287–294. [CrossRef] [PubMed]

66. European Association for the Study of the Liver. EASL clinical practice guideline: The diagnosis and management of patients with primary biliary cholangitis. *J. Hepatol.* **2017**, *67*, 145–172.

67. Himoto, T.; Yoneyama, H.; Kurokochi, K.; Inukai, M.; Masugata, H.; Goda, F.; Haba, R.; Watanabe, S.; Senda, S.; Masaki, T. Contribution of zinc deficiency to insulin resistance in patients with primary biliary cirrhosis. *Biol. Trace Elem. Res.* **2011**, *144*, 133–142. [CrossRef] [PubMed]

68. Formigari, A.; Santon, A.; Irato, P. Efficacy of zinc treatment against iron-induced toxicity in rat hepatoma cell line H4-II-E-C3. *Liver Int.* **2007**, *27*, 120–127. [CrossRef] [PubMed]

69. Liuzzi, J.P.; Aydemir, F.; Nam, H. Zip14 (Slc39a14) mediates non-transferrin-bound iron uptake into cells. *Proc. Natl. Acad. Sci. USA* **2006**, *103*, 13612–13617. [CrossRef] [PubMed]

70. Fernandez-Real, J.M.; Lopes-Bermejo, A.; Ricart, W. Cross-talk between iron metabolism and diabetes. *Diabetes* **2002**, *51*, 2348–2354. [CrossRef] [PubMed]

71. Mendler, M.H.; Turlin, B.; Moirand, R. Insulin resistance-associated hepatic iron overload. *Gastroenterology* **1999**, *117*, 1155–1163. [CrossRef]

72. Farinati, F.; Cardin, R.; De Maria, N.; Lecis, P.E.; Della Libera, G.; Burra, P.; Marafin, C.; Stumiolo, G.C.; Naccarato, R. Iron storage, lipid peroxidation and glutathione turn over in chronic anti-HCV positive hepatitis. *J. Hepatol.* **1995**, *22*, 449–456. [CrossRef]

73. Conover, C.A. Potentiation of insulin-like growth factor (IGF) action by IGF-binding protein-3: Studies of underlying mechanism. *Endocrinology* **1992**, *130*, 3191–3199. [CrossRef] [PubMed]

74. McNall, A.D.; Etherton, T.D.; Fosmire, G.J. The impaired growth induced by zinc deficiency in rat is associated with decreased expression of the hepatic insulin-like growth factor I and growth hormone receptor genes. *J. Nutr.* **1995**, *125*, 874–879. [PubMed]

75. Mikhail, T.H.; Nicola, W.G.; Ibrahim, K.H.; Salama, S.H.; Eman, M. Abnormal zinc and copper metabolism in hepatic steatosis. *Boll. Chim. Farm.* **1996**, *135*, 591–597. [PubMed]

76. Bao, B.; Prasad, A.S.; Beck, F.W.; Fitzgerald, J.T.; Snell, D.; Bao, G.W.; Singh, T.; Cardozo, L.J. Zinc decreases C-reactive protein, lipid peroxidation, and inflammatory cytokines in elderly subjects: A potential implication of zinc as an atheroprotective agent. *Am. J. Clin. Nutr.* **2010**, *91*, 1634–1641. [CrossRef] [PubMed]

77. Runchery, S.S.; Boyko, E.J.; Ioannou, G.N.; Ultzschneider, K.M. The relationship between serum circulating IGF-1 and liver fat in the United States. *J. Gasroenterol. Hepatol.* **2014**, *29*, 589–596. [CrossRef]

78. Lalioti, V.; Sandoval, I.; Cassio, D.; Duclos-Vallee, J.C. Molecular pathology of Wilson's disease: A brief. *J. Hepatol.* **2010**, *53*, 1151–1153. [CrossRef] [PubMed]

79. Ferenci, P. Wioson's disease. *Ital. J. Gastroenterol. Hepatol.* **1999**, *31*, 416–425. [PubMed]

80. Pietrangelo, A. Hereditary hemochromatosis: Pathogenesis, diagnosis, and treatment. *Gastroenterology* **2010**, *139*, 393–408. [CrossRef] [PubMed]

81. Vayenas, D.V.; Repanti, M.; Vassilopoulos, A.; Papanastasiou, D.A. Influence of iron overload on manganese, zinc, and copper concentration in rat tissues in vivo: Study of liver, spleen, and brain. *Int. J. Clin. Lab. Res.* **1998**, *28*, 183–186. [CrossRef] [PubMed]

82. Adams, P.C.; Bradley, C.; Frei, J.V. Hepatic zinc in hemochromatosis. *Clin. Invest. Med.* **1991**, *14*, 16–20. [PubMed]

83. Beckett, J.M.; Ball, M.J. Effect of hereditary haemochromatosis genotypes and iron overload on other trace elements. *Eur. J. Nutr.* **2013**, *52*, 255–261. [CrossRef] [PubMed]

84. Himoto, T.; Hosomi, N.; Nakai, S.; Deguchi, A.; KInekawa, F.; Matsuki, M.; Yachida, M.; Masaki, T.; Kurokochi, K.; Watanabe, S.; et al. Efficacy of zinc administration in patients with hepatitis C virus-related chronic liver disease. *Scand. J. Gastroenterol.* **2007**, *42*, 1078–1087.

85. Takagi, H.; Nagamine, T.; Abe, T.; Takayama, H.; Sato, K.; Otsuka, T.; Kakizaki, S.; Hashimoto, Y.; Matsumoto, T.; Kojima, A.; et al. Zinc supplementation enhances the response to interferon therapy in patients with chronic hepatitis C. *J. Viral. Hepat.* **2001**, *8*, 367–371. [CrossRef] [PubMed]

86. Murakami, Y.; Koyabu, T.; Kawashima, A.; Kakibuchi, N.; Kawakami, T.; Takaguchi, K.; Kita, K.; Okita, M. Zinc supplementation prevents the increase of transaminase in chronic hepatitis C patients during combination therapy with pegylated interferon α -2b and ribavirin. *J. Nutr. Sci. Vitaminol.* **2007**, *53*, 213–218. [CrossRef] [PubMed]

87. Yoshikawa, Y.; Adachi, Y.; Sakurai, H. A new type of orally active anti-diabetic Zn (II)-dithiocarbamate complex. *Life. Sci.* **2007**, *80*, 759–766. [CrossRef] [PubMed]

88. Jayawardena, R.; Ranasinghe, P.; Galappatthy, P.; Malkanthi, R.; Constantine, G.; Katulanda, P. Effects of zinc supplementation on diabetes mellitus: a systematic review and meta-analysis. *Diabetol. Metab. Syndr.* **2012**, *4*, 13. [CrossRef] [PubMed]

89. Marchesini, G.; Bugianesi, E.; Ronchi, M.; Flamia, R.; Thomaseth, K.; Pacini, G. Zinc supplementation improves glucose disposal in patients with cirrhosis. *Metabolism* **1998**, *47*, 792–798. [CrossRef]

90. Sugino, H.; Kumagai, N.; Watanabe, S.; Toda, K.; Takeuchi, O.; Tsunematsu, S.; Morinaga, S.; Tsuchimoto, K. Polaprezinc attenuates liver fibrosis in a mouse model of non-alcoholic steatohepatitis. *J. Gastroenterol. Hepatol.* **2008**, *23*, 1909–1916. [CrossRef] [PubMed]

91. Kang, X.; Zhong, W.; Liu, J.; Song, Z.; McClain, C.J.; Kang, Y.J.; Zhou, Z. Zinc supplementation reverses alcohol-induced steatosis in mice through reactivating hepatocyte nuclear factor-4α and peroxisome proliferator-activated receptor-α. *Hepatology* **2009**, *50*, 1241–1250. [CrossRef] [PubMed]

92. Cave, M.; Deaciuc, I.; Mendez, C.; Sing, Z.; Joshi-Barve, S.; Barve, S.; McClain, C. Nonalcoholic fatty liver disease: Predisposing factors and the role of nutrition. *J. Nutr. Biochem.* **2007**, *18*, 184–195. [CrossRef] [PubMed]

93. Reding, P.; Duchateau, J.; Bataille, C. Oral zinc supplementation improves hepatic encephalopathy. Results of randomized controlled trial. *Lancet* **1984**, *2*, 493–495. [CrossRef]

94. Marchesini, G.; Fabri, A.; Bianchi, G.; Brizi, M.; Zoil, M. Zinc supplementation and amino acid-nitrogen metabolism in patients with advanced cirrhosis. *Hepatology* **1996**, *23*, 1084–1092. [CrossRef] [PubMed]

95. Grüngreiff, K.; Grüngreiff, S.; Reinhold, D. Zinc deficiency and hepatic encephalopathy: Results of a long-term follow-up on zinc supplementation. *J. Trace. Elem. Exp. Med.* **2000**, *13*, 21–31. [CrossRef]

96. Takuma, Y.; Nouso, K.; Makino, Y.; Hayashi, M.; Takahashi, H. Clinical trial: Oral zinc in hepatic encephalopathy. *Aliment. Pharmacol. Ther.* **2010**, *32*, 1080–1090. [CrossRef] [PubMed]

97. Katayama, K.; Saito, M.; Kawaguchi, T.; Endo, R.; Sawara, K.; Nishiguchi, S.; Kato, A.; Kohgo, H.; Suzuki, K.; Sakaida, I.; et al. Effect of zinc on liver cirrhosis with hyperammonia: A preliminary randomized, placebo-controlled double-blinded trial. *Nutrition* **2014**, *30*, 1409–1414. [CrossRef] [PubMed]

98. Kawaguchi, T.; Taniguchi, E.; Sata, M. Effects of oral branched-chain amino acids on hepatic encephalopathy and outcome in patients with liver cirrhosis. *Nutr. Clin. Pract.* **2013**, *28*, 580–588. [CrossRef] [PubMed]

99. Hayashi, M.; Ohnishi, H.; Kawade, Y.; Muto, Y.; Takahashi, Y. Augmented utilization of branched-chain amino acids by skeletal muscle in decompensated liver cirrhosis in special relation to ammonia detoxication. *Gastroenterol. Jpn.* **1981**, *16*, 64–70.

100. Matsumura, H.; Nirei, K.; Nakamura, H.; Arakawa, Y.; Higuchi, T.; Hayashi, J.; Yamagami, H.; Matsuoka, S.; Ogawa, M.; Nakajima, N.; et al. Zinc supplementation therapy improves the outcome of patients with chronic hepatitis C. *J. Clin. Biochem. Nutr.* **2012**, *51*, 178–184. [PubMed]

101. El-Serag, H.B.; Tran, T.; Everhart, J.E. Diabetes increases the risk of chronic liver disease and hepatocellular carcinoma. *Gastroenterology* **2004**, *126*, 460–468. [CrossRef] [PubMed]
102. Kawaguchi, T.; Sata, M. Importance of hepatitis C virus-associated insulin resistance: Therapeutic strategies for insulin sensitization. *World J. Gastroenterol.* **2010**, *16*, 1943–1952. [CrossRef] [PubMed]
103. Mulder, T.P.; Janssens, A.R.; Verspaget, H.W.; van Hattum, J.; Lamers, C.B. Metallothionein concentration in the liver of patients with Wilson's disease, primary biliary cirrhosis, and liver metastasis of colorectal cancer. *J. Hepatol.* **1992**, *16*, 346–350. [CrossRef]
104. Brewer, G.J.; Yuzbasiyan-Gurkan, V.; Lee, D.Y.; Appelman, H. Treatment of Wilson's disease with zinc. VI. Initial treatment studies. *J. Lab. Clin. Med.* **1989**, *114*, 633–638. [PubMed]
105. Sturniolo, G.C.; Mestriner, C.; Irato, P.; Albergoni, V.; Longo, G.; D'Inca, R. Zinc therapy increases duodenal concentrations of metallothionein and iron in Wilson's disease patients. *Am. J. Gastroenterol.* **1999**, *94*, 334–338. [CrossRef] [PubMed]
106. Shimizu, N.; Fujuwara, J.; Ohnishi, S.; Sato, M.; Kodama, H.; Kohsaka, T.; Inui, A.; Fujisawa, T.; Tamai, H.; Ida, S.; et al. Effects of long-term zinc treatment in Japanese patients with Wilson disease: Efficacy, stability, and copper metabolism. *Trans. Res.* **2010**, *156*, 350–357. [CrossRef] [PubMed]
107. Duncan, A.; Yacoubian, C.; Watson, N.; Morrison, I. The risk copper deficiency in patients prescribed zinc supplementation. *J. Clin. Pathol.* **2015**, *68*, 723–725. [CrossRef] [PubMed]
108. Gammoh, N.Z.; Rink, L. Zinc in infection and inflammation. *Nutrients* **2017**, *9*, 624. [CrossRef] [PubMed]
109. Hartman, H.J. Copper-thionein from fetal bovine liver. Biochim. *Biophys. Acta.* **1977**, *491*, 211–222.
110. Milne, D.B.; Davis, C.D.; Nielsen, F.H. Low dietary zinc alters indices of copper function and status in postmenopausal women. *Nutrition* **2001**, *17*, 701–708. [CrossRef]
111. Garafalo, J.A.; Ashiraki, H.; Menendez-Botet, C.; Cunningham-Rundles, S.; Schwartz, M.K.; Good, R.A. Serum zinc, copper, and the copper/zinc ratio in patients with benign and malignant breast lesions. *Cancer* **1980**, *46*, 2682–2685. [CrossRef]
112. Stepien, M.; Hughes, D.J.; Hybsier, S.; Bamia, C.; Tjønneland, A.; Overvad, K.; Affret, A.; His, M.; Boutron-Ruault, M.C.; Katzke, V.; et al. Circulating copper and zinc levels and risk of hepatobiliary cancers in Europeans. *Br. J. Cancer* **2017**, *116*, 688–696. [CrossRef] [PubMed]
113. Guo, C.H.; Chen, P.C.; Ko, W.S. Status of essential trace minerals and oxidative stress in viral hepatitis C patients with nonalcoholic fatty liver disease. *Int. J. Med.Sci.* **2013**, *10*, 730–737. [CrossRef] [PubMed]
114. Himoto, T.; Yoneyama, H.; Kurokohchi, K.; Inukai, M.; Masugata, H.; Goda, F.; Haba, R.; Watanabe, S.; Kubota, S.; Senda, T.; et al. Selenium deficiency is associated with insulin resistance in patients with hepatitis C virus-related chronic liver disease. *Nutr. Res.* **2011**, *31*, 829–835. [CrossRef] [PubMed]
115. Thuluvath, P.J.; Triger, D.R. Selenium in chronic liver disease. *J. Hepatol.* **1992**, *14*, 176–182. [CrossRef]
116. Fatmi, W.; Kechrid, Z.; Naziroglu, M.; Flores-Arce, M. Selenium supplementation modulates zinc levels and antioxidant values in blood and tissues of diabetic rats fed zinc-deficient diet. *Biol. Trace. Elem. Res.* **2013**, *152*, 243–250. [CrossRef] [PubMed]
117. Schölmerich, J.; Becher, M.S.; Köttgen, E.; Rauch, N.; Haussinger, D.; Löhle, E.; Vulleumier, J.P.; Gerok, W. The influence of portosystemic shunting on zinc and vitamin A metabolism in liver cirrhosis. *Hepatogastroenterology* **1983**, *30*, 143–147. [PubMed]
118. Smith, J.C., Jr. The vitamin A-zinc connection: A review. *Ann. N.Y. Acad. Sci.* **1980**, *355*, 62–75. [CrossRef]
119. Solomons, N.W.; Russell, R.M. The interaction of vitamin A and zinc: Implications for human nutrition. *Am. J. Clin. Nutr.* **1980**, *33*, 2031–2040. [PubMed]
120. Petta, S.; Camma, C.; Scazzone, C.; Tripodo, C.; Di Marco, V.; Bono, A.; Cabibi, D.; Licata, G.; Porcasi, R.; Marchesini, G. Low vitamin D serum level is related to severe fibrosis and low responsiveness to interferon-based therapy in genotype 1 chronic hepatitis C. *Hepatology* **2010**, *51*, 1158–1167. [CrossRef] [PubMed]
121. Reda, R.; Abbas, A.A.; Mohammed, M.; El Fedawy, S.F.; Ghareeb, H.; El Kabarity, R.H.; Abo-Shady, R.A.; Zakaria, D. The interplay between zinc, vitamin D and, IL-17 in patients with chronic hepatitis C liver disease. *J Immunol. Res.* **2015**, *2015*, 846348. [CrossRef] [PubMed]
122. Kebapcilar, A.G.; Kulaksizoglu, M.; Kebapcilar, L.; Gonen, M.S.; Unlü, A.; Topcu, A.; Demirci, F.; Taner, C.E. Is there a link between premature ovarian failure and serum concentration of vitamin D, zinc, and copper? *Menopause* **2013**, *20*, 94–99. [CrossRef] [PubMed]

123. Fukushima, H.; Miwa, Y.; Shiraki, M.; Gomi, I.; Toda, K.; Kuriyama, S.; Nakamura, H.; Wakahara, H.; Era, S.; Moriwaki, H. Oral branched-chain amino acid supplementation improves the oxidized/reduced albumin ratio in patients with liver cirrhosis. *Hepatol. Res.* **2007**, *37*, 765–770. [CrossRef] [PubMed]

124. Faure, H.; Leverve, X.; Amaud, J.; Boujet, C.; Favier, A. Zinc changes in blood and urine during cyclic parenteral nutrition: Relationships with amino acid metabolism. *Br. J. Nutr.* **1994**, *72*, 763–773. [CrossRef] [PubMed]

125. Prasad, A.S. Impact of the discovery of human zinc deficiency on health. *J. Am. Coll. Nutr.* **2009**, *28*, 257–265. [CrossRef] [PubMed]

126. Fuse, H.; Kazama, T.; Ohta, S.; Fujiuchi, Y. Relationship between zinc concentrations in seminal plasma and various sperm parameters. *Int. Urol. Nephrol.* **1999**, *31*, 401–408. [CrossRef] [PubMed]

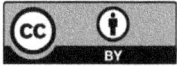

Article

Assessment of Validity and Reproducibility of the Zinc-Specific Dietary Intake Questionnaire Conducted for Young Polish Female Respondents

Dominika Głąbska [1,*], Aleksandra Staniec [1] and Dominika Guzek [2]

[1] Department of Dietetics, Faculty of Human Nutrition and Consumer Sciences, Warsaw University of Life Sciences (WULS-SGGW), 159c Nowoursynowska Str., 02-776 Warsaw, Poland; aleksandra_staniec@sggw.pl

[2] Department of Organization and Consumption Economics, Faculty of Human Nutrition and Consumer Sciences, Warsaw University of Life Sciences (WULS-SGGW), 159c Nowoursynowska Str., 02-776 Warsaw, Poland; dominika_guzek@sggw.pl

* Correspondence: dominika_glabska@sggw.pl; Tel.: +48-22-593-71-26

Received: 15 December 2017; Accepted: 17 January 2018; Published: 19 January 2018

Abstract: One of the brief methods enabling the assessment of the zinc intake and identification of individuals characterized by insufficient zinc intake, is zinc-specific food frequency questionnaire. The aim of the study was to assess the validity and reproducibility of the elaborated zinc-specific food frequency questionnaire ZINC-FFQ (Zinc INtake Calculation—Food Frequency Questionnaire) in a group of young Polish female respondents. The validity was assessed in comparison with 3-day dietary records, while reproducibility was assessed for the ZINC-FFQ filled in twice (FFQ1 and FFQ2—six weeks apart). Bland–Altman indexes in the assessment of validity were 5.5% (FFQ1) and 6.7% (FFQ2), while in assessment of reproducibility it was 3.3%. In the assessment of reproducibility, 83% of respondents were classified into the same category of zinc intake adequacy and 72% of respondents were classified into the same tertile, that contributed to weighted κ statistic of 0.65 (substantial agreement). It may be concluded, that ZINC-FFQ is characterized by a validity on a satisfactory and reproducibility on a very good level, in a group of young Polish female respondents, and may be applied to indicate individuals characterized by the risk of insufficient intake.

Keywords: zinc; validation study; ZINC-FFQ; food frequency questionnaire; validity; reproducibility

1. Introduction

In spite of the fact that severe zinc deficiency is rare, according to the World Health Organization (WHO) [1], mild-to-moderate zinc deficiency is commonly stated throughout the world. Each third individual of the world population is affected by its deficiency of various severities, while in some regions the frequency is even 73% [2]. Each year, in the global population of children under five years of age, zinc deficiency results in about 800 thousand of deaths, that are attributed to diarrhea, pneumonia and malaria [3], as zinc intake reduces related mortality [4].

The zinc delivered during pregnancy results in fetal accumulation and newborn zinc status, as well as zinc intake during lactation results in child zinc status, that was proven in the systematic review and meta-analysis of Petry et al. [5] for low-dose of supplementation. Taking it into account, it must be indicated, that for zinc status in children, the maternal zinc intake, both from diet and supplementation, may be crucial. In the systematic review of Chaffee and King [6], it was indicated, that zinc supplementation in pregnant women may contribute to the reduced risk of the preterm birth, but the currently available information does not support the routine use of zinc supplementation during pregnancy [7], unless emergency supplementation in the low-income countries is needed [8].

Despite the fact, that on the basis of the food supply, it is estimated, that zinc deficiency risk is decreasing [9], the prevalence rate of inadequate zinc intake for general population of Central and

Eastern Europe is still 10% [10]. It indicates the need for appropriate interventions, that should be implemented both in the developing and developed countries, in groups of young women characterized by the risk of zinc deficiency [11].

The pregnant and lactating women zinc requirement is associated with the amount of zinc retained in newly accrued tissues and the zinc secreted in breast milk [12], but the education should include both pregnant or lactating women, and those in preconception period, in order to prevent the deficiency during pregnancy. Among the methods of intervention allowing to educate and change the nutrient intake, are food frequency questionnaires [13]. However, due to the lack of the available validated brief questionnaires enabling rapid assessment of the zinc intake in European countries, there is a need to elaborate and validate such questionnaire.

The aim of the study was to assess the validity and reproducibility of the elaborated zinc-specific food frequency questionnaire ZINC-FFQ (Zinc INtake Calculation—Food Frequency Questionnaire) in a group of young Polish female respondents.

2. Materials and Methods

The study was approved by the Bioethical Commission of the National Food and Nutrition Institute in Warsaw (No. 0701/2015), while it was conducted in compliance with the guideline statements of the Declaration of Helsinki.

2.1. Designing the ZINC-FFQ

The designed ZINC-FFQ included products being sources of zinc (content of 0.01 mg per 100 g or higher [14]), while other products were not included, due to the fact, that it was to be a brief questionnaire to estimate the zinc intake, but not the intake of the other nutrients. All food products included in the designed questionnaire were clustered into 13 groups and 46 food product items, while the typical serving sizes were presented in grams and described [15], as the same approach was applied as in the previous studies [16–18]. To not influence the answers of respondents, the elaborated ZINC-FFQ (Table 1) did not contain the zinc content information that was presented only in the questionnaire calculation key (Table 2).

Table 1. The designed ZINC-food frequency questionnaire (FFQ).

Group of Products	Products	Serving Size	Number of Servings Per Week *
Meat and offals	Pork	100 g (palm of small hand)	
	Poultry		
	Beef		
	Veal		
	Lamb		
	Veal liver		
	Pork and beef liver		
	Other offals		
Cold cuts	Poultry cold cuts	15 g (thin slice of ham, 3 slices of sausage, 1/3 of wiener)	
	Dry sausages		
	Ham, loin, gammon, other sausages		
	Wieners, spam, pate		

Table 1. *Cont.*

Group of Products	Products	Serving Size	Number of Servings Per Week *
Eggs		50 g (1 egg)	
Fish and fish products	Eel, herring, sardine	100 g (palm of small hand)	
	Other fish		
	Fish products from herrings, sprats, sardines	50 g (3 sprats, 1 rollmop)	
	Other fish products	50 g (half of a small can of tuna)	
Milk, dairy beverages, cream		300 g (large glass)	
Cheeses	Emmenthaler, gouda, cheddar, tilsiter, trappist, smoked cheeses	20 g (thin slice)	
	Parmesan, camembert, Roquefort, brie, edam cheese		
	Cottage cheese, curd cheese	30 g (thin slice, tablespoon)	
	Fromage frais, dairy desserts	150 g (packaging)	
	Feta, processed cheese	25 g (slice, triangle serving)	
Breads	Wholemeal, dark breads, breads with grains, graham, pumpernickel bread	30 g (slice, half of a roll)	
	White bread, wheat bread, baguette, rolls, toast bread, confectionery bread		
	Crispbread	10 g (1 slice)	
Other cereal products	Pasta	100 g of cooked (1 glass)	
	Rice		
	Buckwheat, millet		
	Other groats		
	Corn flakes	10 g (1 tablespoon)	
	Other cereals		
	Wheat bran	5 g (tablespoon)	
	Wheat germ		
	Graham flour	10 g (1 tablespoon)	
	Other flours		
Fruits		100 g (half of a glass)	
Vegetables	Legumes	100 g (1 glass of leafy vegetables, half of a glass of the other)	
	Other vegetables		
Potatoes		50 g (2 tablespoons of puree)	
Nuts and seeds	Pumpkin and flax seeds	30 g (handful)	
	Pistachios, coconuts, coconut shreds		
	Other nuts and seeds		
Chocolate products	Cocoa	10 g (1 tablespoon)	
	Plain chocolate	20 g (3–4 chocolate bar squares)	
	Other chocolates and chocolate bars		

* Column to be completed by the respondent. ZINC = Zinc INtake Calculation; FFQ = Food Frequency Questionnaire.

Table 2. The designed ZINC-FFQ calculation key.

Group of Products	Products	Serving Size	Zinc Content (mg)
Meat and offals	Pork	100 g (palm of small hand)	2.54
	Poultry		1.68
	Beef		3.24
	Veal		2.44
	Lamb		3.09
	Veal liver		8.40
	Pork and beef liver		8.31
	Other offals		2.27
Cold cuts	Poultry cold cuts	15 g (thin slice of ham, 3 slices of sausage, 1/3 of wiener)	0.18
	Dry sausages		0.49
	Ham, loin, gammon, other sausages		0.32
	Wieners, spam, pate		0.21
Eggs		50 g (1 egg)	0.88
Fish and fish products	Eel, herring, sardine	100 g (palm of small hand)	1.12
	Other fish		0.54
	Fish products from herrings, sprats, sardines	50 g (3 sprats, 1 rollmop)	0.62
	Other fish products	50 g (half of a small can of tuna)	0.28
Milk, dairy beverages, cream		300 g (large glass)	1.05
Cheeses	Emmenthaler, gouda, cheddar, tilsiter, trappist, smoked cheeses	20 g (thin slice)	0.77
	Parmesan, camembert, Roquefort, brie, edam cheese		0.52
	Cottage cheese, curd cheese	30 g (thin slice, tablespoon)	0.30
	Fromage frais, dairy desserts	150 g (packaging)	0.92
	Feta, processed cheese	25 g (slice, triangle serving)	0.50
Breads	Wholemeal, dark breads, breads with grains, graham, pumpernickel bread	30 g (slice, half of a roll)	0.66
	White bread, wheat bread, baguette, rolls, toast bread, confectionery bread		0.31
	Crispbread	10 g (1 slice)	0.41
Other cereal products	Pasta	100 g of cooked (1 glass)	0.89
	Rice		1.21
	Buckwheat, millet		3.45
	Other groats		0.90
	Corn flakes	10 g (1 tablespoon)	0.01
	Other cereals		0.13
	Wheat bran	5 g (tablespoon)	0.44
	Wheat germ		0.75
	Graham flour	10 g (1 tablespoon)	0.33
	Other flours		0.08

Table 2. *Cont.*

Group of Products	Products	Serving Size	Zinc Content (mg)
Fruits		100 g (half of a glass)	0.17
Vegetables	Legumes	100 g (1 glass of leafy vegetables, half of a glass of the other)	1.61
	Other vegetables		0.45
Potatoes		50 g (2 tablespoons of puree)	0.17
Nuts and seeds	Pumpkin and flax seeds	30 g (handful)	2.29
	Pistachios, coconuts, coconut shreds		0.27
	Other nuts and seeds		0.87
Chocolate products	Cocoa	10 g (1 tablespoon)	0.66
	Plain chocolate	20 g (3–4 chocolate bar squares)	0.43
	Other chocolates and chocolate bars		0.22

ZINC-FFQ = Zinc INtake Calculation—Food Frequency Questionnaire.

In the ZINC-FFQ, respondents were asked about the number of servings of food items consumed typically during a week, while both products consumed separately and as an element of the recipe of dishes were to be included and decimal parts were allowed. The same approach to calculate the typical daily zinc intake was applied as in the previous questionnaires [16–18].

2.2. The ZINC-FFQ Validation Procedure

For the validation of the ZINC-FFQ, the same approach was applied as in previous studies [16–18]. The convenience sampling of women living in Warsaw was applied. The validation was conducted in the same group of young Polish female respondents, as the validation of IOdine Dietary INtake Evaluation-Food Frequency Questionnaire (IODINE-FFQ) designed to assess the iodine intake [18], so the inclusion criteria, exclusion criteria, characteristics of respondents and recruitment procedure (Figure 1) as well as validation approach [19] were previously presented [18].

According to the Biomarkers of Nutrition for Development (BOND) Zinc Expert Panel [20], the assessment of the dietary zinc intake is one of the recommended methods to assess the zinc status. Moreover, the ZINC-FFQ was planned to be validated against the other method enabling calculation of intake on the basis of the self-reported data, so the 3-day dietary record was chosen as the reference method. The record was applied according to the same rules as in the previous studies [16–18], while the zinc intake was analyzed using the Polish database of the nutritional value of products [14], applying Polish dietician software.

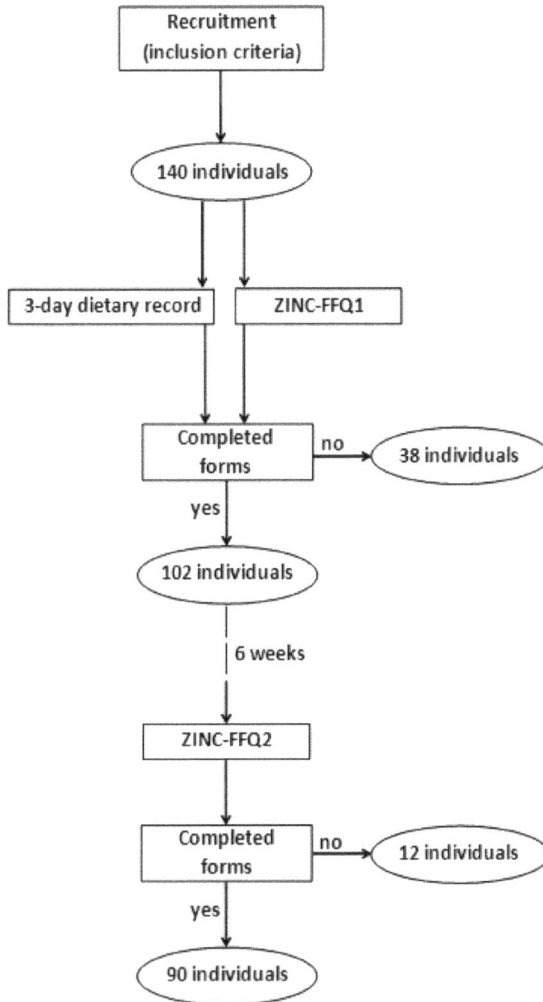

Figure 1. Participant recruitment to the validation of the questionnaire. ZINC-FFQ = Zinc INtake Calculation—Food Frequency Questionnaire.

2.3. Statistical Analysis

The statistical approach included assessment of validity (while results of the ZINC-FFQ1 and ZINC-FFQ2 were compared with the results of the 3-day dietary record) and of reproducibility (while results of the ZINC-FFQ1 and ZINC-FFQ2 were compared). The analysis included Bland–Altman plot, tertiles distribution, weighted κ statistic, adequacy assessment in comparison with Estimated Average Requirement (EAR) level of 6.8 mg [21], as well as supplementary methods, while analysis was conducted as in the previous study [22].

3. Results

Zinc intake observed in the group of young female respondents is presented in Table 3. While using both methods it was stated that the majority of young female individuals were characterized by adequate zinc intake (higher than the EAR level of 6.8 mg per day).

Table 3. The observed zinc intake and the assessment of its adequacy.

Parameters		3-Day Dietary Record	ZINC-FFQ1	ZINC-FFQ2
Mean ± standard deviation (mg)		8.55 ± 3.42	8.61 ± 3.23	8.98 ± 3.45
Median (mg)		8.09 *	8.30 *	8.65 *
Minimum (mg)		3.17	3.00	2.77
Maximum (mg)		22.42	20.97	22.05
Individuals characterized by adequate intake in	*n*	69	61	66
comparison with EAR level [21]	(%)	76.67	67.78	73.33
Individuals characterized by inadequate intake	*n*	21	29	24
in comparison with EAR level [21]	(%)	23.33	32.22	26.67

* Distribution different than normal (Shapiro–Wilk test—$p \leq 0.05$). ZINC-FFQ1 = first food frequency questionnaire. ZINC-FFQ2 = second food frequency questionnaire. EAR = Estimated Average Requirement.

The validation of the ZINC-FFQ including tertiles distribution, weighted κ statistic and adequacy assessment are presented in Table 4. In comparison with 3-day dietary record, over 65% of young female respondents were classified in the same category of zinc intake adequacy and less than 50% were classified into the same tertile. At the same time, in the comparison between ZINC-FFQ1 and ZINC-FFQ2, over 80% of young female respondents were classified in the same category of zinc intake adequacy and almost 75% were classified into the same tertile, that contributed to weighted κ statistic of 0.65 (substantial agreement).

Table 4. The validation of the ZINC-FFQ including tertiles distribution, weighted κ statistic and adequacy assessment.

Parameters			ZINC-FFQ1 vs. 3-Day Dietary Record	ZINC-FFQ2 vs. 3-Day Dietary Record	ZINC-FFQ1 vs. ZINC-FFQ2
Individuals classified into the same tertile		*n*	39	42	65
		%	43.33	46.67	72.22
Individuals misclassified (classified into opposite tertiles)		*n*	15	18	3
		%	16.67	20.00	3.33
Weighted κ statistic			0.175	0.175	0.65
Individuals of the	same zinc intake adequacy category	*n*	60	59	75
		%	66.67	65.56	83.33
	conflicting zinc intake adequacy category	*n*	30	31	15
		%	33.33	34.44	16.67

ZINC-FFQ1 = first food frequency questionnaire. ZINC-FFQ2 = second food frequency questionnaire.

The assessment of the validity of the ZINC-FFQ conducted using the Bland–Altman plot for the ZINC-FFQ1 is presented in Figure 2. The mean absolute difference of the zinc intake was 0.4329, while the agreement limit was observed to be from −7.022 to 7.888 and a Bland–Altman index of 5.5% was obtained.

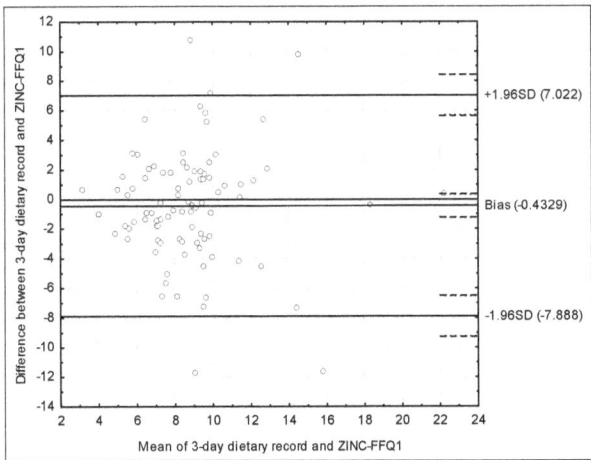

Figure 2. The assessment of the validity of the ZINC-FFQ conducted using the Bland–Altman plot for the ZINC-FFQ1 (Bland–Altman index of 5.5%). ZINC-FFQ1 = first food frequency questionnaire. SD = Standard deviation.

The assessment of the validity of the ZINC-FFQ conducted using the Bland–Altman plot for the ZINC-FFQ2 is presented in Figure 3. The mean absolute difference of the zinc intake was 0.3756, while the agreement limit was observed to be from −7.056 to 7.808 and a Bland–Altman index of 6.7% was obtained.

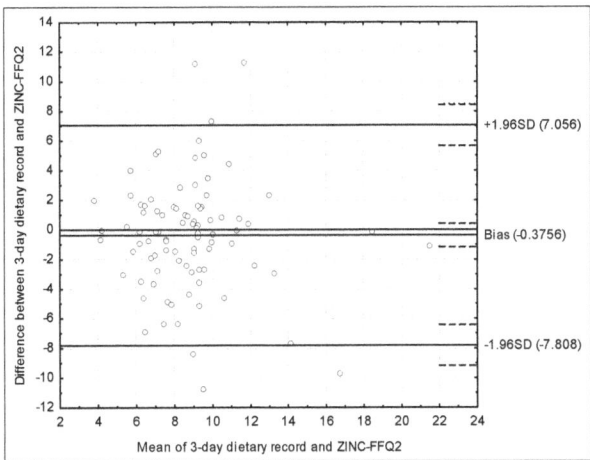

Figure 3. The assessment of the validity of the ZINC-FFQ conducted using the Bland–Altman plot for the ZINC-FFQ2 (Bland–Altman index of 6.7%). ZINC-FFQ2 = second food frequency questionnaire.

The assessment of the reproducibility of the ZINC-FFQ conducted using the Bland–Altman plot is presented in Figure 4. The mean absolute difference of the zinc intake was 0.05732, while the agreement limit was observed to be from −5.055 to 5.170 and a Bland–Altman index of 3.3% was obtained.

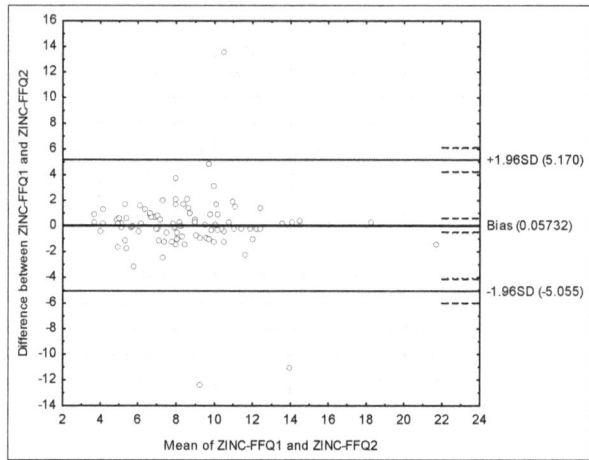

Figure 4. The assessment of the reproducibility of the ZINC-FFQ conducted using the Bland–Altman plot (Bland–Altman index of 3.3%). ZINC-FFQ1 = first food frequency questionnaire. ZINC-FFQ2 = second food frequency questionnaire.

In the assessment of reproducibility, the Root Mean Square Errors of Prediction (RMSEP) of zinc intake estimation in a group of young women was 2.44 mg, the Median Absolute Percentage Errors (MdAPE) was 9.98%, while the correlation was significant ($p = 0.0000$; $R = 0.7440$).

4. Discussion

The most important consequences of zinc deficiency include the adverse fetal effects, as well as increased newborn [7] and children death rate [3]. However, the influence on the offspring is not the only effect proven for young women, as in the systematic review of Lomagno et al. [23], conducted for young and premenopausal women, the better zinc status was indicated as associated with improved emotional and cognitive functioning. Taking it into account, not only pregnant women and those in preconception period would benefit from the control of the zinc intake, but also those who do not intend to be pregnant.

4.1. Food Frequency Questionnaires for Pregnant Women

A number of applied multiple-nutrients food frequency questionnaires include zinc intake assessment, while some of them were designed for a specific group of pregnant women. Such pregnancy questionnaires were validated e.g., in United States of America [24,25], China [26,27], Brasil [28], or Japan [29], but also in European countries—Great Britain [30], Norway [31], and Spain [32].

It is indicated by authors that the intake during pregnancy changes significantly—it may change within each trimester, as well as it is in general less stable than in the case of non-pregnant women, so a significant day-to-day variation is observed [24]. It may result from the appetite fluctuation, caused by nausea or vomiting, changing food preferences, as well as energy requirements [27]. As the diet during pregnancy may change, the season of the year when women is pregnant is also important, as the summer to autumn period is indicated as characterized by the highest seasonal variation, resulting from the fruit and vegetables intake [26].

Regarding the above-mentioned, it must be emphasized that a constant monitoring of intake during pregnancy is needed and food frequency questionnaires enabling assessment of multiple nutrients may be a good option. The dietary record may not be a better method than food frequency questionnaire, as Brantsæter et al. [31] indicated that in their study pregnant women were omitting snacks which were considered as unhealthy, in spite of the fact, that they were asked not to change their typical dietary habits.

However, the indicated questionnaires were designed to assess the intake of many nutrients and, as a result, many questions are included. Consequently, it is indicated, that in the case of validation conducted by Brunst et al. [25], it took about 20–30 min to complete the interviewer-administered modified Block98 Food Frequency Questionnaire [33]. As a result, while only the zinc intake is to be assessed, rather a zinc-specific brief questionnaire should be applied.

4.2. Food Frequency Questionnaires Assessing Zinc Intake

In the review of Serra-Majem et al. [34] it was indicated, that for the zinc assessment, applied using food frequency questionnaires, the methods analyzing intake, such as records and recalls, had an acceptable correlation with validated food frequency questionnaires. Simultaneously, correlations were increased while weighted dietary records were applied and while the assessment of applied supplementation was included [34].

At the same time, the validations conducted using biomarkers often are not so positive. For the electronic semi-quantitative food frequency questionnaire, including 235 items, adapted from the Blue Mountains Eye Study Food Frequency Questionnaire [35], assessing inter alia zinc intake, it was observed, that between zinc intake and serum zinc concentration, there was no significant trend [36]. The lack of association between zinc intake assessed using food frequency questionnaire and zinc biomarkers was explained by many authors. Fayet et al. [36], interpreted it as resulting from the number of other dietary factors that affect zinc absorption [37]. Simultaneously, Brunst et al. [25] indicated the fact that serum zinc concentration reflects the recent intake from food products and supplementation, while the intake from questionnaire reflects the typical intake from diet and sometimes also from supplementation. Moreover, Brantsæter et al. [31], validating food frequency questionnaire for pregnant women in the Norwegian Mother and Child Cohort Study (MoBA) indicated that just a few biological markers are directly related to the nutrients intake, so biomarkers use is limited, mainly due to the high cost [38]. In the conducted study, the blood samples were not collected, as the aim of the study included validation in comparison with the other method of the dietary intake assessment, but it must be indicated, that in the following analysis, the validation in comparison with biomarkers of the zinc status will be needed.

In the review analyzing assessment methods for zinc intake [34], the correlation coefficients for the food frequency questionnaires, validated using methods assessing the dietary intake, were analyzed and it was indicated, that the correlation coefficients for zinc depend on the food items number in food frequency questionnaires. It was stated, that the number of food items lower than 100 is associated with a slightly higher values of correlation coefficient than for higher number of items [34].

The length of the form and a number of questions may be a crucial issue and, as was revealed by Serra-Majem et al. [34], the lower number of questions in the form may be not only easier for respondents, but also associated with a higher validity. Regarding the above-mentioned, the constant analysis of questionnaires is necessary, while redundant food items should be excluded to simplify the questionnaire [39].

For the zinc, it was observed by Samman et al. [40], in the study conducted in Australia, that assessed the validity of the short food frequency questionnaire while the various number of food products from the questionnaire were included into calculation. In the indicated study, it was observed, that the number of food product items in the questionnaire may be successfully reduced from 74 to 37 (food products contributing to 80% of the total zinc intake), as the similar results in the validation were still observed [40].

4.3. Validations Conducted Using Bland–Altman Index

The Bland–Altman plot is recommended to be used instead of the other methods of assessment, in spite of the fact, that in practice it is applied by researchers less often than the other methods [13].

In the present study, the assessment of validity and reproducibility of the ZINC-FFQ, conducted using the Bland–Altman plot indicates a positive validation, or borderline positive validation, on the basis of the commonly applied criteria [41]. In general, a Bland–Altman index of 5% is indicated as a borderline [41]. Such level of a maximum of 5% was observed for the ZINC-FFQ in the assessment of reproducibility (3.3%), while for the validity, the level of 5.5% was observed for FFQ1, but also 6.7%—for FFQ2. The lower validity level for FFQ2 may be associated with the fact, that FFQ2 was filled in 6 weeks after the FFQ1, while FFQ1 was filled in at the similar time as the 3-day dietary record.

However, other authors validating their brief food frequency questionnaires to assess the zinc intake, often observe even higher levels of Bland–Altman index, but they still interpret the questionnaires as a good methods in the assessment. Samman et al. [40], analyzing a food frequency questionnaire of a various number of items, administrated during a personal interview, in a group of 22 young women, being validated against a 7-day weighted dietary record, for the number of 37-item, indicated the successful validation. The number of 20 individuals, out of 22, within the limit of agreement, indicated a Bland–Altman index of 9.1%, being both higher than 5% indicated as a borderline in the assessment [41] and higher than Bland–Altman indexes observed in the validation of ZINC-FFQ in the present study.

Similarly, the Bland–Altman plot was analyzed in the study of Alsufiani et al. [42], in the assessment of the 64-item food frequency questionnaire adapted from the questionnaire previously validated by Samman et al. [40], by adjusting food products list to the nutritional habits in the population of Saudi Arabia. The number of 95 individuals, out of the diverse population of 100, within the limit of agreement, both in the assessment of reproducibility and validity, indicated a Bland–Altman index of 5.0%. The indicated Bland–Altman index may be interpreted as a borderline significant, that was confirmed by authors, who stated, that the reasonable validity and a high repeatability was observed [42].

In spite of the fact that the validity observed in the present study (especially in the case of FFQ2) was lower than recommended, the reproducibility of 3.3% was higher than for the indicated studies of Samman et al. [40] and Alsufiani et al. [42]. As a result, it may be supposed, that ZINC-FFQ may be particularly useful in the repeated measurements, while the researcher may benefit from the high reproducibility.

The observed higher reproducibility than in the mentioned study [42] may result from the different procedure chosen during designing the questionnaire. In the study of Samman et al. [40] food items of a zinc content no lower than 0.5 mg/100 g were chosen and afterwards, during analysis, they removed food product items, until they obtained 37 items contributing 80% of total zinc intake in the assessed group. Alsufiani et al. [42] adapted the questionnaire previously validated by Samman et al. [40], so the procedure was similar. At the same time, in the present study of the ZINC-FFQ, food items characterized by zinc content of 0.01 mg per 100 g or higher were chosen and afterwards they were clustered into 46 food product items. Such procedure may result in a higher accuracy of estimation, as no products were removed from the questionnaire during the designing procedure.

4.4. Validations Conducted Using Other Methods

In spite of the fact, that the Bland–Altman plot is the major method in the validation of questionnaires, it is allowed to use the κ statistic in the assessment of reproducibility and validity, for a small numbers of ordered categories [13]. It is very rarely applied by researchers, but in the present study of the ZINC-FFQ, it confirmed the substantial agreement in the case of reproducibility and a slight agreement (values lower than 0.20) in the assessment of validity.

Authors more often use the analyses of the tertiles or quartiles distribution and adequacy assessment. According to the criteria of Masson et al. [43], when more than 50% of individuals are equally classified, using the compared methods, and less than 10% of individuals are classified into opposite categories, the validity is confirmed. In the present study, the criteria were fulfilled in the assessment of reproducibility of ZINC-FFQ (72.22% correctly classified and 3.33% grossly misclassified), but not in the assessment of validity (43–47% and 16–20% correctly classified and grossly misclassified, respectively, for FFQ1 and FFQ2). It confirms as previously indicated a very good reproducibility, but a minor validity.

The criteria of Masson et al. [43] were fulfilled in the previously mentioned assessment conducted by Alsufiani et al. [42], as in the comparison with the 3-day dietary record for zinc intake, 62% of individuals were correctly classified into tertiles and 2% were grossly misclassified, that confirmed a positive validation. The criteria were also fulfilled in the assessment conducted by Heath et al. [44], while the Meal-Based Intake Assessment Tool (MBIAT) was analyzed (consisting of 630 food products sorted into 16 groups) in healthy male individuals and 60% of individuals were correctly classified into quartiles, while there was no grossly misclassified individuals.

However, similarly as in the case of the Bland–Altman index, in other validation studies are also observed values, that do not fulfill the criteria of Masson et al. [42]. In the study of Fayet et al. [36], in the assessment of electronic semi-quantitative food frequency questionnaire, including 235 items, in young female adults, in comparison with the results of zinc intake obtained on the basis of repeated 24-h dietary recall, 26.4% of individuals were correctly classified into quartiles and 11.3% were grossly misclassified, while questionnaire was interpreted as a relatively valid.

The criteria of Masson et al. [42] are also formulated for the analysis of correlation and it is indicated, that while the correlation coefficient is higher than 0.5, the validity is confirmed. In the present study of ZINC-FFQ, it was analyzed and confirmed in the assessment of reproducibility ($p = 0.0000$; $R = 0.7440$). Similarly, it was confirmed in the reproducibility assessment of the questionnaire conducted by Heath et al. [44] ($R = 0.64$ and $R = 0.73$, for various periods between repeated measurements), as well as in the assessment of validity of the questionnaire conducted by Samman et al. [40] ($p < 0.001$; $R = 0.81$ and $p < 0.001$; $R = 0.76$ for 74-item and 37-item questionnaire, respectively).

However, similarly as in the previously indicated cases of the Bland–Altman index and analysis of tertiles/quartiles, in other validation studies are also observed values that do not fulfill the criteria of Masson et al. [43]. It was observed in the study of Alsufiani et al. [42], that the criteria of Masson et al. [43] were fulfilled in the assessment of reproducibility ($R = 0.758$), but not in the assessment of validity ($R = 0.410$), for the questionnaire interpreted as characterized by a high repeatability and a reasonable validity. Similarly, in the study of Lacey [45], for a Zinc Assessment Tool (ZAT), validated in United States of America, in male and female students, the validity was observed, while compared with the 3-day dietary record, only for female ($p < 0.001$; $R = 0.30$), but not for male respondents ($R = 0.21$), while for both cases correlation coefficient was lower than 0.5.

5. Conclusions

In comparison with the validation studies of other zinc-specific food frequency questionnaires, for the ZINC-FFQ an average validity, but a better reproducibility were observed. It may be concluded, that ZINC-FFQ is characterized by a satisfactory level of validity and very good reproducibility in young Polish female respondents and may be applied to indicate individuals characterized by the risk of insufficient intake.

Moreover, ZINC-FFQ may be adjusted for other populations from European countries, due to the lack of the available validated brief questionnaire enabling rapid assessment of the zinc intake for them. The further studies of the ZINC-FFQ are needed in order to indicate the redundant food items, to improve the questionnaire.

Acknowledgments: Research financed by Polish Ministry of Science and Higher Education within funds of Faculty of Human Nutrition and Consumer Sciences, Warsaw University of Life Sciences (WULS), for scientific research. This research received no specific grant from any funding agency, commercial or not-for-profit sectors.

Author Contributions: Dominika Głąbska made study conception and design; Dominika Głąbska, Aleksandra Staniec and Dominika Guzek performed the research; Dominika Głąbska analyzed the data; Dominika Głąbska, Aleksandra Staniec and Dominika Guzek wrote the paper. All the authors read and approved the final manuscript.

Conflicts of Interest: The authors declare no conflict of interest.

References

1. World Health Organization. *The World Health Report 2002—Reducing Risks, Promoting Healthy Life*; World Health Organization: Geneva, Switzerland, 2002; pp. 1–250.
2. Sandstead, H.H. Zinc deficiency: A public health problem? *Am. J. Dis. Child.* **1991**, *145*, 853–859. [CrossRef] [PubMed]
3. Caulfield, L.E.; Black, R.E. *Comparative Quantification of Health Risks: Global and Regional Burden of Disease Attribution to Selected Major Risk Factors*; Ezzati, M., Lopez, A., Rodgers, A., Murray, C.J., Eds.; World Health Organization: Geneva, Switzerland, 2004; pp. 257–279.
4. Yakoob, M.Y.; Theodoratou, E.; Jabeen, A.; Imdad, A.; Eisele, T.P.; Ferguson, J.; Jhass, A.; Rudan, I.; Campbell, H.; Black, R.E.; et al. Preventive zinc supplementation in developing countries: Impact on mortality and morbidity due to diarrhea, pneumonia and malaria. *BMC Public Health* **2011**, *13*, 23. [CrossRef] [PubMed]
5. Petry, N.; Olofin, I.; Boy, E.; Donahue Angel, M.; Rohner, F. The Effect of Low Dose Iron and Zinc Intake on Child Micronutrient Status and Development during the First 1000 Days of Life: A Systematic Review and Meta-Analysis. *Nutrients* **2016**, *8*, 773. [CrossRef] [PubMed]
6. Chaffee, B.W.; King, J.C. Effect of Zinc Supplementation on Pregnancy and Infant Outcomes: A Systematic Review. *Paediatr. Perinat. Epidemiol.* **2012**, *26*, 118–137. [CrossRef] [PubMed]
7. Shah, D.; Sachdev, H.P. Zinc deficiency in pregnancy and fetal outcome. *Nutr. Rev.* **2006**, *64*, 15–30. [CrossRef] [PubMed]
8. WHO/WFP/UNICEF. Preventing and Controlling Micronutrient Deficiencies in Populations Affected by an Emergency. Joint Statement by the World Health Organization, the World Food Programme and the United Nations Children's Fund. Available online: www.who.int/nutrition/publications/WHO_WFP_UNICEFstatement.pdf (accessed on 15 December 2017).
9. Kumssa, D.B.; Joy, E.J.M.; Ander, E.L.; Watts, M.J.; Young, S.D.; Walker, S.; Broadley, M.R. Dietary calcium and zinc deficiency risks are decreasing but remain prevalent. *Sci. Rep.* **2015**, *5*. [CrossRef] [PubMed]
10. Wessells, K.R.; Brown, K.H. Estimating the Global Prevalence of Zinc Deficiency: Results Based on Zinc Availability in National Food Supplies and the Prevalence of Stunting. *PLoS ONE* **2012**, *7*, e50568. [CrossRef] [PubMed]
11. Shrimpton, R.; Gross, R.; Darnton-Hill, I.; Young, M. Zinc deficiency: What are the most appropriate interventions? *BMJ* **2005**, *330*, 347–349. [CrossRef] [PubMed]
12. Roohani, N.; Hurrell, R.; Kelishadi, R.; Schulin, R. Zinc and its importance for human health: An integrative review. *J. Res. Med. Sci.* **2013**, *18*, 144–157. [PubMed]
13. Cade, J.; Thompson, R.; Burley, V.; Warm, D. Development, validation and utilisation of food-frequency questionnaires—A review. *Public Health Nutr.* **2002**, *5*, 567–587. [CrossRef] [PubMed]
14. Kunachowicz, H.; Nadolna, J.; Przygoda, B.; Iwanow, K. *Food Composition Tables*; PZWL Państwowy Zakład Wydawnictw Lekarskich (State Publishing House for Medicine): Warsaw, Poland, 2005. (In Polish)
15. Szponar, L.; Wolnicka, K.; Rychlik, E. *Atlas of Food Products and Dishes Portion Sizes*; National Food and Nutrition Institute: Warsaw, Poland, 2012. (In Polish)
16. Głąbska, D.; Guzek, D.; Sidor, P.; Włodarek, D. Vitamin D Dietary intake questionnaire validation conducted among young Polish women. *Nutrients* **2016**, *8*, 36. [CrossRef] [PubMed]
17. Głąbska, D.; Guzek, D.; Ślązak, J.; Włodarek, D. Assessing the validity and reproducibility of an iron dietary intake questionnaire conducted in a group of young Polish women. *Nutrients* **2017**, *9*, 199. [CrossRef] [PubMed]
18. Głąbska, D.; Malowaniec, E.; Guzek, D. Validity and Reproducibility of the Iodine Dietary Intake Questionnaire Assessment Conducted for Young Polish Women. *Int. J. Environ. Res. Public Health* **2017**, *29*, 700. [CrossRef] [PubMed]
19. Willett, W.; Lenart, E. *Nutritional Epidemiology*, 3rd ed.; Oxford University Press: Oxford, UK, 1985.
20. King, J.C.; Brown, K.H.; Gibson, R.S.; Krebs, N.F.; Lowe, N.M.; Siekmann, J.H.; Raiten, D.J. Biomarkers of Nutrition for Development (BOND)-Zinc Review. *J. Nutr.* **2016**, 220079. [CrossRef]
21. Jarosz, M. (Ed.) *Human Nutrition Recommendations for Polish Population*; National Food and Nutrition Institute: Warsaw, Poland, 2012. (In Polish)

22. Głąbska, D.; Książek, A.; Guzek, D. Development and Validation of the Brief Folate-Specific Food Frequency Questionnaire for Young Women's Diet Assessment. *Int. J. Environ. Res. Public Health* **2017**, *14*, 1574. [CrossRef] [PubMed]

23. Lomagno, K.A.; Hu, F.; Riddell, L.J.; Booth, A.O.; Szymlek-Gay, E.A.; Nowson, C.A.; Byrne, L.K. Increasing iron and zinc in pre-menopausal women and its effects on mood and cognition: A systematic review. *Nutrients* **2014**, *14*, 5117–5141. [CrossRef] [PubMed]

24. Baer, H.J.; Blum, R.E.; Rockett, H.R.; Leppert, J.; Gardner, J.D.; Suitor, C.W.; Colditz, G.A. Use of a food frequency questionnaire in American Indian and Caucasian pregnant women: A validation study. *BMC Public Health* **2005**, *5*, 135. [CrossRef] [PubMed]

25. Brunst, K.J.; Kannan, S.; Ni, Y.-M.; Gennings, C.; Ganguri, H.B.; Wright, R.J. Validation of a Food Frequency Questionnaire for Estimating Micronutrient Intakes in an Urban US Sample of Multi-Ethnic Pregnant Women. *Matern. Child Health J.* **2016**, *20*, 250–260. [CrossRef] [PubMed]

26. Cheng, Y.; Yan, H.; Dibley, M.J.; Shen, Y.; Li, Q.; Zeng, L. Validity and reproducibility of a semi-quantitative food frequency questionnaire for use among pregnant women in rural China. *Asia Pac. J. Clin. Nutr.* **2008**, *17*, 166–177. [PubMed]

27. Zhang, H.; Qiu, X.; Zhong, C.; Zhang, K.; Xiao, M.; Yi, N.; Xiong, G.; Wang, J.; Yao, J.; Hao, L.; et al. Reproducibility and relative validity of a semi-quantitative food frequency questionnaire for Chinese pregnant women. *Nutr. J.* **2015**, *4*, 56. [CrossRef] [PubMed]

28. Barbieri, P.; Crivellenti, L.C.; Nishimura, R.Y.; Sartorelli, D.S. Validation of a food frequency questionnaire to assess food group intake by pregnant women. *J. Hum. Nutr. Diet.* **2015**, *28*, 38–44. [CrossRef] [PubMed]

29. Ogawa, K.; Jwa, S.C.; Kobayashi, M.; Morisaki, N.; Sago, H.; Fujiwara, T. Validation of a food frequency questionnaire for Japanese pregnant women with and without nausea and vomiting in early pregnancy. *J. Epidemiol.* **2017**, *27*, 201–208. [CrossRef] [PubMed]

30. Mouratidou, T.; Ford, F.; Fraser, R.B. Validation of a food-frequency questionnaire for use in pregnancy. *Public Health Nutr.* **2006**, *9*, 515–522. [CrossRef] [PubMed]

31. Brantsæter, A.L.; Haugen, M.; Alexander, J.; Meltzer, H.M. Validity of a new food frequency questionnaire for pregnant women in the Norwegian Mother and Child Cohort Study (MoBa). *Matern. Child Nutr.* **2008**, *4*, 28–43. [CrossRef] [PubMed]

32. Vioque, J.; Navarrete-Muñoz, E.M.; Gimenez-Monzó, D.; García-de-la-Hera, M.; Granado, F.; Young, I.S.; Ramón, R.; Ballester, F.; Murcia, M.; Rebagliato, M.; et al. INMA-Valencia Cohort Study. Reproducibility and validity of a food frequency questionnaire among pregnant women in a Mediterranean area. *Nutr. J.* **2013**, *19*, 26. [CrossRef] [PubMed]

33. Block, G.; Hartman, A.M.; Dresser, C.M.; Carroll, M.D.; Gannon, J.; Gardner, L. A data-based approach to diet questionnaire design and testing. *Am. J. Epidemiol.* **1986**, *124*, 453–469. [CrossRef] [PubMed]

34. Serra-Majem, L.; Pfrimer, K.; Doreste-Alonso, J.; Ribas-Barba, L.; Sánchez-Villegas, A.; Ortiz-Andrellucchi, A.; Henríquez-Sánchez, P. Dietary assessment methods for intakes of iron, calcium, selenium, zinc and iodine. *Br. J. Nutr.* **2009**, *102*, 38–55. [CrossRef] [PubMed]

35. Smith, W.; Mitchell, P.; Reay, E.M.; Webb, K.; Harvey, P.W. Validity and reproducibility of a self-administered food frequency questionnaire in older people. *Aust. N. Z. J. Public Health* **1998**, *22*, 456–463. [CrossRef] [PubMed]

36. Fayet, F.; Flood, V.; Petocz, P.; Samman, S. Relative and biomarker-based validity of a food frequency questionnaire that measures the intakes of vitamin B(12), folate, iron, and zinc in young women. *Nutr. Res.* **2011**, *31*, 14–20. [CrossRef] [PubMed]

37. Gibson, R.S.; Heath, A.L.; Ferguson, E.L. Risk of suboptimal iron and zinc nutriture among adolescent girls in Australia and New Zealand: Causes, consequences, and solutions. *Asia Pac. J. Clin. Nutr.* **2002**, *11*, 543–552. [CrossRef]

38. Bates, J.C.; Thurnham, D.I.; Bingham, S.A.; Margetts, B.M.; Nelson, M. Biochemical markers of nutrient intake. In *Design Concepts in Nutritional Epidemiology*; Margetts, B.M., Nelson, M., Eds.; Oxford University Press: Oxford, UK, 1997; pp. 170–240.

39. Huybrechts, I.; De Backer, G.; De Bacquer, D.; Maes, L.; De Henauw, S. Relative Validity and Reproducibility of a Food-Frequency Questionnaire for Estimating Food Intakes among Flemish Preschoolers. *Int. J. Environ. Res. Public Health* **2009**, *6*, 382–399. [CrossRef] [PubMed]

40. Samman, S.; Herbert, J.; Petocz, P.; Lyons-Wall, P.M. Development and validation of a short questionnaire for estimating the intake of zinc. *Biol. Trace Elem. Res.* **2010**, *134*, 226–234. [CrossRef] [PubMed]

41. Myles, P.S.; Cui, J. Using the Bland-Altman method to measure agreement with repeated measures. *Br. J. Anaesth.* **2007**, *99*, 309–311. [CrossRef] [PubMed]

42. Alsufiani, H.M.; Yamani, F.; Kumosani, T.A.; Ford, D.; Mathers, J.C. The relative validity and repeatability of an FFQ for estimating intake of zinc and its absorption modifiers in young and older Saudi adults. *Public Health Nutr.* **2015**, *18*, 968–976. [CrossRef] [PubMed]

43. Masson, L.F.; McNeill, G.; Tomany, J.O.; Simpson, J.A.; Peace, H.S.; Wei, L.; Bolton-Smith, C. Statistical approaches for assessing the relative validity of a food-frequency questionnaire, use of correlation coefficients and the kappa statistic. *Public Health Nutr.* **2003**, *6*, 313–321. [CrossRef] [PubMed]

44. Heath, A.L.; Roe, M.A.; Oyston, S.L.; Fairweather-Tait, S.J. Meal-based intake assessment tool: Relative validity when determining dietary intake of Fe and Zn and selected absorption modifiers in UK men. *J. Nutr.* **2005**, *93*, 403–416. [CrossRef]

45. Lacey, J.M. Zinc-specific food frequency questionnaire. *Can. J. Diet. Pract. Res.* **2007**, *68*, 150–152. [CrossRef] [PubMed]

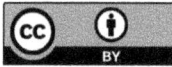

nutrients

MDPI

Protocol

Study Protocol for a Randomized, Double-Blind, Community-Based Efficacy Trial of Various Doses of Zinc in Micronutrient Powders or Tablets in Young Bangladeshi Children

M. Munirul Islam [1,*], Christine M. McDonald [2], Nancy F. Krebs [3], Jamie Westcott [3], Ahmed Ehsanur Rahman [4], Shams El Arifeen [4], Tahmeed Ahmed [1], Janet C. King [2] and Robert E. Black [5]

[1] Nutrition and Clinical Services Division, International Centre for Diarrhoeal Disease Research, Bangladesh (icddr,b), Dhaka 1212, Bangladesh; tahmeed@icddrb.org
[2] Children's Hospital Oakland Research Institute, Oakland, CA 94609, USA; chmcdonald@chori.org (C.M.M.); jking@chori.org (J.C.K.)
[3] Department of Pediatrics, University of Colorado Denver Anschutz Medical Campus, Aurora, CO 80045, USA; Nancy.Krebs@ucdenver.edu (N.F.K.); Jamie.Westcott@ucdenver.edu (J.W.)
[4] Maternal and Child Health Division, International Centre for Diarrhoeal Disease Research, Bangladesh (icddr,b), Dhaka 1212, Bangladesh; ehsanur@icddrb.org (A.E.R.); shams@icddrb.org (S.E.A.)
[5] Institute for International Programs, Bloomberg School of Public Health, Johns Hopkins University, Baltimore, MD 21205, USA; rblack1@jhu.edu
* Correspondence: mislam@icddrb.org; Tel.: +880-2-982-7001-10 (ext. 2352)

Received: 6 December 2017; Accepted: 16 January 2018; Published: 26 January 2018

Abstract: Zinc is essential to supporting growth in young children especially for tissues undergoing rapid cellular differentiation and turnover, such as those in the immune system and gastrointestinal tract. Therapeutic zinc supplementation has been initiated in low-income countries as part of diarrhea treatment programs to support these needs for young children, but the effects of preventive supplemental zinc as a tablet or as a multiple micronutrient powder (MNP) on child growth and diarrheal disease are mixed and pose programmatic uncertainties. Thus, a randomized, double-blind community-based efficacy trial of five different doses, forms, and frequencies of preventive zinc supplementation vs. a placebo was designed for a study in children aged 9–11 months in an urban community in Dhaka, Bangladesh. The primary outcomes of this 24-week study are incidence of diarrheal disease and linear growth. Study workers will conduct in-home morbidity checks twice weekly; anthropometry will be measured at baseline, 12 weeks and 24 weeks. Serum zinc and other related biomarkers will be measured in a subsample along with an estimate of the exchangeable zinc pool size using stable isotope techniques in a subgroup. Therapeutic zinc will be provided as part of diarrhea treatment, in accordance with Bangladesh's national policy. Therefore, the proposed study will determine the additional benefit of a preventive zinc supplementation intervention. The protocol has been approved by the Institutional Review Boards (IRBs) of icddr,b and Children's Hospital Oakland Research Institute (CHORI). The IRB review process is underway at the University of Colorado Denver as well.

Keywords: zinc; multiple micronutrient powder; diarrhea; linear growth; infants; exchangeable zinc pool size

---

1. Introduction

Zinc is an essential mineral in humans [1]. Zinc deficiency is common in low- and middle-income countries (LMICs), thought to be primarily due to an inadequate zinc intake [2]. A large number of randomized controlled trials of daily supplementation with zinc in the form of dispersible tablets or syrups have been conducted in children in LMIC; meta-analyses of these trials have demonstrated a significant reduction in diarrhea and improved linear growth [3,4]. Some trials have also reported reductions in pneumonia, hospitalizations, and deaths [3,5,6].

Zinc is a component of multiple micronutrient powders (MNPs), which are added to complementary foods consumed by older infants and young children [7]. MNPs are intended to improve vitamin and mineral intakes and address key micronutrient gaps including zinc and iron [8]. MNPs currently contain 5 mg or 4.1 mg of zinc, in the standard 5-component or 15-component MNP, respectively [7].

MNP programs are rapidly being scaled up globally for delivering iron to older infants and young children [9]. However, concerns about potential adverse outcomes with MNPs have been expressed. For example, MNP supplementation of Pakistani children under 2 years of age increased in the number of days with diarrhea compared to controls even in the group consuming an MNP with 10 mg of zinc [10]. This finding was supported by a systematic review of 17 studies, which showed that MNPs significantly increased the incidence of diarrhea [11]. The deleterious effects of MNPs may be due to iron, as several studies have reported that iron supplementation increased the incidence of diarrhea [10,12–14]. Research has also shown that the administration of MNPs to children under 2 years of age in LMICs had no effect on anthropometric indices [15]. The effect of MNPs containing zinc and iron on serum zinc concentrations is inconclusive [10,12–14]. The bioavailability of these trace elements from MNPs may be impaired by components such as phytate in the foods to which the MNPs are added. However, a recent study showed that giving iron and zinc together in MNPs did not reduce zinc absorption [16].

The objectives of this research are to determine the optimal physical form (i.e., powder or dispersible tablet), dose, and frequency of preventive zinc supplementation and the best way to co-administer zinc with iron for reducing diarrhea and improving growth in older infants and young children. To achieve these objectives, we propose to compare the following groups of children in a randomized, partially double-blind, controlled, community-based efficacy trial in a low-income urban population of Dhaka, Bangladesh: (1) standard 15-component MNPs consumed daily; (2) high-zinc, low-iron MNPs containing the same micronutrients as study group 1, except with 10 mg instead of 4.1 mg of zinc and 6 mg instead of 10 mg of iron, consumed daily; (3) high-zinc (10 mg instead of 4.1 mg) MNPs with low iron (6 mg instead of 10 mg) and high-zinc, iron-free MNPs consumed on alternating days; (4) dispersible tablet with 10 mg zinc only, consumed daily; (5) dispersible tablet with 10 mg zinc only, consumed daily for two weeks at the beginning and at the 3-month point of the trial and placebo tablets on all other days; and (6) placebo MNP consumed daily. Rationales for selection of the aforementioned intervention groups have been detailed in Section 2.3. Additionally, we also will measure the exchangeable zinc pool (EZP) size in response to supplementation in a sub-group of children from the study population who will be randomly allocated to groups 2, 4 and 6, and to measure serum zinc, serum ferritin, serum transferrin receptor (sTfR), serum retinol binding protein (RBP), serum alpha 1-acid glycoprotein (AGP), serum c-reactive protein (CRP) and hemoglobin in all six groups.

Incidence of diarrhea and change in length-for-age z-score (LAZ) are the primary outcomes of the trial. EZP size, a measure of zinc nutrition, and biomarkers of zinc and iron status will be secondary outcomes to be evaluated in subgroups of study participants. Since therapeutic zinc supplementation is recommended by the World Health Organization (WHO) and Bangladesh's national policy as part of treatment for diarrhea, all children will receive therapeutic zinc supplementation along with Oral Rehydration Solution (ORS) for treatment of diarrhea as part of the study protocol [17]. As such, the proposed study will examine the incremental benefit of preventive zinc supplementation on the study outcomes over and above what is currently afforded by therapeutic zinc supplementation for treating diarrhea.

2. Methods

2.1. Study Setting

The study will be conducted in the peri-urban, low-income area of Mirpur in Dhaka, Bangladesh. This area was selected for the study given that it is only ~10 km from the icddr,b, and the prevalences of zinc deficiency (serum zinc < 9.9 mmol/L), diarrhea and stunting among preschool-aged children in the urban slums of Dhaka reported in the National Micronutrient Survey 2011–2012, were 51.7%, 10% and 51.1%, respectively [18]. The population of Mirpur is approximately 500,000; therefore, it will be possible to enroll the desired number of participants from this study site within 12 months. This area in Dhaka is served by a Community Health Centre/Research Field Office (CHC/RFO) operated by the icddr,b and several other scientific research projects are currently being conducted there as well. The study will recruit a total of 2886 children as study participants.

2.2. Study Participants

Children will be eligible to participate in the trial if they are 9–11 months of age at the time of enrolment and have a weight-for-length z-score (WLZ) ≥ -3 according to the 2006 WHO Growth Standards [19]. Children will be excluded from the trial if they have any of the following conditions: (1) Severe Acute Malnutrition, defined as WLZ < -3 and/or the presence of bipedal edema and/or mid-upper arm circumference (MUAC) < 115 mm; (2) Congenital anomalies (e.g., cardiac defects, cleft lip or palate) or any other conditions that interfere with feeding; and (3) Chromosomal anomalies and other organic problems (e.g., jaundice, tuberculosis, etc.). The 9–11 month age range was chosen for study because the beneficial impact of zinc supplementation on growth and on the incidence of diarrhea appears to be greatest during the second year of life (i.e., 12–24 months). Furthermore, maximal growth responses are usually seen among children less than 2 years of age. In addition, children under 2 years of age are a high-risk group for zinc deficiency in Bangladesh and other South Asian countries, given their usual dietary practices primarily of plant-origin [20].

2.3. Study Interventions

The study will have six intervention groups with varying doses, forms and/or frequencies of zinc supplementation; the duration of the intervention is 24 weeks for all arms. Table 1 lists the details of the supplement in each study group. All powder formulations will be manufactured by the DSM India Private Limited (Haryana, India). The dispersible zinc and placebo tablets will be manufactured by Nutriset (Malaunay, France). Study group 1 will consume the standard, 15-component MNP, which is currently recommended for areas where the prevalence of anemia is $\geq$20% [21]. Because this standard MNP formulation with 4.1 mg zinc has not been shown to affect linear growth, as occurs with higher zinc supplementation doses, and because MNPs containing 10 mg of iron have been associated with an increase in the incidence of diarrhea [15], study group 2 will consume a high-zinc, low-iron MNP formulation to determine if a MNP formulation with a lower iron: zinc ratio (3:5 in group 2 versus 10:4.1 in group 1) improves growth while reducing diarrhea. Participants assigned to study group 3 will consume the high-zinc, low-iron MNP formulation and a high-zinc, no-iron MNP formulation on alternating days (i.e., on day 1 consumes high-zinc, low iron MNP formulation then on day 2 will consume high zinc, no iron MNP formulation, then on day 3 again the same formulation as on day 1 and so on) to determine the impact of giving iron and zinc on alternate days on growth and diarrhea prevention. Since several studies have documented the positive impact of preventive zinc supplementation in the form of a dispersible tablet [3,22], study group 4 will receive a 10 mg dispersible zinc tablet, which will serve as the positive control. Study group 5 will assess whether intermittent consumption of 10 mg of preventive zinc supplements for 14 days immediately following enrolment, for 14 days at 3 months and placebo tablets on all other days' results in sustained benefits on diarrhea prevention and growth. Finally, study group 6 will receive a placebo powder.

Table 1. Characteristics of study interventions.

Study Group	Description	Form	Micronutrient Content	Frequency of Supplementation
1	Standard Micronutrient Powder (MNP)	Powder	Vitamin A: 400 µg Vitamin D: 5 µg Vitamin E: 5 mg Vitamin C: 30 mg Thiamine: 0.5 mg Riboflavin: 0.5 mg Niacin: 6 mg Pyridoxine: 0.5 mg Vitamin B12: 0.9 mg Folate: 150 µg Iron: 10 mg Zinc: 4.1 mg Copper: 0.56 mg Selenium: 17.0 µg Iodine: 90 µg	Daily for 24 weeks
2	High zinc, low iron MNP	Powder	Same as study group 1, except with 10 mg zinc and 6 mg iron	Daily for 24 weeks
3	High zinc, low iron MNP; high-zinc, no-iron MNP on alternating days	Powder	Same as study group 1, except with 10 mg zinc, and 6 mg iron and no iron on alternating days	Daily for 24 weeks
4	Dispersible zinc supplement	Dispersible tablet	10 mg zinc	Daily for 24 weeks
5	Intermittent zinc supplement	Dispersible tablet	10 mg zinc	Daily for 14 days at baseline and 3 months, placebo tablet on all other days
6	Placebo powder	Powder	None	Daily for 24 weeks

2.4. Screening and Enrollment

Trained study workers will survey the communities and the surrounding households close to the study site to identify children who are between 9 and 11 months of age and to screen for the exclusion criteria mentioned above. Surveys will be repeated during the study period as required until enough participants are identified to meet the specified sample size. Children will be screened for exclusion criteria, and then the parents of eligible children will be invited to bring their child to the Research Field Office (RFO) so that a study physician can verify eligibility and consent can be obtained. If more than one eligible child is present in each household, both children will be enrolled in the same trial group; however, one of the two children will be randomly designated as the "study child", and only his/her data will be entered into the database.

In a dedicated room in the RFO, a study physician will explain the study objectives to the caregivers in detail and perform a thorough physical examination of the potential study participants to assess their health status including presence of any congenital anomalies and acute or chronic illness(s), as mentioned above. The child's age will be verified against documentation (birth certificate or immunization card, if available) or the caregiver's report of the child's birth date; it will also be cross-checked with religious or major social events, if necessary. A trained study anthropometrist assisting the study physician will measure the child's length and weight using standard methods described below. LAZ and WLZ will be calculated following the 2006 WHO Growth Standards [17].

After the physician has confirmed the child's eligibility, written informed consent will be sought from one or both parents or the primary caregiver by the study staff.

2.5. Consent Procedures

The consent process will be in Bangla, the national language of Bangladesh that is universally spoken and understood in Bangladesh. The Field Research Supervisors will be primarily responsible for the informed consent process, and in all cases will confirm consent and respond to any questions from participants prior to completion of the process. The initial components of the consent process overlap with detailed eligibility assessment, and thus will be overseen by the physician. However, other trained study workers (i.e., Field Research Assistants (FRAs)) may assist in providing detailed explanations of study procedures, risks, and benefits to the prospective participants.

Literate women or their family members will be encouraged to read the consent form aloud, under the supervision of study personnel. Alternatively, because of variable levels of literacy, consent documents will be read to prospective participants by study personnel if necessary. If a woman is interested in enrolling her child in the study, she will be given a consent form and asked to review it with her husband and/or family members. Prospective participants may take several days to consider participation, if they would like to. A copy of the model consent form is provided in Appendixs A and B.

If a participant's caregiver withdraws consent at any point of the study, all study procedures will be stopped. Data on participants/caregivers who refuse to continue in the study will be included in the analysis on an intention-to-treat basis. However, the primary outcome data for such participants, if missing, will not be imputed.

2.6. Follow-Up Procedures

Trained FRAs will visit the study child and his/her caregiver at their home twice per week throughout the 24-week study period. At one of these twice-weekly visits, the FRA will provide the child's caregiver with the prescribed study supplement for seven days. If the child is in study groups 1, 2, 3, or 6, the FRA will instruct the mothers to mix the daily dose of MNP or placebo powder into the first few portions (preferably 1–2 tablespoons) of the child's food in a single meal each day of the week. If the child is in study groups 4 or 5, respective mothers will be instructed to place the dispersible tablets in approximately one half tablespoon (5–10 mL) of expressed breast milk or clean water, wait until the tablet dissolves, and then feed the entire amount of the liquid in one spoonful to the child. The mothers will be instructed to follow this process daily for the 24-week study.

If a child enrolled in the trial develops diarrhea, he/she will receive standard treatment, including a 20 mg therapeutic zinc supplementation in the form of a dispersible tablet for 10 days. The mother will be instructed how to give the 20 mg zinc supplement in one of two ways. If the study worker diagnoses diarrheal disease during one of the household visits, (1) the study worker will provide therapeutic zinc and ORS to the child's caregiver and instruct the caregiver to withhold the usual study regimen until the diarrheal treatment course has been completed (which is typically 10 days); (2) if a child experiences diarrhea (or any other illness) between the semi-weekly household visits, the child's caregiver will be instructed to bring the child to the day clinic at the Field Research Office, which will be staffed by a study physician. This physician will provide the child with therapeutic zinc and ORS for diarrhea treatment and will instruct the caregiver to withhold the usual study regimen. The physician will inform the study worker who normally visits the child's home and the corresponding supervisor, so the child's treatment can be monitored and the study regimen can be resumed upon completion of treatment.

The zinc and iron content of all study interventions and placebo products will be analyzed at three time points (i.e., at the beginning of the study, at the middle of the recruitment and at the end of the study), in order to document that the iron and zinc content of the supplements are consistent with the study protocol. At least 10 random samples will be analyzed at each time point. The results will not be provided to study investigators to maintain blinding unless any of the six study regimens contain ±5% of the desired amount of zinc. This laboratory analysis will be performed using flame atomic absorption spectrophotometry with a deuterium arc background correction lamp (AAS, Perkin-Elmer Corporation, model AAnalyst 400, Norwalk, CT, USA) at the Pediatric Nutrition Laboratory at the University of Colorado Denver.

2.7. Study Outcomes

The first primary outcome variable is the diarrheal incidence over the study period of 24 weeks. Diarrheal incidence will be expressed as the number of episodes (as defined above) per child during the 24-week study period. Secondary outcomes linked to diarrhea include the prevalence of diarrhea, incidence of dysentery, incidence of diarrhea with dehydration, and all hospitalizations. The other primary outcome variable will be change in linear growth defined by LAZ over the 24-week study period, i.e., the absolute change in LAZ from enrolment to the end of the 24-week study period.

2.8. Participant Recruitment Plans and Study Timeline

Study participants will be recruited and enrolled on a monthly basis. Given the sample size described below, our targeted enrolment rate is 241 children per month; we anticipate completing enrolment in 12 months. Each participant will be studied 24 weeks. The total timeline for the study will be approximately 27 months, excluding time for manuscript publication in peer-reviewed journals. A schematic of the proposed timeline is provided in Appendix B.

2.9. Sample Size Calculations

Diarrheal incidence over a 24-week period is expected to follow an overdispersed Poisson distribution; the mean incidence from 9 to 15 months is expected to be 2.1 episodes, and the overdispersion parameter is 1.56 (based on prior data from the same study area); the statistical test will involve comparing six means simultaneously at a 5% level of significance. In order to detect a 20% difference between the mean diarrheal incidence in any two groups with 80% power, a sample size of 418 participants per group will be needed. When this is inflated by 15% to account for possible attrition and sub-optimal adherence to the study interventions, the final sample size is 481 participants per group (i.e., 2886 participants total).

The sample size of 481 children per group allows for the detection of an effect size of 0.25 Standard Deviation (SD) for all other continuous outcomes, including linear growth, with 80% power and a maximum attrition rate of 15%. Assuming that the change in LAZ has a standard deviation of about 0.7, this equates to a difference of 0.175 z-score between any two groups.

The sample size calculation for the biochemistry subgroups was based on an expected standard deviation of serum zinc of no more than 3 μmol/L, 80% power, and a potential loss of 15% of samples due to attrition, sampling errors or insufficient blood collection. With these parameters, 58 children are required per group (i.e., 174 children total) to detect a difference of 1.68 μmol/L between any two sub-groups. With a sample size of 58 children per sub-group (i.e., 174 children total), we will have 80% power to detect a difference in EZP size of 0.67 mg/kg body weight, assuming a one-sided test, alpha of 0.05, standard deviation of 1.2, and potential loss of 15% of samples due to attrition or sampling errors. This effect size is consistent with findings from a study of zinc supplementation in Pakistani infants, which reported an effect size of 0.8 mg/kg body weight for EZP size [22].

2.10. Randomization and Double-Blinding

Children meeting the eligibility criteria and whose caregivers provided informed consent will be stratified by sex and then randomized into one of six groups using block randomization, in order to ensure even distribution of groups across time. Sealed opaque envelopes bearing the subject number and containing a paper with the group assignment and any subgroup assignments will be prepared by a person not involved in any study activities and codes will be stored in a secure computer file accessible only by two persons not involved in the project working at icddr,b.

At the time of allocation, the study personnel will open the envelope as per the specific child's study identification numbers in a chronological way, and will record the specific code allocation in the infant's clinical record forms and also in a register. Then, she/he will request the appropriate supplement from a person responsible for dispensing of supplements. All individuals involved in the trial (including parents, research staff and investigators) will be unaware of the intervention group assignment until the code is revealed when the data analysis is complete.

Given the distinct differences between powders and dispersible tablets, it will not be possible to blind study groups 1, 2, 3, and 6 from study groups 4 and 5. However, complete double-blinding will occur among study groups 1, 2, 3, and 6, and between study groups 4 and 5. Since participants in study group 3 will be required to consume different formulations on alternating days, and, because this characteristic distinguishes them from groups 1, 2, and 6, the powders for each of these groups will be packaged in two distinct colors. All participants in study groups 1, 2, 3, and 6 will be asked to consume the powders in different-colored sachets on alternating days. Neither the study personnel nor the participants will know the meaning of the different colors. Similarly, the dispersible zinc and placebo tablets will be manufactured with different codes marked directly on the tablets, and will be packaged in color-coded blister packs, so that participants in study group 5 consume tablets with a specific code/color for two weeks at baseline and 3 months, and tablets with a different code/color on all other days. Since this schedule distinguishes study group 5 from study group 4, all participants in study group 4 will also consume different marked/color-coded tablets for 2 weeks at baseline and 3 months; however, for this group, both types of tablets will contain 10 mg zinc.

2.11. Data Collection: Sociodemographics, Morbidity, and Anthropometry

At enrolment, trained study workers will collect data on background, socioeconomic status, household characteristics, assets, household composition, education, and food security using pretested questionnaires. The study workers will visit each study participant's household twice weekly (i.e., Sunday/Wednesday or Monday/Thursday) to inquire about and record any morbidity that took place in the previous three to four days. It is necessary to visit the households twice weekly to document any diarrhea that occurred in the past 3 or 4 days and how it is being treated. If treatment was not initiated, the health worker will evaluate the health status of the child and make further recommendations as per the national strategy [17].

Diarrhea will be defined as three or more loose, liquid, or watery stools over a 24-hour period, separated in time from an earlier or subsequent episode by at least 2 consecutive diarrhea-free days [23,24]. Dysentery will be defined as any diarrheal episode in which the loose or watery stools contain visible blood [24,25]. Dehydration will be assessed using a standardized method established by the icddr,b [26]. Fever will be defined as an axillary temperature above 38.3 °C reported either by the caregiver or the study workers, who will be carrying thermometers. Acute upper respiratory infection will be defined as pharyngitis or rhinitis, both without rapid respiratory rate or chest in-drawing [27]. Acute lower respiratory infection will be defined as cough or difficulty breathing, rapid respiratory rate (>50 breaths/minute in infants 9–11 months of age and >40 breaths per minute among infants 12 months of age and older), and either a fever of >38.3 °C or chest retractions [27]. Hospitalization will be defined as an overnight stay in the hospital due to illness.

During the home visits, the study worker will inquire about the supplement consumption during the previous 3 or 4 days and continuous supplement consumption in the future will be encouraged. Leftover supplements (if any) along with the tablet strips/used sachets will be collected. The number consumed along with the number prescribed will be recorded.

Study anthropometrists who are trained in the anthropometry procedures will conduct all of the measurements at three central measurement sites at three individual field offices. Body weight and length of each child will be measured at enrolment and at 12 and 24 weeks. Body weight will be measured on a balance sensitive to 2 g (SECA, model No. 7281321009, Hamburg, Germany) and length will be measured to 0.1 cm using an infantometer (SECA, model No. 4161721009, Hamburg, Germany). The measurements will be performed in triplicate following standard procedures [28]. Workshops will be conducted every 6 months to standardize the methods used by the anthropometrist; workshops are also scheduled whenever any new anthropometrists are hired.

2.12. Data Collection: Biochemistry Sub-Group

The first 58 participants in all the six study groups will be enrolled in a biochemistry subgroup for measuring serum zinc, ferritin, sTfR, RBP, CRP, AGP and hemoglobin will be compared. At baseline and upon completion of the 24-week study period, a trained phlebotomist will collect 5 mL of venous whole blood from the antecubital vein using universal procedures and aseptic techniques. The tubes will be placed on ice immediately after drawing and sent to the local icddr,b laboratory for serum separation within 60 min for centrifugation at 3000 rpm for 10 min. Each serum sample will be aliquoted into two separate tubes (one for serum zinc, one for ferritin, sTfR, RBP, AGP, and CRP) and stored at −20 °C. The first set of frozen serum samples will later be shipped to Children's Hospital Oakland Research Institute (CHORI) where serum zinc concentrations will be measured using Inductively Coupled Plasma Optical Emission Spectrometry (ICP-OES). The second set of frozen serum samples will be shipped to the VitMin Lab, Willstaett, Germany where ferritin, sTFR, RBP, AGP, and CRP will be measured by sandwich ELISA [29]. Hemoglobin concentration will be measured at the RFO using a Hemocue, HB 301 Analyzer (Hemocue AB, Angelholm, Sweden).

2.13. Data Collection: Exchangeable Zinc Pool (Ezp) Size Estimation

The EZP size will also be measured in the children in the biochemistry subgroup at baseline and at the end of the 24-week study period. The children will come to the iccddr,b's Clinical Trial Unit (CTU) in Dhaka for this measurement. On the morning of the study day, a zinc isotopic tracer will be administered intravenously in the ante-cubital vein (~300 µg of ^{67}Zn at baseline and ~400 µg ^{70}Zn at endline). Half of the children will be randomized to receive one of these isotopes at baseline and the other one at the endline and vice versa. A 3-way stopcock will be attached to the end of the butterfly tubing and the zinc isotope solution will be infused over 2–3 min. To ensure that the entire isotope dose is infused, the syringe and tubing will be rinsed twice with equal volumes of normal saline. Precautions to avoid zinc contamination will be used for all of the biochemical procedures. The participants' body weight at the time of isotope infusion at baseline and endline will also be recorded.

On the 3rd day after isotope infusion (day 4), ~20 mL urine samples will be collected at the homes of the participants by the mothers with assistance from the study personnel. Morning and evening samples will be collected for 4 consecutive days (days 4–7) for a total of 8 urine samples/participant. After thoroughly cleaning the child's perineum, urine will be collected in zinc-free standard adhesive pediatric urine collection bags (Briggs Health Care, Des Moines, IA, USA and then transferred to zinc-free Nalgene bottles (Thermo Fisher Scientific, Waltham, MA, USA) and stored at −20 °C at the CTU of icddr,b. Urine samples, along with any dose losses, will be shipped to the University of Colorado Denver for analysis of isotope ratios and enrichment via Inductively Coupled Plasma-Mass-Spectrometry (ICP-MS).

Stable isotope enrichment data processing: the size of the EZP will be calculated by dividing the dose of the intravenous isotope (^{67}Zn or ^{70}Zn) infused by the enrichment value at the y-intercept of the linear regression of a semi-log plot of urine enrichment data from d 4–7 (4 days) [30,31]. EZP will be expressed both in absolute mass (mg) and relative to body weight (mg/kg).

3. Data Management and Analysis

3.1. Data Management

Study workers and their designated supervisor will review all pre-coded data collection forms on a daily basis before submitting the forms to the data entry team at icddr,b. All data will be entered by two or three Data Management Assistants and verified by the Data Management Officer. Any differences between entries, as identified by the database program, will be resolved by rechecking the original forms against both datasets. A common dataset will then be generated. The Data Management Officer will develop programs in Microsoft Access to check for inconsistent or implausible values of variables in the common dataset. Any aberrant values will be forwarded to the field office and resolved by checking the original data collection form or by a repeat home visit whenever possible.

Outliers will be identified by visually inspecting box plots and/or histograms of individual continuous variables, and scatterplots of related variables. Outliers, which are clearly impossible or implausible values, will be corrected if possible, or recoded to missing if correction is not possible. Outliers, which are plausible or possible, will be maintained.

3.2. Data Analysis Principles

A participant flow diagram will be prepared in accordance with the 2010 CONSORT guidelines [32]. The primary analysis will be conducted on a 'complete-case intention to treat' basis (i.e., results for all children will be analysed according to the study group to which they were randomized regardless of any protocol violations). Data from participants who were lost to follow-up because of death, travel from the study site, or refusal to continue the trial will be included in the analysis if available. However, there will also be a secondary set of analyses, which will be restricted to the sub-set of participants who adhere well to the protocol (i.e., a "per protocol" analysis).

All statistical analyses will be two-sided, at 5% level of significance other than the variables related to EZP, which will be one-sided. Where more than 10% of observations are missing for a dependent variable, we will report the number of observations used in the analysis. We will also compare the baseline characteristics of participants who are lost to follow-up with those who remained in the trial for the duration of the follow-up period to identify any possible biases and include such characteristics as covariates in the statistical analysis if bias is detected.

With the exception of analyzing severe adverse events throughout the course of the trial, formal interim analyses that examine study progress for futility issues will not be conducted. If enrolment is slower than anticipated, the study/screening area will be expanded or other corrective measures will be taken.

All analyses will be performed using SAS version 9.4 (SAS Institute, Cary, NC, USA) or Stata version 14 (Stata Corp., College Station, TX, USA). The WHO 2006 Child Growth Standards will be used for age- and sex-standardization of child weight, length, arm circumference, and WLZ.

3.3. Monitoring of Data Collection

Previously established and validated standard operating procedures for data collection, monitoring and quality control measures will be used throughout the study [33]. Supervisors will conduct quality control checks by repeating 10% of the visits by the supervisors on the same day as the FRA for the morbidity surveillance as per the definitions as outlined in the manual of procedures. These visits will be carried out without informing the respective FRAs. For the anthropometry, if the measurements with the supervisors are found to be greater than 1 cm in length or 500 g in weight [26], then the measurements will be unacceptable and a newer episode of measurements will be conducted on the same day. If the same anthropometrist is found to make mistakes repeatedly, then the supervisor will ensure that a refresher training is completed by the anthropometrists. All weighing scales will be calibrated daily and infantometers weekly [26], and three measurements will be taken and the average value will be recorded.

3.4. Data Analysis Methods

All variables measured at the time of enrolment (i.e., prior to the first intake of the study supplement) will be considered background or baseline characteristics. These variables include: infant sex, infant anthropometry, i.e., LAZ, WLZ, and weight-for-age, z-score (WAZ); proportion stunting, wasting and underweight), breastfeeding status, morbidity occurrence in the previous two weeks, hemoglobin concentration, concentrations of biochemical measures (i.e., ferritin, sTfR, CRP, AGP, RBP, serum zinc) among infants in the biochemistry subgroup, maternal age, maternal marital status, maternal education, maternal Body Mass Index (BMI), parity, household size and composition, household food security status, household characteristics needed to calculate a wealth index. These treatment-group baseline characteristics will be presented in a table. Frequencies and percentages will be reported for categorical data, and Pearson's chi-square test of homogeneity will be used to compare differences between groups. The mean and standard deviation or the median and range will be reported for continuous variables, and differences will be compared using ANOVA or the Kruskal–Wallis test. If more than 10% of data are missing, the number of participants included in the analysis will be indicated. The following variables will be considered as effect modifiers: (1) LAZ at enrolment; (2) serum zinc concentration at enrolment; (3) iron status (i.e., ferritin corrected for inflammation and sTfR) at enrolment; (4) sex of infant; (5) household socioeconomic status, primarily wealth and maternal education; and (6) household food security status.

The incidence of diarrhea between groups will be compared using Poisson regression (SAS GENMOD procedure). Following the initial test of equality of all group means, pairwise comparisons between all groups will be conducted with the Tukey-Kramer test. Additionally, we will compare the difference in incidence of diarrhea among all participants in study groups 1–5 vs. group 6 using Scheffe's test. The change in LAZ from enrolment to study completion will be compared between groups using analysis of covariance (ANCOVA, SAS General Linear Model (GLM) procedure). Following the initial test of equality of all group means, pairwise comparisons between all groups will be conducted with the Tukey–Kramer test. Additionally, we will compare the difference in incidence of diarrhea and changes in LAZ among all participants in study groups 1–5 vs. group 6 using Scheffe's test. Baseline LAZ will be included as a covariate in these models.

Other secondary efficacy outcomes will be examined using the same approach. Logistic regression models (SAS LOGISTIC procedure) will be used to compare any dichotomous variables at specific time points. For repeated measures of continuous outcome variables, a linear mixed model (SAS MIXED or HPMIXED procedure) will be used to compare patterns in the variable across time among the groups. For categorical variables, a variant mixed model logistic regression (SAS GLIMMIX procedure) will be used.

All statistical models will include any baseline characteristics as covariates that were not equally distributed between study groups at enrolment or which can be assumed to be associated with the outcome. The effects of potential effect modifiers listed above will be assessed with an interaction term in the ANOVA/ANCOVA model. Interactions with a p-value < 0.05 will be further explored with stratified analyses.

4. Safety and Ethics

4.1. Data Safety Monitoring

A Data Safety Monitoring Board (DSMB) will be formed for safety monitoring throughout the trial. The DSMB will consist of three persons (a statistician, a Bangladeshi pediatrician, and an external expert in zinc nutrition of toddlers). The group will meet prior to the start of the trial to define severe adverse events (SAEs) and a procedure for reporting and analysis of SAEs. Preliminary SAEs include: deaths, hospitalizations (i.e., an overnight stay in the hospital because of illness), and severe acute reactions associated with consumption of the supplement. The DSMB will meet three times, at the beginning of the study, 6–9 months after the start of the trial, and a final meeting after all data are collected, cleaned and locked.

4.2. Discontinuation Procedures and Stopping Rules

Because MNPs and zinc supplements have both been proven to be safe and are widely used in Bangladesh (and elsewhere), participants will continue consuming their assigned regimen for the entire 24-week study period unless they no longer meet the inclusion criteria (e.g., a child develops severe acute malnutrition). We propose discontinuing any of the study arms if the number of severe adverse events and hospitalizations is significantly higher ($p < 0.05$) than any of the other study arms. However, the final set of stopping rules will be determined by the DSMB.

4.3. Ethical Approval

Ethical approval has been obtained from Children's Hospital Oakland Research Institute's Institutional Review Board (IRB) as well as the Research Review Committee and Ethical Review

Committee that comprise icddr,b's IRB. The IRB review process is underway at the University of Colorado Denver as well. The trial has been registered with clinicaltrials.gov and the trial registration number is NCT03406793. The protocol version is Version 1.04, 23 May 2017.

4.4. Confidentiality

Privacy, anonymity and confidentiality of data/information identifying the participants will be strictly maintained. All medical information, description of treatment, and results of the laboratory tests performed on the participants will be confidential. No one other than the investigators of this research will have access to the data. Data related to the study may be sent to collaborating institutions outside the country for analysis; however, any personal identifiable information will be withheld.

The parent(s) or legal guardians of the participants will freely be able to communicate with the Principal Investigator of this study (contact address will be provided in the consent form). Absolute confidentiality cannot be guaranteed, since research documents are not protected from subpoena. The Ethical Review Committee of icddr,b, which ensures the right of the study participants, reserves the right to prohibit access those information. The research sponsors (CHORI and the Bill and Melinda Gates Foundation) may also look at the research files and medical records. However, the participants' name or any identity will not be disclosed in publications from this study.

4.5. Declaration of Interests

None of the authors have shown any financial and other competing interests for the overall trial and the study site.

4.6. Dissemination Policy

The data, results and other findings originating from this study will be published after approval by all investigators of the protocol. The International Committee of Medical Journal Editors guidelines will be used to establish authorship on papers.

Project Status: As of 6 December 2017, study site preparation is ongoing.

Acknowledgments: The trial has been funded by a grant from the Bill and Melinda Gates Foundation to the Children's Hospital Oakland Research Institute (CHORI), Oakland, CA, USA (OPP 1150161) and a sub-grant to the International Centre for Diarrhoeal Disease Research, Bangladesh (icddr,b). Funding correspondence: chmcdonald@chori.org.

Author Contributions: R.E.B. originated the idea for the study and led the protocol design and development. M.M.I., C.M.M., N.F.K., J.W., S.E.A., T.A. and J.C.K. participated in the design of the study and development of the protocol. M.M.I., A.E.R., S.E.A. and T.A. will be involved in the study protocol implementation. All authors were involved in study design and the data analysis plan. All authors read and approved the final manuscript.

Conflicts of Interest: The authors declare no conflict of interest.

Appendix A. Consent Form

Protocol Title: A Randomized, Double-blind Community Trial of Supplementation of Varied Doses of Zinc in Micronutrient Powders in Young Bangladeshi Children.

Investigator's name: Dr. Md. Munirul Islam

Organization: icddr,b

Purpose of the Research: The purpose of this study is to determine the optimal physical form (e.g., powder or dispersible tablet), dose, and frequency of preventive zinc supplements for reducing diarrhea and improving growth in older infants and young children.

Background: Zinc is a nutrient that is found in foods and is important for young children to grow and help to prevent diarrhea. We are conducting this study to learn more about the optimal physical form (e.g., powder or dispersible tablet), dose, and frequency of preventive zinc supplements and whether this amount of zinc will be adequate in reducing diarrhea and improving growth of your children. We also will like to know that how much zinc is stored in your children's body. To allow your child to participate in this study, it will be necessary to give your written consent.

This is a research study. Research studies only include participants who choose to participate. As a parent/guardian of the study participant, you have the right to know about the procedures that will be used in this research study so that you can make the decision whether or not to participate. The information presented here is to make you better informed so that you may give or withhold your consent to participate in this research study. Please take your time to make your decision and discuss it with your family and friends.

Why Invited to Participate in the Study?: You are being asked to allow your child to take part in this study because: (1) s/he is between the ages of 9–11 months; (2) s/he is adequately nourished, as indicated by the fact that his/her height and weight are within the normal range and (3) s/he does not have any chronic illness. We know that young children have the greatest benefit from zinc and also at the risk of deficiency in Bangladesh.

Methods and Procedures: If you agree and allow your child to participate in the study, you expect the following procedures during the duration of the intervention, which will be 24 weeks as described below.

(i) Your child will be allocated to any one of the intervention groups as mentioned below by a method like lottery where none of us have any control over it:

1. Study group 1: Standard Micronutrient Powder (MNP) (15 micronutrients) will be supplemented daily. Your child will receive Red package on even days and Green package on odd days.
2. Study group 2: High Zinc low Iron MNP (10 mg zinc instead of 4.1 mg), and decreased iron (6 mg encapsulated iron instead of 10 mg) supplemented daily. Your child will receive Blue package on odd days and Yellow package on even days.
3. Study group 3: MNP with or without iron on alternating days. On alternating days, children will consume (Day 1) the High Zinc low Iron MNP described above (i.e., Group 2) followed by (Day 2) the same MNP composition but without iron. Your child will receive Orange package on odd days and Purple package on even days.
4. Study group 4: Daily zinc tablet: Dispersible tablet with 10 mg zinc only will be supplemented daily.
5. Study group 5: Intermittent zinc tablets. Dispersible tablet with 10 mg zinc daily for 2 weeks at the beginning and at the 3 month-point of the trial. Placebo dispersible tablets will be given on all other days to ensure study participants are blinded.
6. Study group 6: Placebo control group: Placebo powder will be supplemented daily. Your child will receive Brown package on odd days and White package on even days.

(ii) At the beginning of the study, we will ask you about your socioeconomic status, household characteristics, assets, household composition, education, and household food security. We will also measure your child's height and body weight at this time, at 12 weeks and at 24 weeks or end of the study period.

(iii) We will visit your home twice a week throughout the study and will enquire about his/her wellbeing during preceding three days.

(iv) Every week, at one of these semi-weekly visits, we will provide the child's caregiver with 7 days worth of the study regimen. If the child is in Study Groups 1, 2, 3, or 6, then we will ask you to feed the daily dose of MNP or placebo powder after mixing with the first few portions (preferably 1–2 tablespoons) of the food in a single meal 7 days a week. If the child is in Study Groups 4 or 5, then we will ask you to place the dispersible tablets in a half spoon of expressed breast milk or clean water, wait until the tablet dissolves, and then feed the whole content at once to the child.

(v) If during any household visits, we can see that your child is having diarrhea then we will provide you with therapeutic zinc and ORS and instruct to withhold the usual study regimen until the course of treatment has been completed (which is typically 10 days).

(vi) If your child experiences diarrhea (or any other illness) between the semi-weekly household visits, we will request you to bring the child to a day clinic at the field office where a doctor will examine your child and will treat with best care possible accordingly.

(vii) One 5 mL (equivalent to one tea-spoon) blood sample each will be collected from a vein in your child's arm at the beginning and at the end of a 24-week intervention period to assess zinc, iron and vitamin A status and presence of infection. In addition, we will also measure the protein and fat contents, immunologic markers like a number of cytokines of your child's body as the same time points.

(viii) Some children will be assigned to a sub-group where the total body zinc of the children will be measured. If your child may be allocated to this sub-group, then we will also measure the total zinc pool size or total body zinc contents by using zinc stable isotopes. For this part of the study, we will request you and your child to visit the Clinical Trial Unit of icddr,b and stay there for 6 h during the day time. During this time, zinc isotope tracer will be administered intravenously (~300 µg of ^{67}Zn at baseline and ~400 µg ^{68}Zn at endline). We will collect your child's spot urine (each ~20 mL equivalent to 4 tea-spoon full) on this day during morning and evening and also on days 4, 5, 6 and 7 from your house during morning and evening on these days. This procedure will take place once at the beginning of the intervention period and the other one at the end of the intervention period.

Risk and Benefits: Your child may have mild side effects while participating in this study. The Investigators may give you medicines to help lessen side effects. Many side effects go away soon after the study interventions or test solutions are stopped. There are no major risks associated with participation in this study. At the time of collection of the blood sample, your child will feel a momentary pain due to the needle prick. There is also a rare chance of bluish discoloration surrounding the prick site due to mild leakage of blood in the skin, and a very distant possibility of local or systemic infections or problems. However, we will take required precautions, including using of disposable syringes and needles, to prevent these problems. All blood samples will be obtained by a qualified health care professional. Five ml of blood (equivalent to one tea-spoonful) two times each will be obtained once from your child during the course of the study.

"Heavy" zinc or zinc isotopes are not radioactive and are non-toxic. There are no known risks associated with ingestion of "heavy" zinc. However, infusion of "heavy" zinc is momentarily uncomfortable and may result in bruising at the puncture site, but rarely causes infection.

You or your child may not benefit from taking part in this research if your child is allocated to Group No. 6. The information we get from this study will help us to understand that what could be the optimal physical form (e.g., powder or dispersible tablet), dose, and frequency of preventive zinc supplements for reducing diarrhea and improving growth in older infants and young children.

Privacy, Anonymity and Confidentiality: We do hereby affirm that privacy, anonymity and confidentiality of data/information identifying you and your child will strictly be maintained. We will keep all medical information, description of treatment, and results of the laboratory tests performed on your child confidential. No one other than the investigators of this research will have access to the data. Data related to the study may be sent outside the country for analysis; however, any personal identifiable information will be held and processed under secured conditions, with access to limited appropriate staff of that organization.

You will be able to freely communicate with any investigator of this study (contact address to be provided). Absolute confidentiality cannot be guaranteed, since research documents are not protected from subpoena. Ethical Review Committee of icddr,b, who ensures the right of the study participants, reserves the right to access those information. The research sponsor (*Children's Hospital Oakland Research Institute and Bill and Melinda Gates Foundation*) may also look at your research files and medical record. Your child's name or any identity will not be disclosed while publishing the results of this study.

Future Use of Information: If there is any other future use of the data or biological samples for this study, we are asking for your permission now in doing so, and, if you agree, we affirm the privacy, anonymity and confidentiality of any data/information identifying your child. The blood and urine samples of your child will be shipped to Germany and USA for laboratory analysis. The samples will be preserved for five years there, if the blood and urine analysis is required to repeat.

Right Not to Participate and Withdraw: Your participation in the study is voluntary, and you are the sole authority to decide for and against your child's participation in this study. You will also be able to withdraw your child's participation any time during the study. Refusal to take part in or withdrawal from the study will involve no penalty or loss of benefits or attention.

Principle of Compensation: There are no financial benefits for participating in this study. However, you and your child shall be provided the best possible free treatment for any condition requiring treatment or any research related injuries.

Answering Your Questions/Contact Persons: We will happily provide you further information about the study, if any, now or at a later time. You may communicate with the principal investigators of the study or her/his designated person at the contact address given below. If you have additional questions later, you may physically contact Dr. Md. Munirul Islam at the Dhaka Hospital of icddr,b (*Mohakhali Cholera Hospital*) or call him at the telephone No. +880-2-982-7001 to 10. Ext. 2352 or mobile No. +880-1-755-6286-24.

If you agree to our proposal of enrolling you/your child in our study, please indicate that by putting your signature or your left thumb impression at the specified space below

Thank you for your cooperation

_____   _____
Signature or left thumb impression of   Date
Parent/ Guardian/ Attendant

_____   _____
Signature or left thumb impression of the witness   Date

_____   _____
Signature of the PI or his/her representative   Date

(NOTE: In case of representative of the PI, she/he shall put her/his full name and designation and then sign)
(Name and contact phone of IRB Secretariat, RA, M. A. Salam Khan, Phone No: +880-2-988-6498 or PABX: +880-2-982-7001-10 (ext. 3206)

Appendix B. Study Timeline

Study Activities / Months	Year 1												Year 2									Year 3		
	1	2	3	4	5	6	7	8	9	10	11	12	13	14	15	16	17	18	19	20	21	22	23	24	25	26	27
Institutional Review Board (IRB) Approval			▓																								
Staff Recruitment and Training				▓	▓																						
Study Preparation					▓	▓																					
Participant Enrollment							▓	▓	▓	▓	▓	▓	▓	▓	▓	▓	▓										
Study Procedure/Follow-Up										▓	▓	▓	▓	▓	▓	▓	▓	▓	▓	▓	▓	▓	▓				
Laboratory Analysis												▓	▓	▓	▓	▓	▓	▓	▓	▓	▓	▓	▓	▓	▓	▓	
Sample Shipping								▓																			
Data Entry and Analysis																									▓	▓	▓
Report Writing																									▓	▓	▓

References

1. King, J.C.; Brown, K.H.; Gibson, R.S.; Krebs, N.F.; Lowe, N.M.; Siekmann, J.H.; Raiten, D.J. Biomarkers of Nutrition for Development (BOND)—Zinc Review. *J. Nutr.* **2016**, *146*, 858S–885S. [CrossRef] [PubMed]
2. International Zinc Nutrition Consultative Group. Assessment of the risk of zinc deficiency in populations and options for its control. *Food Nutr. Bull.* **2004**, *25*, S94–S203.
3. Brown, K.H.; Peerson, J.M.; Baker, S.K.; Hess, S.Y. Preventive zinc supplementation among infants, preschoolers, and older prepubertal children. *Food Nutr. Bull.* **2009**, *30* (Suppl. 1), S12–S40. [CrossRef] [PubMed]
4. Brown, K.H.; Peerson, J.M.; Rivera, J.; Allen, L.H. Effect of supplemental zinc on the growth and serum zinc concentrations of prepubertal children: A meta-analysis of randomized controlled trials. *Am. J. Clin. Nutr.* **2002**, *75*, 1062–1071. [CrossRef] [PubMed]
5. Bhutta, Z.A.; Black, R.E.; Brown, K.H.; Gardner, J.M.; Gore, S.; Hidayat, A.; Khatun, F.; Martorell, R.; Ninh, N.X.; Penny, M.E.; et al. Prevention of diarrhea and pneumonia by zinc supplementation in children in developing countries: Pooled analysis of randomized controlled trials. Zinc Investigators' Collaborative Group. *J. Pediatr.* **1999**, *135*, 689–697. [CrossRef]
6. Brown, K.H.; Hess, S.Y.; Vosti, S.A.; Baker, S.K. Comparison of the estimated cost-effectiveness of preventive and therapeutic zinc supplementation strategies for reducing child morbidity and mortality in sub-Saharan Africa. *Food Nutr. Bull.* **2013**, *34*, 199–214. [CrossRef] [PubMed]
7. Zlotkin, S.H.; Schauer, C.; Christofides, A.; Sharieff, W.; Tondeur, M.C.; Hyder, S.M. Micronutrient sprinkles to control childhood anaemia. *PLoS Med.* **2005**, *2*, e1. [CrossRef] [PubMed]
8. Ward, E. Addressing nutritional gaps with multivitamin and mineral supplements. *Nutr. J.* **2014**, *13*. [CrossRef] [PubMed]
9. Reerink, I.; Namaste, S.M.; Poonawala, A.; Nyhus Dhillon, C.; Aburto, N.; Chaudhery, D.; Kroeun, H.; Griffiths, M.; Haque, M.R.; Bonvecchio, A.; et al. Experiences and lessons learned for delivery of micronutrient powders interventions. *Matern. Child Nutr.* **2017**, *13* (Suppl. 1). [CrossRef] [PubMed]
10. Soofi, S.; Cousens, S.; Iqbal, S.P.; Akhund, T.; Khan, J.; Ahmed, I.; Zaidi, A.K.; Bhutta, Z.A. Effect of provision of daily zinc and iron with several micronutrients on growth and morbidity among young children in Pakistan: A cluster-randomised trial. *Lancet* **2013**, *6*, 29–40. [CrossRef]
11. Salam, R.A.; MacPhail, C.; Das, J.K.; Bhutta, Z.A. Effectiveness of Micronutrient Powders (MNP) in women and children. *BMC Public Health* **2013**, *13* (Suppl. 3), S22.
12. Adu-Afarwuah, S.; Lartey, A.; Brown, K.H.; Zlotkin, S.; Briend, A.; Dewey, K.G. Randomized comparison of 3 types of micronutrient supplements for home fortification of complementary foods in Ghana: Effects on growth and motor development. *Am. J. Clin. Nutr.* **2007**, *86*, 412–420. [PubMed]
13. Zlotkin, S.; Arthur, P.; Schauer, C.; Antwi, K.Y.; Yeung, G.; Piekarz, A. Home-fortification with iron and zinc sprinkles or iron sprinkles alone successfully treats anemia in infants and young children. *J. Nutr.* **2003**, *133*, 1075–1080. [CrossRef] [PubMed]
14. Jack, S.J.; Ou, K.; Chea, M.; Chhin, L.; Devenish, R.; Dunbar, M.; Eang, C.; Hou, K.; Ly, S.; Khin, M.; et al. Effect of micronutrient sprinkles on reducing anemia: A cluster-randomized effectiveness trial. *Arch. Pediatr. Adolesc. Med.* **2012**, *166*, 842–850. [CrossRef] [PubMed]
15. De-Regil, L.M.; Suchdev, P.S.; Vist, G.E.; Walleser, S.; Peña-Rosas, J.P. Home fortification of foods with multiple micronutrient powders for health and nutrition in children under two years of age (Review). *Evid. Based Child Health* **2013**, *8*, 112–201. [CrossRef] [PubMed]
16. Esamai, F.; Liechty, E.; Ikemeri, J.; Westcott, J.; Kemp, J.; Culbertson, D.; Miller, L.V.; Hambidge, K.M.; Krebs, N.F. Zinc absorption from micronutrient powder is low but is not affected by iron in Kenyan infants. *Nutrients* **2014**, *6*, 5636–5651. [CrossRef] [PubMed]
17. World Health Organization (WHO). Implementing the New Recommendations on the Clinical Management of Diarrhoea: Guidelines for Policy Makers and Programme Managers. Geneva. 2006. Available online: http://apps.who.int/iris/bitstream/10665/44651/1/9789241502047_eng.pdf (accessed on 19 November 2017).
18. National Micronutrient Survey, 2011–2012. Available online: http://www.icddrb.org/publications/cat_view/52-publications/10043-icddrb-documents/10058-icddrb-reports-and-working-papers/14275-survey-reports (accessed on 19 November 2017).

19. De Onis, M.; Onyango, A.W.; Van den Broeck, J.; Chumlea, W.C.; Martorell, R. Measurement and standardization protocols for anthropometry used in the construction of a new international growth reference. *Food Nutr. Bull.* **2004**, *25* (Suppl. 1), S27–S36. [CrossRef] [PubMed]

20. Arsenault, J.E.; Yakes, E.A.; Islam, M.M.; Hossain, M.B.; Ahmed, T.; Hotz, C.; Lewis, B.; Rahman, A.S.; Jamil, K.M.; Brown, K.H. Very low adequacy of micronutrient intakes by young children and women in rural Bangladesh is primarily explained by low food intake and limited diversity. *J. Nutr.* **2013**, *143*, 197–203. [CrossRef] [PubMed]

21. World Health Organization (WHO). *Guideline: Use of Multiple Micronutrient Powders for Home Fortification of Foods Consumed by Infants and Children 6–23 Months of Age*; WHO: Geneva, Switzerland, 2011.

22. Ariff, S.; Krebs, N.F.; Soofi, S.; Westcott, J.; Bhatti, Z.; Tabassum, F.; Bhutta, Z.A. Absorbed zinc and exchangeable zinc pool size are greater in Pakistani infants receiving traditional complementary foods with zinc-fortified micronutrient powder. *J. Nutr.* **2014**, *144*, 20–26. [CrossRef] [PubMed]

23. Penny, M.E. Zinc supplementation in public health. *Ann. Nutr. Metab.* **2013**, *62* (Suppl. 1), 31–42. [CrossRef] [PubMed]

24. Kotloff, K.L.; Nataro, J.P.; Blackwelder, W.C.; Nasrin, D.; Farag, T.H.; Panchalingam, S.; Wu, Y.; Sow, S.O.; Sur, D.; Breiman, R.F.; et al. Burden and aetiology of diarrhoeal disease in infants and young children in developing countries (the Global Enteric Multicenter Study, GEMS): A prospective, case-control study. *Lancet* **2013**, *20*, 209–222. [CrossRef]

25. Chang, S.; El Arifeen, S.; Bari, S.; Wahed, M.A.; Rahman, K.M.; Rahman, M.T.; Mahmud, A.B.; Begum, N.; Zaman, K.; Baqui, A.H.; et al. Supplementing iron and zinc: Double blind, randomized evaluation of separate or combined delivery. *Eur. J. Clin. Nutr.* **2010**, *64*, 153–160. [CrossRef] [PubMed]

26. Chisti, M.J.; Salam, M.A.; Bardhan, P.K.; Sharifuzzaman; Ahad, R.; La Vincente, S.; Duke, T. Influences of dehydration on clinical features of radiological pneumonia in children attending an urban diarrhoea treatment centre in Bangladesh. *Ann. Trop. Paediatr.* **2010**, *30*, 311–316. [CrossRef] [PubMed]

27. World Health Organization. Revised WHO Classification and Treatment of Pneumonia in Children at Health Facilities: Evidence Summaries. 2014. Available online: http://apps.who.int/iris/bitstream/10665/137319/1/9789241507813_eng.pdf (accessed on 19 November 2017).

28. Cogill, B. *Anthropometric Indicators Measurement Guide. Food and Nutrition Technical Assistance Project*; Academy for Educational Development: Washington, DC, USA, 2003.

29. Erhardt, J.G.; Estes, J.E.; Pfeiffer, C.M.; Biesalski, H.K.; Craft, N.E. Combined measurement of ferritin, soluble transferrin receptor, retinol binding protein, and C-reactive protein by an inexpensive, sensitive, and simple sandwich enzyme-linked immunosorbent assay technique. *J. Nutr.* **2004**, *134*, 3127–3132. [CrossRef] [PubMed]

30. Krebs, N.F.; Westcott, J.E.; Culbertson, D.L.; Sian, L.; Miller, L.V.; Hambidge, K.M. Comparison of complementary feeding strategies to meet zinc requirements of older breastfed infants. *Am. J. Clin. Nutr.* **2012**, *96*, 30–35. [CrossRef] [PubMed]

31. Miller, L.V.; Hambidge, K.M.; Naake, V.L.; Hong, Z.; Westcott, J.L.; Fennessey, P.V. Size of the zinc pools that exchange rapidly with plasma zinc in humans: Alternative techniques for measuring and relation to dietary zinc intake. *J. Nutr.* **1994**, *124*, 268–276. [PubMed]

32. Schulz, K.F.; Altman, D.G.; Moher, D. CONSORT 2010 statement: Updated guidelines for reporting parallel group randomised trials. *BMJ* **2010**, *340*, c332. [CrossRef] [PubMed]

33. Kosek, M.; Guerrant, R.L.; Kang, G.; Bhutta, Z.; Yori, P.P.; Gratz, J.; Gottlieb, M.; Lang, D.; Lee, G.; Haque, R. Assessment of environmental enteropathy in the MAL-ED cohort study: Theoretical and analytic framework. *Clin. Infect. Dis.* **2014**, *59* (Suppl. 4), S239–S247. [CrossRef] [PubMed]

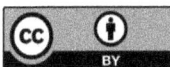

nutrients

MDPI

Review

Zinc, Carnosine, and Neurodegenerative Diseases

Masahiro Kawahara *, Ken-ichiro Tanaka and Midori Kato-Negishi

Department of Bio-Analytical Chemistry, Faculty of Pharmacy, Musashino University, 1-1-20 Shinmachi, Nishitokyo-shi, Tokyo 202-8585, Japan; k-tana@musashino-u.ac.jp (K.-i.T.); mnegishi@musashino-u.ac.jp (M.K.-N.)
* Correspondence: makawa@musashino-u.ac.jp; Tel./Fax: +81-42-468-8299

Received: 14 November 2017; Accepted: 23 January 2018; Published: 29 January 2018

Abstract: Zinc (Zn) is abundantly present in the brain, and accumulates in the synaptic vesicles. Synaptic Zn is released with neuronal excitation, and plays essential roles in learning and memory. Increasing evidence suggests that the disruption of Zn homeostasis is involved in various neurodegenerative diseases including Alzheimer's disease, a vascular type of dementia, and prion diseases. Our and other numerous studies suggest that carnosine (β-alanyl histidine) is protective against these neurodegenerative diseases. Carnosine is an endogenous dipeptide abundantly present in the skeletal muscles and in the brain, and has numerous beneficial effects such as antioxidant, metal chelating, anti-crosslinking, and anti-glycation activities. The complex of carnosine and Zn, termed polaprezinc, is widely used for Zn supplementation therapy and for the treatment of ulcers. Here, we review the link between Zn and these neurodegenerative diseases, and focus on the neuroprotective effects of carnosine. We also discuss the carnosine level in various foodstuffs and beneficial effects of dietary supplementation of carnosine.

Keywords: zinc; copper; synapse; amyloid; apoptosis; ER stress; food analysis

1. Introduction

Zinc (Zn) is an essential trace element abundantly present after iron (Fe). It is a co-factor of more than 300 enzymes or metalloproteins, and plays a critical role in many functions including cell division, immune system, protein synthesis, and DNA synthesis [1,2]. Increasing evidence suggests that Zn acts as a second messenger in various biological systems, similar to calcium (Ca) [3]. Zn reportedly binds with a Zn-binding motif or metal-responsive element of about 10% of all proteins and regulates their levels of expression by recent bioinformatics research of the human genome [4].

Given these crucial functions in humans, Zn deficiency causes various adverse effects [5–8]. Zn deficiency in childhood causes the retardation of mental and physical development, learning disabilities, dwarfism, and dysfunction of the immunological system in humans. Because Zn is essential for olfaction and taste, Zn deficiency leads to learning, taste, and olfactory disorders in adults. Moreover, Zn deficiency is related to levels of depression and stress.

It was recommended that the estimated average requirement (EAR) of Zn is 12 mg/day for adult males and 9 mg/day for adult females by the Japanese Ministry of Health, Labour and Welfare. Although daily intake of Zn is estimated to be 10–15 mg, many patients suffer from a mild Zn deficiency because Zn intake and absorption are distinctive. The bioavailability of Zn is influenced by many food constituents such as phytates and fibers in plants, which form poorly soluble complexes with Zn and inhibit its gastrointestinal absorption [9]. Yasuda and Tsutui reported that approximately 20% or more of the elderly and children in Japan suffers from Zn deficiency [10]. The World Health Organization reported that 1.4% (0.8 million) of deaths worldwide are attributed to Zn deficiency [11]. Therefore, supplementation is important for the prevention and treatment of Zn deficiency. Zn supplementation therapy is used in the treatment of pressure ulcers, measles, and taste disorders [12–14]. A complex of

Zn and carnosine (β-alanyl histidine), termed polaprezinc, is widely used for this purpose [15]. Polaprezinc is also used for protecting the mucosa against ulcerations and for the treatment of Helicobacter pylori-associated gastritis [16,17].

Carnosine is an endogenou dipeptide [18]. Carnosine is small and water-soluble. Carnosine and its analogues (homocarnosine and anserine) (Figure 1) exist in many organisms such as birds, fish, and mammals, including humans. It is abundantly present in skeletal muscles, but is also observed in the stomach, kidneys, cardiac muscle, and brain. Thus, daily foods such as meats or fish contain considerable amounts of carnosine.

Carnosine has various advantageous characteristics, such as anti-glycation, anti-stress, and antioxidant properties, hydroxyl radical scavenging, maintenance of pH-balance, and chelation of metals including divalent zinc ion (Zn^{2+}) and bivalent copper ion (Cu^{2+}) (Figure 2) [19]. Carnosine is one of the most abundant small-molecule compounds in skeletal muscle, with concentrations similar to those of creatine and adenosine triphosphate (ATP). Carnosine contributes to the physicochemical buffering of lactate caused by exercise in skeletal muscles and has anti-fatigue effects. It is possible that carnosine contributes to the regulation of Zn availability in the brain [9]. Ours and other numerous studies indicate that carnosine is neuroprotective against various neurodegenerative diseases such as Alzheimer's disease (AD) [20], the vascular type of senile dementia (VD) [21], prion diseases [22], autism spectrum disorder [23], and Gulf War syndrome [24]. Furthermore, supplementation therapy with carnosine and anserine is reported to be effective for improving cognitive impairment in the elderly [25].

Here, with a focus on the neuroprotective functions of carnosine, we review the link between Zn and neurodegenerative diseases, and investigate the neuroprotective roles of carnosine in terms of nutrients as a drug for these neurodegenerative diseases. We also discuss the levels of carnosine in foodstuffs based on our developed convenient quantitative analysis method using high performance liquid chromatography (HPLC).

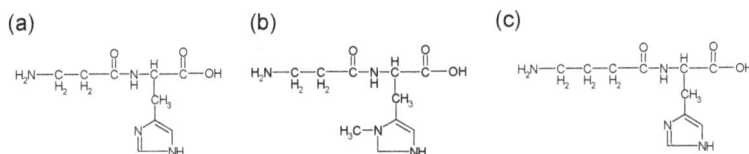

Figure 1. Structures of carnosine and its analogues: (**a**) carnosine (**b**) anserine (**c**) homocarnosine.

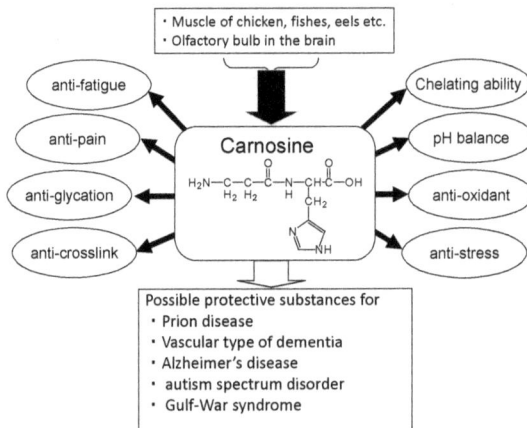

Figure 2. Beneficial effects of carnosine.

2. Roles of Zinc in the Brain

Zn is abundantly present in the testes, muscle, liver, and brain tissues, and total Zn content is approximately 2 g. Zn is accumulated in the hippocampus, amygdala, cerebral cortex, thalamus, and olfactory cortex in the brain [26]. Zn is estimated to be present as 70–90 ppm (~20 μM) in the hippocampus [27]. Zn in the brain binds to metalloproteins or enzymes; however, approximately 10% or more Zn is stored in the presynaptic vesicles of glutamatergic excitatory neurons as free zinc ions (Zn^{2+}). During neuronal excitation, the chelatable Zn^{2+} is secreted into synaptic clefts from vesicles with glutamate. The secreted Zn reportedly regulates the overall excitability of the brain by binding with various neurotransmitter receptors such as *N*-methyl-D-aspartate (NMDA)-type glutamate receptors, amino-3-hydroxy-5-methyl-4-isoxazolepropionic acid (AMPA)-type glutamate receptors, γ-aminobutyric acid (GABA) receptors, and glycine receptors [28]. Ueno et al. reported that secreted Zn^{2+} modulates spatio-temporal information in the hippocampus [29]. Thus, the secreted Zn is essential for synaptic plasticity, information processing, and memory formation. Indeed, Zn is reported to be essential for the induction of long-term potentiation (LTP) in the mossy fiber, a form of synaptic information storage [30]. It is possible that secreted Zn^{2+} has neuromodulators roles. Since Zn has been shown to generate neural inhibition, Zn can modulate the activity of the neighboring synapses by diffusing into synaptic clefts to the adjacent synapses in a distance-dependent manner. A similar phenomenon was reported as 'lateral inhibition', which caused the contrast of signals underlying the mechanism of synaptic plasticity [31].

Similar to Zn^{2+}, Cu^{2+} was also reported to exist in synaptic vesicles. During neuronal excitation, Cu^{2+} is secreted into the synaptic cleft [32]. The secreted Cu^{2+} modulates neuronal excitability by binding to various receptors, including the GABA receptor, AMPA-type glutamate receptor, and NMDA-type glutamate receptor. The size of the synaptic cleft is estimated to be 20 nm in height and 120 nm in width, and is composed of ~1% of the total extracellular volume in the brain [33]. Considering its small size, it is more than plausible that the levels of neurotransmitters or metals are high in the synapse. Indeed, the concentration of glutamate is estimated to reach the mM range after neuronal depolarization in the synaptic cleft. Although the level of Zn in cerebrospinal fluid (CSF) is less than 1 μM, its level in the synaptic clefts is reported to be 1–100 μM [34]; meanwhile, the level of Cu^{2+} in the synaptic clefts is reported to be 2–15 μM [35]. Since Zn^{2+} and Cu^{2+} compete for entry into the body or for many binding proteins, it is possible that excess Zn can also lead to Cu dyshomeostasis.

Carnosine is reported to be synthesized in astrocytes and oligodendrocytes. It exists in olfactory bulb neurons and in glial cells, and is secreted from glial cells into the synaptic cleft [36]. Thus, it is highly possible that carnosine regulates Zn and Cu homeostasis in synaptic clefts. The hypothetical roles of Zn^{2+} and Cu^{2+} in the synapse are displayed in Figure 3.

Zn homeostasis is regulated by three factors, besides carnosine; metallothioneins, Zn transporters (ZnT), and Zrt-, Irt-like protein (ZIP) Zn transporters [37,38]. Metallothioneins are ubiquitous metal-binding proteins composed of 68 amino acids. These proteins possess 20 cysteine residues, and bind seven metal atoms including Cu, cadmium (Cd), and Zn. Among three types of metallothioneins: MT-1, MT-2, and MT-3, MT-3 is mainly observed in the central nervous system. However, MT-1 and MT-2 generally exist in the whole body.

There are 14 types of ZnTs in mammals. ZnTs decrease intracellular Zn by facilitating Zn efflux from cells. They are encoded with the solute carrier (*SLC30*) gene family. ZnT-1 has a pivotal role in Zn efflux and is involved in protection from excess Zn. ZnT-1 and ZnT-3 are co-localized with chelatable Zn in the brain. ZnT-3 transports Zn into synaptic vesicles, and maintains high Zn concentrations in these vesicles.

ZIP Zn transporters transport Zn from extracellular compartments to those which are intracellular and increase cytosolic Zn. ZIP Zn transporters are encoded by fourteen *SLC39* genes. ZIP transporters are also located in the membranes of the Golgi apparatus or the endoplasmic reticulum (ER), and regulate Zn in subcellular organelles. Genetic defects of Zn transporter mutations produce severe diseases such as Ehlers-Danlos syndrome [39].

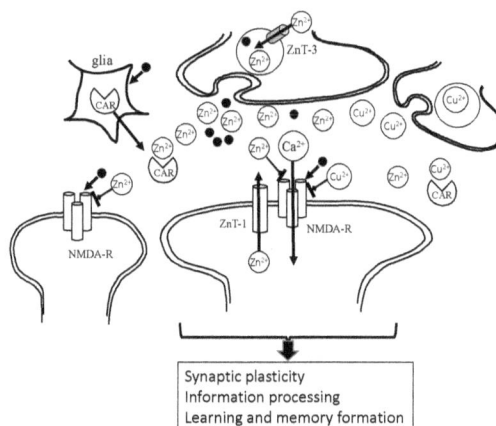

Figure 3. Under physiological conditions, Zn^{2+} and glutamate are released from presynaptic vesicles, and inhibit NMDA-type glutamate receptors (NMDA-Rs) and regulate other receptors. Zn^{2+} spilled over into the neighboring synapse, modulating excitability. It is possible that Zn is essential in the maintenance of synaptic plasticity and the formation of memory. Cu^{2+} is also secreted and acts in a similar manner to Zn^{2+}. Carnosine binds to Zn^{2+}, as well as Cu^{2+}, and regulates these concentrations at the synapse. Zn^{2+}: divalent zinc ion; Cu^{2+}: bivalent copper ion; Ca^{2+}: divalent calcium ion; CAR: carnosine; ZnT-1: zinc transporter 1, ● glutamate.

Furthermore, the excess or deficiency of Zn, namely, the dyshomeostasis of Zn in the brain, is considered to have relationships with the pathogenesis of several neurodegenerative diseases including AD, VD, prion diseases, and amyotrophic lateral sclerosis (ALS) [40–43].

3. Zinc, Carnosine and Alzheimer's Disease

3.1. The Amyloid Hypothesis

In Japan, elderly adults aged more than 75 years represented 10% of the total population in 2013. Therefore, approximately 4 million people are affected by senile dementia and this is a number that continues to grow annually.

Most senile dementia is divided into AD, VD, and dementia with Lewy bodies (DLB). AD accounts for more than half the cases of senile dementia. Although AD was first reported in 1906, the number of AD patients was estimated to be more than 5 million in the U.S. in 2016. AD is characterized by the deposition termed senile plaques and neurofibrillary tangles (NFTs). The selective loss of synapses and neurons in the hippocampal and cerebral cortical regions is also observed [44]. The major component of NFTs is phosphorylated tau protein, and that of senile plaques is β-amyloid protein (AβP). The primary factor of AD pathogenesis remains controversial. The accumulation of tau protein and/or the degeneration of cholinergic neurons might occur during the pathogenesis. However, the idea of the amyloid cascade hypothesis, which suggests that the accumulation of AβP and the consequent neurodegeneration play a central role in AD is supported by many researchers [45,46]. AβP is a small peptide composed of 39–43 amino acid residues. AβP is secreted from a large precursor protein (amyloid precursor protein; APP) in the N-terminal by β-secretase (β-site APP cleaving enzyme; BACE), which is followed by the intra-membrane cleavage of its C-terminal by γ-secretase. The truncated AβPs, such as AβP (1−40), the first 40 amino acid residues, or AβP (1–42) are produced by the different C-terminal cleavage of APP (Figure 4). Secreted AβP is generally degraded by specific proteases such as neprilysin. It was reported that APP mutations and AβP metabolism are associated with AD from genetic studies of early-onset cases of familial AD indicated in [47]. It was also revealed that mutations in the presenilin genes account for the majority of cases of early-onset familial AD. Presenilins are reported to be one of the γ-secretases. Their mutations also influence the production of truncated AβP and its neurotoxicity.

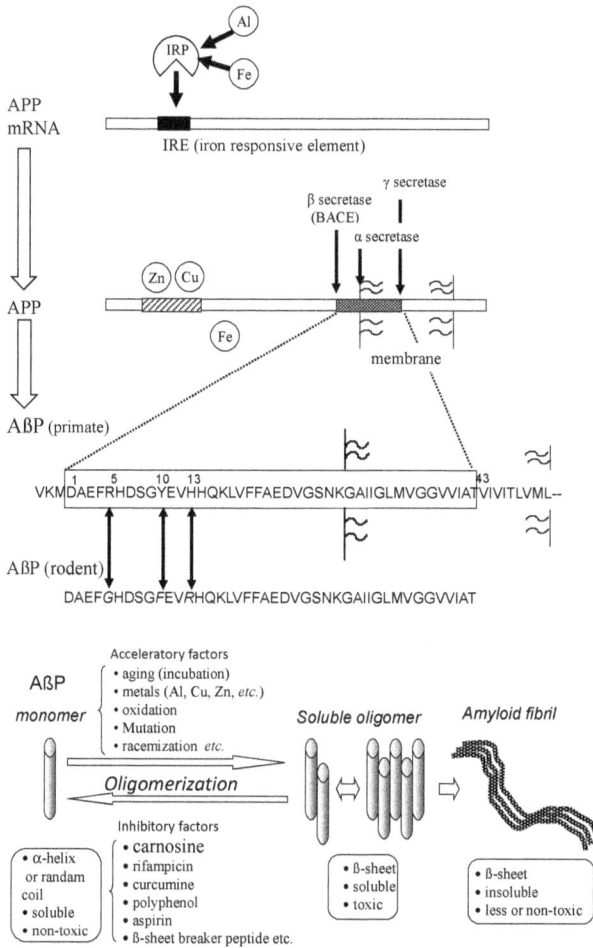

Figure 4. Secretion and oligomerization of AβP. AβP is secreted from APP by β-secretase (BACE) and by γ-secretase. The expression of APP is regulated by Fe and may be influenced by Al. APP also binds to Cu and Zn. Three amino acids (Arg^5, Tyr^{10}, and His^{13}) of human AβP are substituted in rodent AβP. Under aging conditions or in the presence of acceleratory factors, monomeric AβP with random or α-helix structures self-aggregates and forms several types of oligomers (SDS-soluble oligomers, amyloid β-derived diffusible ligands, globulomers, protofibrils) before finally forming insoluble aggregates (amyloid fibrils). The monomeric and fibril aggregates are relatively nontoxic; however, oligomeric soluble AβPs are toxic. APP: amyloid precursor protein; mRNA: messenger ribonucleic acid; AβP: β-amyloid protein; Al: aluminum; Fe: iron; IRP: iron regulatory protein.

In 1990, Yankner et al. found that AβP (1–40) caused the toxicity of cultured rat hippocampal neurons [48]. Although these findings were controversial, the neurotoxicity of AβP was demonstrated to be influenced by its oligomerization and subsequent conformational change [49]. AβP has a tendency to self-aggregate into oligomers. AβP exists as a monomeric protein when freshly prepared and dissolved in an aqueous solution, and exhibits a random coil structure. However, AβP forms aggregates (oligomers) after incubation at 37 °C for several days (aging). The oligomer AβP possess β-pleated sheet structures and finally forms insoluble aggregates (amyloid fibrils). Neurotoxicity of AβP was reported to be enhanced during the aging process [50].

3.2. Metals and Amyloid

AβP is reportedly secreted in the CSF of non-dementia aged individuals, as well as young individuals [51]. Therefore, not only the amount of AβP, acceleratory factors, or inhibitory factors of its oligomerization may be essential in AD pathogenesis. AβP oligomerization is influenced by peptide concentrations, pH, solvent composition, and temperature. The oxidation, mutation, and racemization of AβP can affect it [52]. Zn and other trace elements such as aluminum (Al), Cu, and iron (Fe) are important accelerating factors. The amino acid sequences of humans and rodents AβP are similar, and rodent AβP is different from primate AβP by only three amino acids (Arg^5, Tyr^{10}, and His^{13}). However, the accumulation of AβP is rarely observed in the rodent brains. Indeed, rodent AβP has less of a tendency to aggregate compared with primate AβP in vitro [53]. Interestingly, all of these three amino acids have the ability to bind metals. Bush et al. found that Zn induced the oligomerization of AβP, even the low concentrations (300 nM) [54]. They also reported that Cu remarkably enhanced the AβP aggregation [55]. Zn binds to three histidine residues (His^6, His^{13}, and His^{14}) and/or to carboxyl group of Asp^1 of AβP [56].

However, the oligomerization of AβP by metals is still controversial. The morphologies of AβP oligomers with Al, Cu, Fe, and Zn are quite different [57]. Metals such as Al, Cu, Fe, and Zn alter the oligomerization and toxicity of AβP in a different manner [58]. Cu-oligomerized AβP is more toxic compared with Zn-oligomerized AβP [59]. We found that Al caused more marked oligomerization than other metals, such as Zn, Cu, Fe, and cadmium (Cd) [60]. Furthermore, Al-aggregated AβPs bind tightly to the surfaces of cultured neurons and form fibrillary deposits several days after exposure, compared to Zn-aggregated AβPs.

Meanwhile, Zn can attenuate AβP-induced neurotoxicity and contributes to AD as a protector [40]. Various adverse effects after AβP exposure are reported, such as the induction of cytokines, the induction of ER stress, the production of reactive oxygen species, and the abnormal increase of intracellular calcium levels ($[Ca^{2+}]_i$) [61]. Although these effects may interact with each other, the disruption of Ca^{2+} homeostasis could be the primary adverse event of AβP neurotoxicity given that Ca^{2+} is involved in numerous cellular functions [62]. Arispe et al. first demonstrated that AβP forms pore-like channel structures on artificial lipid bilayers, which are permeable to Ca^{2+} and other cations, multilevel, voltage-independent, and long-lasting [63]. We found that AβP forms pore-like channels on neuronal membranes [64], and demonstrated that AβP caused the increase of intracellular Ca^{2+} levels of cultured neurons using fura-2 Ca^{2+} imaging [65]. Based on these results, the 'amyloid channel hypothesis' was demonstrated; which suggests that the direct incorporation of AβPs on neuronal membranes and the subsequent increase of intracellular Ca^{2+} through the amyloid channels might be the primary event in AβP neurotoxicity [66]. AβP might share the similar mechanism underlying the toxicity of various antimicrobial or antifungal peptides that also exhibit channel-forming activity and cell toxicity in this respect [67]. We and other researchers found that the channel activity was inhibited by the exposure to Zn^{2+}, and recovered by *o*-phenanthroline, a Zn chelator [64,68]. Since His residues are exposed to inner surfaces of amyloid channels, Zn can bind to these His residues and protect neurons from AβP-induced Ca dyshomeostasis [69]. Therefore, the role of Zn in the pathogenesis of AD is still controversial and Zn may act as a contributor of AD pathogenesis, as well as a protector. In this context, Zn might play a role like Janus, the ancient Roman god of doorways, who is depicted with two different faces [40].

Moreover, APP is a metal binding protein that has two Cu and/or Zn binding domains in its N-terminal. APP possesses the ability to reduce Cu^{2+} to Cu^+. Cu and Zn influence the expression and processing of APP and enhance AβP production [70,71]. Cu induces the dimerization and trafficking of APP from the ER to neurites. APP also regulates Fe homeostasis. APP mRNA possesses an iron responsive element (IRE). It means that the expression of APP is regulated by Fe, as well as ferritin (iron storage protein) [72]. In contrast, APP binds to ferroportin, which controls Fe efflux [73]. Therefore, APP is suggested to regulate the homeostasis of metals including Zn, Cu, and Fe.

3.3. Carnosine as an Anti-Crosslinker of AβP

Molecules that inhibit the oligomerization of AβP may be candidates for preventive AD therapeutics. Several compounds such as rifampicin, curcumin, and transthyretin have been reported to inhibit the oligomerization of AβP [52]. A small peptide composed of five amino acids, called a β-sheet breaker peptide, markedly blocks AβP oligomerization [74].

Carnosine has an anti-crosslinking ability, as shown in Figure 2, and inhibits the oligomerization of proteins such as α-crystalline [75]. Thus, *N*-acetyl carnosine has been used for the treatment of cataracts [76]. Increasing evidence indicates that carnosine inhibits the oligomerization of AβP and blocks its neurotoxicity [77,78]. Corona et al. demonstrated that orally administered carnosine inhibits the accumulation of AβP, and prevents learning deficits in a murine model of AD [20]. Moreover, histidine and carnosine are significantly reduced in the CSF of AD patients [79]. Therefore, carnosine may well play neuroprotective roles against AD.

4. Zinc, Carnosine, and Vascular Type of Dementia

4.1. Zinc and Ischemia-Induced Neuronal Death

VD accounts for about one-third of senile dementia cases in Japan. Its risk factors are high blood pressure and diabetes. The interruption of blood flow causes the oxygen-glucose deprivation and membrane depolarization after transient global ischemia or stroke [80]. Thereafter, an excess release of glutamate into synaptic clefts causes the overstimulation of the glutamate receptor and the entry of large quantities of Ca^{2+} into neurons, and triggers the death of pyramidal neurons in the hippocampus, which are crucial in memory formation.

Zn plays a crucial role in the neuronal death after ischemia and the pathogenesis of VD [81,82]. Excess Zn can be neurotoxic in spite of its importance in the brain. The concentration of Zn in synaptic clefts is estimated to be 1–100 μM. However, a considerable amount of Zn (up to 300 μM) is co-released with glutamate into synaptic clefts during ischemic conditions [27]. Koh et al. demonstrated that Zn accumulates in apoptotic neurons in the hippocampus after ischemia [83]. The membrane-impermeable Zn chelator (calcium ethylene diamine tetraacetic acid (Ca-EDTA)) protects hippocampal neurons after ischemia and reduces infarct volume [84]. Zn can cause mitochondrial failure and oxidative stress [85].

4.2. Molecular Mechanism of Zn-Induced Neurotoxicity: GT1–7 Cells as an In Vitro Model System

We investigated the molecular mechanism underlying Zn neurotoxicity and the protective mechanism of carnosine in immortalized hypothalamic neurons (GT1–7 cells). We found that Zn causes the death of GT1–7 cells in a dose-dependent manner [86]. The degenerated GT1–7 cells exhibited apoptotic characteristics including DNA fragmentation, as well as terminal deoxynucleotidyl transferase-mediated biotinylated uridine triphosphate (UTP) nick-end labeling (TUNEL)-positive. GT1–7 cells were revealed to be much more sensitive to Zn and exhibited much lower viability after Zn exposure compared with other neuronal cells, such as primary cultured rat hippocampal neurons, B-50 neuroblastoma cells, and PC-12 cells [87]. The GT1–7 cells were developed by Mellon et al. from mouse hypothalamic neurons by genetically targeted tumorigenesis [88]. The cells possess neuronal characteristics, such as the extension of neurites and expression of neuron-specific proteins or receptors. Meanwhile, the GT1–7 cells possess low levels of ionotropic glutamate receptors and are not subject to glutamate toxicity. These properties imply that the GT1–7 cell line is a good model system for the investigation of Zn-induced neurotoxicity.

Using GT1–7 cells, it was found that pyruvate, citrate, the antagonists of Ca^{2+} channels (nifedipine, conotoxine), and Al^{3+} blocked the Zn-induced death of GT1–7 cells [86,87,89]. We also found that intracellular Ca^{2+} levels ($[Ca^{2+}]_i$) are increased after exposure to Zn. The preadministration of Al^{3+}, a Ca^{2+} channel blocker, inhibited the Zn-induced rise in $[Ca^{2+}]_i$ and attenuated Zn-induced neurotoxicity. Thus, it is highly possible that Ca^{2+} homeostasis is implicated in Zn neurotoxicity pathways.

4.3. Protective Substances against Zn-Induced Neuronal Death

Considering the significance of Zn in the pathogenesis of VD, it is highly possible that substances that inhibit Zn-induced neurotoxicity may become candidate drugs for the prevention or treatment of VD. Thus, we developed an assay system for screening such substances using GT1–7 cells and examined various agricultural products (such as fruits, vegetables, fish, and sea-products) [90]. Among the compounds tested, we found that the water-soluble extract of muscle tissue of Japanese eel (*Anguilla japonica*) exerted marked protective activity [91]. This activity was not diminished when the extract was boiled at 95 °C for 30 min. We separated the heated extract using HPLC and determined the structure of the active fraction as that of carnosine using liquid chromatography mass spectrometry (LC-MS). Moreover, we found the protective activities in the extract of mango fruits (*Mangifera indica*) and in the extract of round herring (*Etrumeus teres*), and determined the active fraction as pyruvate and histidine, respectively [92,93].

4.4. The Protective Roles of Carnosine

We investigated the neuroprotective mechanism of carnosine, and firstly focused on Zn translocation since carnosine can chelate Zn. First, we analysed intracellular Zn^{2+} levels ($[Zn^{2+}]_i$) in Zn-treated GT1–7 cells using Zn-specific fluorescent dye, ZnAF-2. However, neither carnosine nor anserine inhibited Zn influx into GT1–7 cells, whereas treatment with Ca-EDTA, a membrane impermeable chelator, decreased $[Zn^{2+}]_i$ [94]. Thus, it is plausible that carnosine did not act as a Zn chelator and protect neurons from Zn-induced neurotoxicity.

Second, we have analyzed the genetic changes induced by Zn, and our real-time polymerase chain reaction (RT-PCR) analysis revealed that Zn caused the upregulation of several genes, including metal-related genes (*MT-1*, *MT-2*, *ZnT-1*), ER-stress related genes (*GADD* (growth-arrest- and DNA-damage-inducible gene) 34, *GADD45*, *p8*, *CHOP* (CCAAT-enhancer-binding protein homologous protein)), and a Ca^{2+}-related gene (*Arc*). Although carnosine is able to chelate Zn^{2+}, we demonstrated that carnosine did not influence the intracellular concentration of Zn nor the Zn-induced upregulation of *MT-1* or *ZnT-1*. Meanwhile, carnosine was found to inhibit the upregulation of ER stress-related genes such as *GADD34*, *GADD45*, *CHOP*, Ca^{2+} homeostasis-related genes such as activity-regulated cytoskeleton-associated protein (*Arc*). We also found that carnosine attenuated neurodegenerations induced by the ER-stressor such as thapsigargin and tunicamycin, and/or induced by hydrogen peroxide (H_2O_2). We demonstrated that anserine also attenuated Zn-induced neurotoxicity, as well as carnosine. Furthermore, we recently found that sub-lethal concentrations of Cu^{2+} strongly enhance Zn^{2+}-induced neurotoxicity and the expression of ER stress-related genes [95]. The Cu^{2+} enhanced Zn^{2+}-induced neurotoxicity was attenuated by pyruvate and thioredoxin-albumin fusion protein [96,97]. Taken together, we hypothesize the possible molecular mechanisms underlying Zn neurotoxicity and the action of carnosine (Figure 5). After exposure to Zn, intracellular Zn levels increase for at least 30 min. Chelators such as Ca-EDTA block this process. Zn leads to an increase in intracellular Ca^{2+} levels and then triggers ER stress. This process is inhibited by Al^{3+} and other Ca^{2+} channel blockers. Zn triggers the inhibition of the energy production machinery in the mitochondria and the production of oxidative stress. The energy substrates pyruvate and citrate prevent this process. The oxidative stress was attenuated by the thioredoxin-albumin fusion protein. Finally, these three processes trigger neurodegenerative pathways and lead to the neuronal death observed in VD. Carnosine, released from glial cells, enters neurons by peptide transporters and inhibits Zn-induced ER stress. Numerous in vivo studies have suggested that carnosine is protective against ischemia-induced neurodegeneration using experimental animals [98–100]. We have published a patent for carnosine to prevent or treat senile dementia based on the activities of carnosine [101].

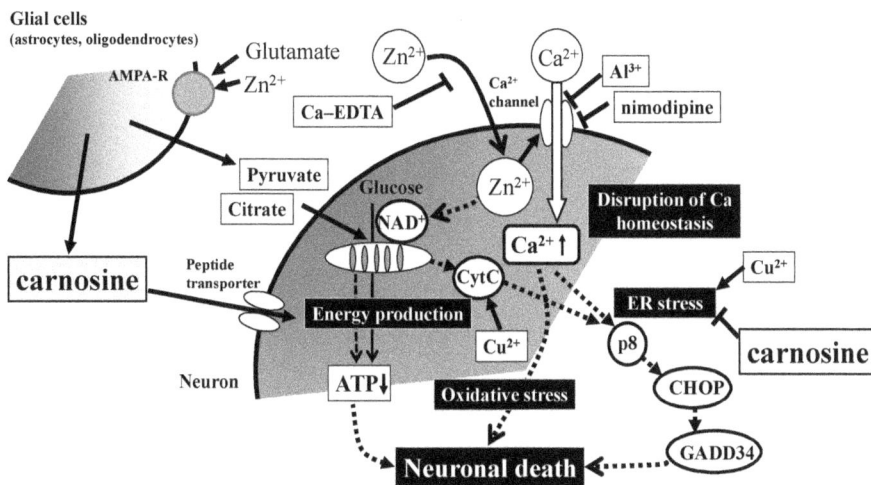

Figure 5. Possible molecular mechanisms underlying the protective effects of carnosine in preventing the neuronal death induced by Zn. Secreted excess amounts of Zn can translocate into cells and cause the disruption of Ca^{2+} homeostasis, energy failure in mitochondria, the induction of ER (reticulum) stress as well as oxidative stress, and apoptotic neuronal death. Carnosine is released into the synaptic cleft and is transported into cell bodies, where it can inhibit ER stress-related and/or Arc-related apoptotic pathways activated by Zn. Details are shown in the text. Ca-EDTA: calcium ethylene diamine tetraacetic acid; NAD^+: nicotinamide adenine dinucleotide; CytC: cytochrome C; ATP: adenosine triphosphate; *CHOP*: CCAAT-enhancer-binding protein homologous protein; *GADD34*: growth-arrest- and DNA-damage-inducible gene 34. AMPA-R: AMPA-type glutamate receptor.

5. Zinc, Carnosine, and Prion Diseases

5.1. Zinc, Copper and Prion Diseases

Zn and carnosine are also involved in prion diseases. Prion diseases include Creutzfeldt-Jakob disease (CJD), Gerstmann-Straussler-Scheinker syndrome (GSS), and Kuru disease in humans. They also include bovine spongiform encephalopathy (BSE) in cattle and scrapie in sheep [102]. Prion diseases are characterized by the spongiform degeneration of neurons and glial cells and the accumulation of amyloidogenic prion protein (PrP). The administration of pathogenic tissue causes the characteristic infections, and thus, prion diseases are also called transmissible spongiform encephalopathies. During the transmissible infections, a normal prion protein (PrP^C) is converted to an abnormal scrapie-type isoform (PrP^{Sc}). Although both of PrP^C and PrP^{Sc} have the same primary sequence, PrP^C differs from PrP^{Sc} in that PrP^{Sc} possesses a high content of β-sheet secondary structure compared to PrP^C, and therefore has resistance to protease digestion. PrP^C is ubiquitously expressed throughout the entire body (Figure 6). It is speculated that the misfolded PrP^{Sc} administrated from contaminated food induces normal PrP^C molecules in the brain to misfold and aggregate.

Therefore, prion diseases are considered to be protein-misfolding diseases (conformational diseases), namely, the conformational change from PrP^C to PrP^{Sc} is crucial for the pathogenesis of prion diseases [103]. These features are similar to AD. PrP^C is reported to be a metalloprotein and regulates metal homeostasis [41]. PrP^C is a 30–35-kDa glycoprotein and contains 208 amino acid residues. In its N-terminal, PrP^C possesses an octa-repeat domain composed of multiple tandem copies of the eight-residue sequence –PHGGGWGQ– The octa-repeat domain can bind four metal ions (including Cu^{2+}, Zn^{2+}, and other divalent ions), and two other histidine residues, His^{96} and His^{111}, can bind two metal ions [104]. The levels of Cu in the brains of PrP-knockout mice were decreased compared with wild-type mice [105]. PrP^C possesses protective roles against oxidative stress as Cu/Zn superoxide dismutase (Cu/Zn SOD) [106].

Zn^{2+} also binds PrP, and can influence Cu binding to PrP^C. Moreover, prion genes and genes encoding ZIP transporters possess evolutionary sequence similarities [107]. Watt et al. hypothesized that PrP^C acts as a 'Zn sensor' and facilitates the uptake of Zn into neurons by binding with AMPA receptors [108].

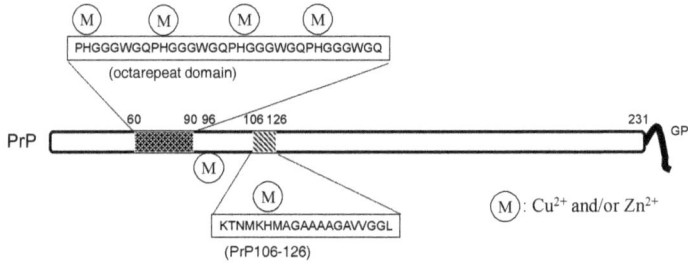

Figure 6. The structure of the prion protein. PrP: prion protein.

5.2. Carnosine and PrP^{Sc}-Induced Neurotoxicity

Normal PrP^C has regulatory and neuroprotective functions such as regulating Cu homeostasis and antioxidant. Thus, loss of the protective functions by converting to PrP^{Sc} will lead to neurodegeneration. Meanwhile, PrP^{Sc} is neurotoxic. Since PrP^{Sc} has strongly infectious characteristics, using a full-length prion protein is difficult [109]. Thus, we and other researchers have used synthetic fragment peptides of PrP (PrP106–126) in the study of PrP^{Sc} neurotoxicity, owing to its similar characteristics with PrP^{Sc} such as β-sheet formation, neurotoxicity, and metal-binding ability.

Our results using primary cultured rat hippocampal neurons and the thioflavin T (ThT) fluorescence method exhibited that PrP106–126 forms β-sheet structures during the "aging" process (incubation at 37 °C for several days), and that aged PrP106–126 causes significant neurotoxicity. These characteristics are quite similar to AβP [22]. Either Zn^{2+} or Cu^{2+} significantly attenuates PrP106–126 neurotoxicity. Furthermore, either Zn^{2+} or Cu^{2+} inhibits the oligomerization of PrP106–126 during the aging process, observed by thioflavin T fluorescence and atomic force microscopy observation.

Although chelators such as clioquinol and deferoxamine did not influence PrP106–126 neurotoxicity, we found that carnosine attenuates the neurotoxicity of PrP106–126 and inhibits oligomerization (Figure 7). Therefore, it is possible that carnosine acts as an anti-crosslinker of PrP106–126. Carnosine also inhibits the oligomerization of α-synuclein, which is a major player in DLB and Parkinson's disease [110], and α-crystalline in lens [111]. In this respect, the anti-crosslinking activity of carnosine is important for the protective functions of carnosine against these diseases.

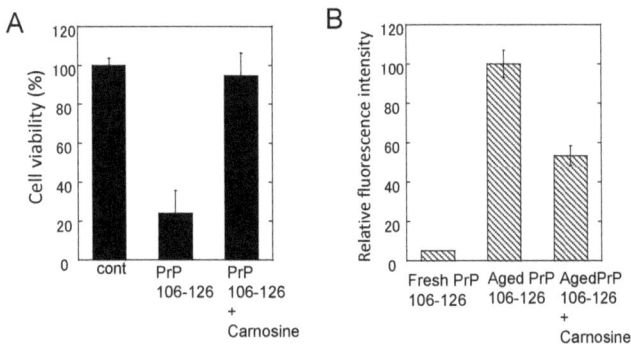

Figure 7. Effects of carnosine on the neurotoxicity and the conformational changes of PrP106–126. (**A**) Effects of carnosine on the neurotoxicity of PrP106–126. The viability of cultured rat hippocampal neurons was analyzed using the lactate dehydrogenase (LDH) method after three days of exposure to 50 μM PrP106–126 aged alone or with 1 mM carnosine. Data are presented as mean ± S.E.M. (*n* = 6); (**B**) Effects of carnosine on the thioflavin T (ThT) fluorescence of PrP106–126. The ThT fluorescence (ex. 490 nm, em. 520 nm) of 25 μM of fresh PrP106–126 or aged PrP106–126 with 1 mM carnosine was analyzed. Data are presented as mean ± S.E.M. (*n* = 7).

6. Crosstalk of Metals and Amyloidogenic Proteins at Synapse

6.1. Colocalization of APP and PrP at Synapse

Synapses are small but critical nodes for information processing and memory formation in neural networks. Since synaptic plasticity is essential to memory formation, synaptic degenerations are primary observed in many neurodegenerative diseases. As discussed in the previous sections, metals (Zn^{2+} or Cu^{2+}) as well as neurotransmitters are co-released from synaptic vesicles into synaptic clefts. They bind to receptors at postsynaptic densities.

Two amyloidogenic proteins, APP and PrP^C, are localized in the synapse, and play essential roles in the regulation of metal homeostasis. APP is in the presynaptic region and AβP is secreted into synaptic clefts in the presence of neuronal stimuli [112]. PrP^C is coupled to glutamate receptors in the postsynaptic membranes [113]. Considering the short distance across the synaptic cleft (approximately 20 nm), APP can interact with PrP^C in this small compartment surrounded by a considerable amount of Zn^{2+} and Cu^{2+}. Indeed, PrP^C reportedly binds to AβP oligomers and attenuates its neurotoxicity.

Given that the homeostasis of metals regulated by APP and PrP^C is disrupted, it triggers the degeneration of synapses, causing neurodegeneration and finally leading to the pathogenesis of these diseases. ZnT-1 is also localized in postsynaptic membranes and regulates Zn homeostasis by enhancing Zn efflux to the extracellular compartment [114]. ZnT-1 also regulates the activity of NMDA-type glutamate receptors. Meanwhile, PrP^C controls Zn^{2+} influx into cells as an analogue of ZIP transporters, with AMPA-type glutamate receptors regulating synaptic Zn^{2+} levels. MT-3, brain specific metallothionein, may also regulate Zn homeostasis at synapses [115]. In addition, MT-3 is decreased in the brains of patients with AD [116].

6.2. Carnosine: A Regulator of Zn and Cu in the Synapse

Carnosine is another important contributor to regulating metal homeostasis in the synapse. The concentration of carnosine in the olfactory bulb is as high as 0.5 mM [18]. Carnosine and homocarnosine is synthesized in glial cells, and carnosine-like immunoreactivity was observed in astrocytes or oligodendrocites [117]. Carnosine is reported to be secreted into the synaptic cleft from oligodendrocytes by glutamate in a Zn-dependent manner [36,118]. Therefore, carnosine is suggested to contribute the availability of Zn at the synapse and to control Zn homeostasis and, therefore, provides wide protection against various neurodegenerative disorders. Figure 8 exhibits a hypothetical scheme showing interactions between carnosine, APP, PrP, Zn, and Cu at the synapse.

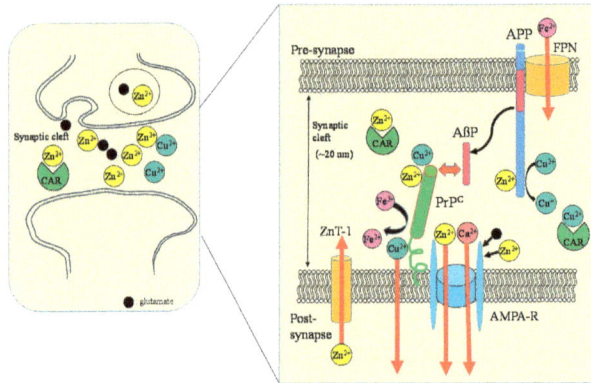

Figure 8. Crosstalk between carnosine, metals, APP, and PrP at the synapse. Zn, Cu, and glutamate accumulate in synaptic vesicles and are released into synaptic clefts during neuronal excitation. Under normal physiological conditions, APP binds Cu and regulates Cu levels by reducing Cu^{2+} to Cu^+. The normal prion protein isoform PrP^C binds to Cu at its N-terminal domain and regulates synaptic Cu levels. It is possible that PrP^C provides Cu to APP or to NMDA-type glutamate receptors, thereby influencing the production of AβP or neuronal excitability. Both APP and PrP^C reportedly attenuate Cu-induced toxicity. PrP^C also controls Zn^{2+} influx into the cells as an analogue of ZIP transporters, with AMPA-type glutamate receptors regulating synaptic Zn^{2+} levels. ZnT-1 is localized to postsynaptic membranes that express NMDA-type glutamate receptors and regulates Zn homeostasis. APP binds ferroportin (FPN) and regulates Fe^{2+} efflux. By contrast, PrP^C acts as ferrireductase to regulate the Fe^{2+}/Fe^{3+} ratio in synapses. The Fe^{2+} ions are transferred to enzymes, including neurotransmitter synthetases. Fe levels also regulate the expression of APP. It is plausible that carnosine binds to Zn^{2+} and Cu^{2+} and regulates homeostasis in these metals. ZnT-1: zinc transporter 1; NMDA-R: NMDA-type glutamate receptor; MT-3: metallothionein 3; CAR: carnosine.

7. Carnosine in Foodstuffs

Considering the beneficial and neuroprotective roles of carnosine, dietary supplementation with carnosine may become important for the prevention of various neurodegenerative diseases. The supplementation with carnosine/anserine improves the cognitive decline of AD model mice [119], or of elderly people [120]. Orally administered carnosine can cause increased carnosine levels in the brain [121]. Moreover, the amount of carnosine is age-dependently decreased [122].

Therefore, the quantitative analysis of carnosine in foods is essential for developing supplementation therapy. For this purpose, we established a convenient system for the analysis of carnosine and anserine in various foods using HPLC [123,124]. However, it is difficult to separate carnosine and anserine by performing reversed phase HPLC with a conventional octadecylsilyl (ODS) column used in ordinary peptide analysis, since carnosine and its analogues are highly hydrophilic and not retained in an ODS column. Thus, we used a carbon column (Hypercarb™ column; Thermo Electron Corp., Waltham, MA, USA) containing porous graphite carbon. The typical chromatograms of standard carnosine and anserine are shown in Figure 9A. Under these conditions, carnosine appeared at 5.7 min and anserine at 7.3 min. We used conventional UV spectroscopy for measuring the absorbance at 215 nm to detect carnosine and anserine. The typical chromatograms of the water extract of chicken breast and the pork shoulder after being heated at 95 °C for 30 min to reduce and remove proteins are shown in Figure 9B,C. The recovery rate of carnosine was determined to be 98.8 ± 6.6% and that of anserine was 99.4 ± 1.8% after this simple pretreatment.

Using this method, the level of carnosine and anserine in food extracts was examined (Figure 10). Our results suggest that relatively high concentrations of carnosine exist in muscles. For example, 1 g of chicken muscle (breast) contained 2.16 ± 0.67 mg/g (i.e., approximately 1 mM) of carnosine. The concentrations of carnosine and anserine were different among species and varied in various regions. These results coincide with previous studies [18].

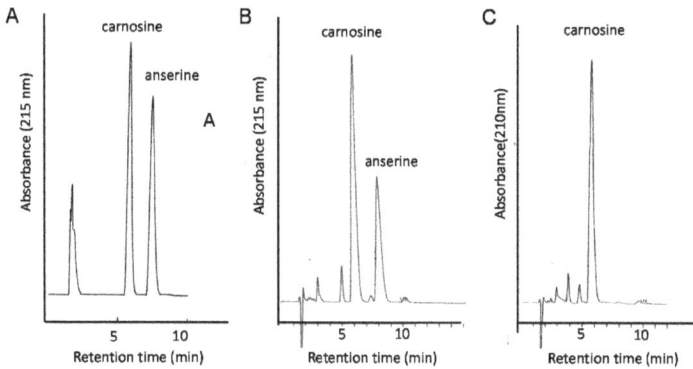

Figure 9. Typical chromatograms of the food extracts examined in this study. Standard solutions carnosine and anserine (**A**); extract of chicken breast (**B**), or extract of pork (**C**) were applied to the HPLC system equipped with a carbon column. Eluent: 0.05% TFA and 7% CH_3CN; flow rate: 1.0 mL/min. The absorbance at 215 nm was observed.

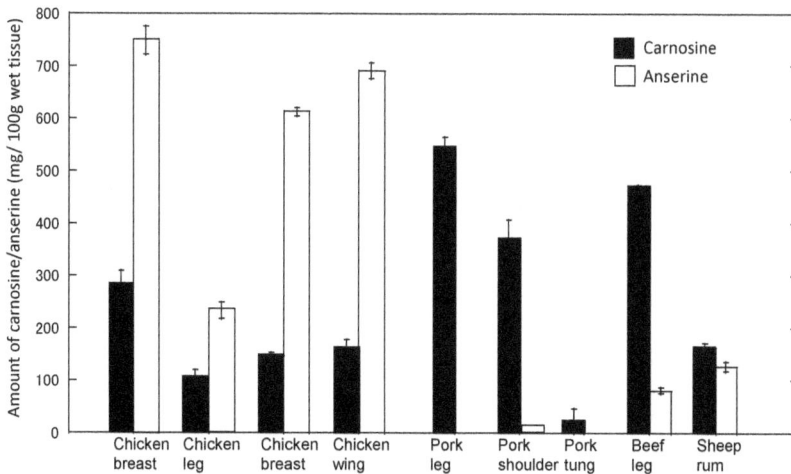

Figure 10. Levels of carnosine and anserine in various foods. The amount of carnosine and anserine of water-soluble extracts of various foods was analyzed by HPLC. Data are expressed as mean $\pm$ S.E.M. ($n = 3$).

Furthermore, we analyzed the amount of carnosine in the muscle of thoroughbred horses and found that the gluteus medius exhibited the highest concentration of carnosine among five muscle tissues (flexor capri radius, triceps branchii, masseter, gluteus medius, sternocleidomastoid). Considering that the gluteus medius is abundant in Type IIa muscles and mainly used in high intensity exercise, carnosine may play essential roles in high intensity exercise. Indeed, the supplementation of β-alanine reportedly increases muscle carnosine concentrations and improves exercise performance, as concluded by the International Society of Sports Nutrition [125].

8. Conclusions and Future Perspectives

Zn plays critical roles in the pathogenesis of neurodegenerative diseases, such as AD, VD, and prion diseases. Although Zn acts as an enhancer of neurotoxicity as well as a protector in AD and VD, it is possible that carnosine, a Zn chelator, acts as a neuroprotector in these diseases owing to its numerous beneficial characteristics including anti-ER stress, antioxidant, and anti-crosslink activities. Additionally, the properties of carnosine such as being water-soluble, heat-inactive, and nontoxic make it a good neuroprotective nutrient beneficial for health. Considering the beneficial characteristics of carnosine, dietary supplementation with carnosine or its component may become useful for health, as carnosine in food plays a critical role in the regulation of Zn homeostasis and the prevention of neurodegenerative diseases. Further research about the molecular mechanism of carnosine in preventing neurotoxicity is required.

Acknowledgments: This work was partially supported by a Grant-in Aid for Scientific Research from the Ministry of Education, Culture, Sports, Science, and Technology of Japan. (JSPS Kakennhi Grant No. 26460177). We thank N. Kobayashi for technical assistance.

Author Contributions: K.-i.T. and M.K. conceived and designed the experiments; K.-i.T. and M.K. conducted experiments. M.K. and M. K.-N. contributed to the writing of the manuscript.

Conflicts of Interest: The authors declare no conflicts of interest.

Abbreviations

AD	Alzheimer's disease
AMPA	amino-3-hydroxy-5-methyl-4-isoxazolepropionic acid
CSF	cerebrospinal fluid
EAR	estimated average
ER	endoplasmic reticulum
GABA	γ-aminobutyric acid
HPLC	high performance liquid chromatography
NMDA	N-methyl-d-aspartate
VD	vascular type of senile dementia
ZIP	Zrt-, Irt-like protein

References

1. Ackland, M.L.; Michalczyk, A.A. Zinc and infant nutrition. *Arch. Biochem. Biophys.* **2016**, *611*, 51–57. [CrossRef] [PubMed]
2. Wessels, I.; Maywald, M.; Rink, L. Zinc as a gatekeeper of immune function. *Nutrients* **2017**, *9*, 1286. [CrossRef] [PubMed]
3. Hojyo, S.; Fukada, T. Roles of Zinc signaling in the immune system. *J. Immunol. Res.* **2016**, *2016*. [CrossRef] [PubMed]
4. Andreini, C.; Banci, L.; Bertini, I.; Rosato, A. Counting the zinc-proteins encoded in the human genome. *J. Proteome Res.* **2006**, *5*, 196–201. [CrossRef] [PubMed]
5. Prasad, A.S. Impact of the discovery of human zinc deficiency on health. *J. Am. Coll. Nutr.* **2009**, *28*, 257–265. [CrossRef] [PubMed]
6. Hambidge, M. Human zinc deficiency. *J. Nutr.* **2000**, *130*, 1344S–1349S. [CrossRef] [PubMed]
7. Takeda, A.; Tamano, H. Subclinical zinc deficiency impairs human brain function. *J. Trace Elem. Med. Biol.* **2012**, *26*, 70–73.
8. Doboszewska, U.; Wlaź, P.; Nowak, G.; Radziwoń-Zaleska, M.; Cui, R.; Młyniec, K. Zinc in the monoaminergic theory of depression: Its relationship to neural plasticity. *Neural Plast.* **2017**, *2017*. [CrossRef] [PubMed]

9. Udechukwu, M.C.; Collins, S.A.; Udenigwe, C.C. Prospects of enhancing dietary zinc bioavailability with food-derived zinc-chelating peptides. *Food Funct.* **2016**, *7*, 4137–4144. [CrossRef] [PubMed]

10. Yasuda, H.; Tsutsui, T. Infants and elderlies are susceptible to zinc deficiency. *Sci. Rep.* **2016**, *6*, 21850. [CrossRef] [PubMed]

11. World Health Organization. Zinc Supplementation and Growth in Children: Biological, Behavioural and Contextual Rationale. Available online: http://www.who.int/elena/bbc/zinc_stunting/en/ (accessed on 21 January 2017).

12. Heintschel, M.; Heuberger, R. The potential role of zinc supplementation on pressure injury healing in older adults: A review of the literature. *Wounds* **2017**, *29*, 56–61. [PubMed]

13. Awotiwon, A.A.; Oduwole, O.; Sinha, A.; Okwundu, C.I. Zinc supplementation for the treatment of measles in children. *Cochrane Database Syst. Rev.* **2017**, *6*, CD011177. [CrossRef] [PubMed]

14. Heyneman, C.A. Zinc deficiency and taste disorders. *Ann. Pharmacother.* **1996**, *30*, 186–187. [CrossRef] [PubMed]

15. Ikeda, M.; Aiba, T.; Ikui, A.; Inokuchi, A.; Kurono, Y.; Sakagami, M.; Takeda, N.; Tomita, H. Taste disorders: A survey of the examination methods and treatments used in Japan. *Acta Otolaryngol.* **2009**, *129*, 1115–1120. [CrossRef]

16. Matsukura, T.; Tanaka, H. Applicability of zinc complex of L-carnosine for medical use. *Biochemistry* **2000**, *65*, 817–823. [PubMed]

17. Suzuki, H.; Mori, M.; Seto, K.; Miyazawa, M.; Kai, A.; Suematsu, M.; Yoneta, T.; Miura, S.; Ishii, H. Polaprezinc attenuates the Helicobacter pylori-induced gastric mucosal leucocyte activation in Mongolian gerbils—A study using intravital videomicroscopy. *Aliment. Pharmacol. Ther.* **2001**, *15*, 715–725. [CrossRef] [PubMed]

18. Boldyrev, A.A.; Aldini, G.; Derave, W. Physiology and pathophysiology of carnosine. *Physiol. Rev.* **2013**, *93*, 1803–1845. [CrossRef] [PubMed]

19. Hipkiss, A.R. On the relationship between energy metabolism, proteostasis, aging and Parkinson's disease: Possible causative role of methylglyoxal and alleviative potential of carnosine. *Aging Dis.* **2017**, *8*, 334–345. [CrossRef] [PubMed]

20. Corona, C.; Frazzini, V.; Silvestri, E.; Lattanzio, R.; La Sorda, R.; Piantelli, M.; Canzoniero, L.M.; Ciavardelli, D.; Rizzarelli, E.; Sensi, S.L. Effects of dietary supplementation of carnosine on mitochondrial dysfunction, amyloid pathology, and cognitive deficits in 3xTg-AD mice. *PLoS ONE* **2011**, *6*, e17971. [CrossRef] [PubMed]

21. Mizuno, D.; Kawahara, M. Carnosine: A possible drug for vascular dementia. *J. Vasc. Med. Surg.* **2014**, *2*, 3. [CrossRef]

22. Kawahara, M.; Koyama, H.; Nagata, T.; Sadakane, Y. Zinc, copper, and carnosine attenuate neurotoxicity of prion fragment PrP106-126. *Metallomics* **2011**, *3*, 726–734. [CrossRef] [PubMed]

23. Chez, M.G.; Buchanan, C.P.; Aimonovitch, M.C.; Becker, M.; Schaefer, K.; Black, C.; Komen, J. Double-blind, placebo-controlled study of L-carnosine supplementation in children with autistic spectrum disorders. *J. Child Neurol.* **2002**, *17*, 833–837. [CrossRef] [PubMed]

24. Baraniuk, J.N.; El-Amin, S.; Corey, R.; Rayhan, R.; Timbol, C. Carnosine treatment for gulf war illness: A randomized controlled trial. *Glob. J. Health Sci.* **2013**, *5*, 69–81. [CrossRef] [PubMed]

25. Rokicki, J.; Li, L.; Imabayashi, E.; Kaneko, J.; Hisatsune, T.; Matsuda, H. Daily carnosine and anserine supplementation alters verbal episodic memory and resting state network connectivity in healthy elderly adults. *Front. Aging Neurosci.* **2015**, *7*, 219. [CrossRef] [PubMed]

26. Frederickson, C.J.; Suh, S.W.; Silva, D.; Frederickson, C.J.; Thompson, R.B. Importance of zinc in the central nervous system: The zinc-containing neuron. *J. Nutr.* **2000**, *130*, 1471S–1483S. [CrossRef] [PubMed]

27. Frederickson, C.J.; Klitenick, M.A.; Manton, W.I.; Kirkpatrick, J.B. Cytoarchitectonic distribution of zinc in the hippocampus of man and the rat. *Brain Res.* **1983**, *27*, 335–339. [CrossRef]

28. Sensi, S.L.; Paoletti, P.; Koh, J.Y.; Aizenman, E.; Bush, A.I.; Hershfinkel, M. The neurophysiology and pathology of brain zinc. *J. Neurosci.* **2011**, *31*, 16076–16085. [CrossRef] [PubMed]

29. Ueno, S.; Tsukamoto, M.; Hirano, T.; Kikuchi, K.; Yamada, M.K.; Nishiyama, N.; Nagano, T.; Matsuki, N.; Ikegaya, Y. Mossy fiber Zn^{2+} spillover modulates heterosynaptic N-methyl-D-aspartate receptor activity in hippocampal CA3 circuits. *J. Cell Biol.* **2002**, *158*, 215–220. [CrossRef] [PubMed]

30. Takeda, A.; Nakamura, M.; Fujii, H.; Tamano, H. Synaptic Zn^{2+} homeostasis and its significance. *Metallomics* **2013**, *5*, 417–423. [CrossRef] [PubMed]

31. Wang, X.; Sommer, F.T.; Hirsch, J.A. Inhibitory circuits for visual processing in thalamus. *Curr. Opin. Neurobiol.* **2011**, *21*, 726–733. [CrossRef] [PubMed]

32. D'Ambrosi, N.; Rossi, L. Copper at synapse: Release, binding and modulation of neurotransmission. *Neurochem. Int.* **2015**, *90*, 36–45. [CrossRef] [PubMed]

33. Schikorski, T.; Stevens, C.F. Quantitative ultrastructural analysis of hippocampal excitatory synapses. *J. Neurosci.* **1997**, *17*, 5858–5867. [PubMed]

34. Vogt, K.; Mellor, J.; Tong, G.; Nicoll, R. The actions of synaptically released zinc at hippocampal mossy fiber synapses. *Neuron* **2000**, *26*, 187–196. [CrossRef]

35. Hopt, A.; Korte, S.; Fink, H.; Panne, U.; Niessner, R.; Jahn, R.; Herms, J. Methods for studying synaptosomal copper release. *J. Neurosci. Methods* **2003**, *128*, 159–172. [CrossRef]

36. Bauer, K. Carnosine and homocarnosine, the forgotten, enigmatic peptides of the brain. *Neurochem. Res.* **2005**, *30*, 1339–1345. [CrossRef] [PubMed]

37. Bolognin, S.; Cozzi, B.; Zambenedetti, P.; Zatta, P. Metallothioneins and the central nervous system: From a deregulation in neurodegenerative diseases to the development of new therapeutic approaches. *J. Alzheimers Dis.* **2014**, *41*, 29–42. [PubMed]

38. Fukada, T.; Kambe, T. Molecular and genetic features of zinc transporters in physiology and pathogenesis. *Metallomics* **2011**, *3*, 662–674. [CrossRef] [PubMed]

39. Bin, B.H.; Fukada, T.; Hosaka, T.; Yamasaki, S.; Ohashi, W.; Hojyo, S.; Miyai, T.; Nishida, K.; Yokoyama, S.; Hirano, T. Biochemical characterization of human ZIP13 protein: A homo-dimerized zinc transporter involved in the spondylocheiro dysplastic ehlers-danlos syndrome. *J. Biol. Chem.* **2011**, *286*, 40255–40265. [CrossRef] [PubMed]

40. Kawahara, M.; Mizuno, D.; Koyama, H.; Konoha, K.; Ohkawara, S.; Sadakane, Y. Disruption of zinc homeostasis and the pathogenesis of senile dementia. *Metallomics* **2013**, *6*, 209–219. [CrossRef] [PubMed]

41. Mizuno, D.; Koyama, H.; Ohkawara, S.; Sadakane, Y.; Kawahara, M. Involvement of trace elements in the pathogenesis of prion diseases. *Curr. Pharam. Biotechnol.* **2014**, *15*, 1049–1057. [CrossRef]

42. Sirangelo, I.; Iannuzzi, C. The role of metal binding in the amyotrophic lateral sclerosis-related aggregation of copper-zinc superoxide dismutase. *Molecules* **2017**, *22*, 1429. [CrossRef] [PubMed]

43. Kawahara, M.; Kato-Negishi, M.; Tanaka, K. Cross talk between neurometals and amyloidogenic proteins at the synapse and the pathogenesis of neurodegenerative diseases. *Metallomics* **2017**, *9*, 619–633. [CrossRef] [PubMed]

44. Selkoe, D.J. The molecular pathology of Alzheimer's disease. *Neuron* **1991**, *6*, 487–498. [CrossRef]

45. Hardy, J.A.; Higgins, G.A. Alzheimer's disease: The amyloid cascade hypothesis. *Science* **1992**, *256*, 184–185. [CrossRef] [PubMed]

46. Wirths, O.; Multhaup, G.; Bayer, T.A. A modified β-amyloid hypothesis: Intraneuronal accumulation of the β-amyloid peptide—The first step of a fatal cascade. *J. Neurochem.* **2004**, *91*, 513–520. [CrossRef] [PubMed]

47. Goate, A.; Chartier-Harlin, M.C.; Mullan, M.; Brown, J.; Crawford, F.; Fidani, L.; Giuffra, L.; Haynes, A.; Irving, N.; James, L.; et al. Segregation of a missense mutation in the amyloid precursor protein gene with familial Alzheimer's disease. *Nature* **1991**, *349*, 704–706. [CrossRef] [PubMed]

48. Yankner, B.A.; Duffy, L.K.; Kirschner, D.A. Neurotropic and neurotoxic effects of amyloid β protein: Reversal by tachykinin neuropeptides. *Nature* **1990**, *250*, 279–282.

49. Kawahara, M.; Negishi-Kato, M.; Sadakane, Y. Calcium dyshomeostasis and neurotoxicity of Alzheimer's beta-amyloid protein. *Expert Rev. Neurother.* **2009**, *9*, 681–693. [CrossRef] [PubMed]

50. Pike, C.J.; Walencewicz, A.J.; Glabe, C.G.; Cotman, C.W. In vitro aging of beta-amyloid protein causes peptide aggregation and neurotoxicity. *Brain Res.* **1991**, *563*, 311–314. [CrossRef]

51. Fukuyama, R.; Mizuno, T.; Mori, S.; Nakajima, K.; Fushiki, S.; Yanagisawa, K. Age-dependent change in the levels of Aβ40 and Aβ42 in cerebrospinal fluid from control subjects, and a decrease in the ratio of Aβ42 to Aβ40 level in cerebrospinal fluid from Alzheimer's disease patients. *Eur. Neurol.* **2000**, *43*, 155–160. [CrossRef] [PubMed]

52. Kawahara, M. Role of calcium dyshomeostasis via amyloid channels in the pathogenesis of Alzheimer's disease. *Curr. Pharm. Des.* **2010**, *16*, 2779–2789. [CrossRef] [PubMed]

53. Dyrks, T.; Dyrks, E.; Masters, C.L.; Beyreuther, K. Amyloidogenicity of rodent and human βA4 sequences. *FEBS Lett.* **1993**, *324*, 231–236. [CrossRef]

54. Bush, A.I.; Pettingell, W.H.; Multhaup, G.; d Paradis, M.; Vonsattel, J.P.; Gusella, J.F.; Beyreuther, K.; Masters, C.L.; Tanzi, R.E. Rapid induction of Alzheimer A-β amyloid formation by zinc. *Science* **1994**, *265*, 1464–1467. [CrossRef] [PubMed]

55. Atwood, C.S.; Moir, R.D.; Huang, X.; Scarpa, R.C.; Bacarra, N.M.; Romano, D.M.; Hartshorn, M.A.; Tanzi, R.E.; Bush, A.I. Dramatic aggregation of Alzheimer Aβ by Cu(II) is induced by conditions representing physiological acidosis. *J. Biol. Chem.* **1998**, *273*, 12817–12826. [CrossRef] [PubMed]

56. Solomonov, I.; Korkotian, E.; Born, B.; Feldman, Y.; Bitler, A.; Rahimi, F.; Li, H.; Bitan, G.; Sagi, I. Zn^{2+}-Aβ40 complexes form metastable quasi-spherical oligomers that are cytotoxic to cultured hippocampal neurons. *J. Biol. Chem.* **2012**, *287*, 20555–20564. [CrossRef] [PubMed]

57. Chen, W.T.; Liao, Y.H.; Yu, H.M.; Cheng, I.H.; Chen, Y.R. Distinct effects of Zn^{2+}, Cu^{2+}, Fe^{3+}, and Al^{3+} on amyloid-beta stability, oligomerization, and aggregation: Amyloid-β destabilization promotes annular protofibril formation. *J. Biol. Chem.* **2011**, *286*, 9646–9656. [CrossRef] [PubMed]

58. Bolognin, S.; Zatta, P.; Lorenzetto, E.; Valenti, M.T.; Buffelli, M. β-Amyloid-aluminum complex alters cytoskeletal stability and increases ROS production in cortical neurons. *Neurochem. Int.* **2013**, *62*, 566–574. [CrossRef] [PubMed]

59. Sharma, A.K.; Pavlova, S.T.; Kim, J.; Kim, J.; Mirica, L.M. The effect of Cu^{2+} and Zn^{2+} on the Aβ42 peptide aggregation and cellular toxicity. *Metallomics* **2013**, *5*, 1529–1536. [CrossRef] [PubMed]

60. Kawahara, M.; Kato, M.; Kuroda, Y. Effects of aluminum on the neurotoxicity of primary cultured neurons and on the aggregation of β-amyloid protein. *Brain Res. Bull.* **2001**, *55*, 211–217. [CrossRef]

61. Small, D.H.; Mok, S.S.; Bornstein, J.C. Alzheimer's disease and Aβ toxicity: From top to bottom. *Nat. Rev. Neurosci.* **2001**, *2*, 595–598. [CrossRef] [PubMed]

62. Demuro, A.; Parker, I.; Stutzmann, G.E. Calcium signaling and amyloid toxicity in Alzheimer disease. *J. Biol. Chem.* **2010**, *285*, 12463–12468. [CrossRef] [PubMed]

63. Arispe, N.; Rojas, E.; Pollard, H.B. Alzheimer disease amyloid β protein forms calcium channels in bilayer membranes: Blockade by tromethamine and aluminum. *Proc. Natl. Acad. Sci. USA* **1993**, *90*, 567–571. [CrossRef] [PubMed]

64. Kawahara, M.; Arispe, N.; Kuroda, Y.; Rojas, E. Alzheimer's disease amyloid β-protein forms Zn^{2+}-sensitive, cation-selective channels across excised membrane patches from hypothalamic neurons. *Biophys. J.* **1997**, *73*, 67–75. [CrossRef]

65. Kawahara, M.; Arispe, N.; Kuroda, Y.; Rojas, E. Alzheimer's β-amyloid, human islet amylin and prion protein fragment evoke intracellular free-calcium elevations by a common mechanism in a hypothalamic GnRH neuronal cell-line. *J. Biol. Chem.* **2000**, *275*, 14077–14083. [CrossRef] [PubMed]

66. Kawahara, M.; Ohtsuka, I.; Yokoyama, S.; Kato-Negishi, M.; Sadakane, Y. Membrane incorporation, channel formation, and disruption of calcium homeostasis by Alzheimer's β-amyloid protein. *Int. J. Alzheimers Dis.* **2011**, *2011*. [CrossRef]

67. Sepulveda, F.J.; Parodi, J.; Peoples, R.W.; Opazo, C.; Aguayo, L.G. Synaptotoxicity of Alzheimer β amyloid can be explained by its membrane perforating property. *PLoS ONE* **2010**, *27*, e11820. [CrossRef] [PubMed]

68. Arispe, N.; Pollard, H.B.; Rojas, E. Zn^{2+} interactions with Alzheimer's amyloid β protein calcium channels. *Proc. Natl. Acad. Sci. USA* **1996**, *93*, 1710–1715. [CrossRef] [PubMed]

69. Lin, H.; Bhatia, R.; Lal, R. Amyloid β protein forms ion channels: Implications for Alzheimer's disease pathophysiology. *FASEB J.* **2001**, *15*, 2433–2444. [CrossRef] [PubMed]

70. Kepp, K.P. Alzheimer's disease due to loss of function: A new synthesis of the available data. *Prog. Neurobiol.* **2016**, *143*, 36–60. [CrossRef] [PubMed]

71. Wild, K.; August, A.; Pietrzik, C.U.; Kins, S. Structure and synaptic function of metal binding to the amyloid precursor protein and its proteolytic fragments. *Front. Mol. Neurosci.* **2017**, *10*, 21. [CrossRef] [PubMed]

72. Rogers, J.T.; Randall, J.D.; Cahill, C.M.; Eder, P.S.; Huang, X.; Gunshin, H.; Leiter, L.; McPhee, J.; Sarang, S.S.; Utsuki, T.; et al. An iron-responsive element type II in the 5′-untranslated region of the Alzheimer's amyloid precursor protein transcript. *J. Biol. Chem.* **2002**, *277*, 45518–45528. [CrossRef] [PubMed]

73. Wong, B.X.; Tsatsanis, A.; Lim, L.Q.; Adlard, P.A.; Bush, A.I.; Duce, J.A. β-Amyloid precursor protein does not possess ferroxidase activity but does stabilize the cell surface ferrous iron exporter ferroportin. *PLoS ONE* **2014**, *9*, e114174. [CrossRef] [PubMed]

74. Soto, C.; Sigurdsson, E.M.; Morelli, L.; Kumar, R.A.; Castaño, E.M.; Frangione, B. β-sheet breaker peptides inhibit fibrillogenesis in a rat brain model of amyloidosis: Implications for Alzheimer's therapy. *Nat. Med.* **1998**, *4*, 822–826. [CrossRef] [PubMed]

75. Babizhayev, M.A. Antioxidant activity of L-carnosine, a natural histidine-containing dipeptide in crystalline lens. *Biochim. Biophys. Acta* **1989**, *1004*, 363–371. [CrossRef]

76. Dubois, V.D.; Bastawrous, A. N-acetylcarnosine (NAC) drops for age-related cataract. *Cochrane Database Syst. Rev.* **2017**, *2*, CD009493. [CrossRef] [PubMed]

77. Aloisi, A.; Barca, A.; Romano, A.; Guerrieri, S.; Storelli, C.; Rinaldi, R.; Verri, T. Anti-aggregating effect of the naturally occurring dipeptide carnosine on Aβ1-42 fibril formation. *PLoS ONE* **2013**, *8*, e68159. [CrossRef] [PubMed]

78. Attanasio, F.; Convertino, M.; Magno, A.; Caflisch, A.; Corazza, A.; Haridas, H.; Esposito, G.; Cataldo, S.; Pignataro, B.; Milardi, D.; et al. Carnosine inhibits Aβ42 aggregation by perturbing the H-bond network in and around the central hydrophobic cluster. *ChemBioChem* **2013**, *14*, 583–592. [CrossRef] [PubMed]

79. Fonteh, A.N.; Harrington, R.J.; Tsai, A.; Liao, P.; Harrington, M.G. Free amino acid and dipeptide changes in the body fluids from Alzheimer's disease subjects. *Amino Acids* **2007**, *32*, 213–224. [CrossRef] [PubMed]

80. Choi, D.W. Calcium: Still center-stage in hypoxic-ischemic neuronal death. *Trends Neurosci.* **1995**, *18*, 58–60. [CrossRef]

81. Choi, D.W.; Koh, J.Y. Zinc and brain injury. *Annu. Rev. Neurosci.* **1998**, *21*, 347–375. [CrossRef] [PubMed]

82. Weiss, J.H.; Sensi, S.L.; Koh, J.Y. Zn^{2+}: A novel ionic mediator of neural injury in brain disease. *Trends Pharmacol. Sci.* **2000**, *21*, 395–401. [CrossRef]

83. Koh, J.Y.; Suh, S.W.; Gwag, B.J.; He, Y.Y.; Hsu, C.Y.; Choi, D.W. The role of zinc in selective neuronal death after transient global cerebral ischemia. *Science* **1996**, *272*, 1013–1016. [CrossRef] [PubMed]

84. Calderone, A.; Jover, T.; Mashiko, T.; Noh, K.M.; Tanaka, H.; Bennett, M.V.; Zukin, R.S. Late calcium EDTA rescues hippocampal CA1 neurons from global ischemia-induced death. *J. Neurosci.* **2004**, *24*, 9903–9913. [CrossRef] [PubMed]

85. Capasso, M.; Jeng, J.M.; Malavolta, M.; Mocchegiani, E.; Sensi, SL. Zinc dyshomeostasis: A key modulator of neuronal injury. *J. Alzheimers Dis.* **2005**, *8*, 93–108. [CrossRef] [PubMed]

86. Kawahara, M.; Kato-Negishi, M.; Kuroda, Y. Pyruvate blocks zinc-induced neurotoxicity in immortalized hypothalamic neurons. *Cell. Mol. Neurobiol.* **2002**, *22*, 87–93. [CrossRef] [PubMed]

87. Koyama, H.; Konoha, K.; Sadakane, Y.; Ohkawara, S.; Kawahara, M. Zinc neurotoxicity and the pathogenesis of vascular-type dementia: Involvement of calcium dyshomeostasis and carnosine. *J. Clin. Toxicol.* **2011**, *S3*. [CrossRef]

88. Mellon, P.L.; Windle, J.J.; Goldsmith, P.C.; Padula, C.A.; Roberts, J.L.; Weiner, R.I. Immortalization of hypothalamic GnRH neurons by genetically targeted tumorigenesis. *Neuron* **1990**, *5*, 1–10. [CrossRef]

89. Konoha, K.; Sadakane, Y.; Kawahara, M. Effects of gadolinium and other metal on the neurotoxicity of immortalized hypothalamic neurons induced by zinc. *Biomed. Res. Trace Elem.* **2004**, *15*, 275–277.

90. Kawahara, M.; Konoha, K.; Nagata, T.; Sadakane, Y. Protective substances against zinc-induced neuronal death after ischemia: Carnosine a target for drug of vascular type of dementia. *Recent Patents CNS Drug Discov.* **2007**, *2*, 145–149. [CrossRef]

91. Sadakane, Y.; Konoha, K.; Nagata, T.; Kawahara, M. Protective activity of the extracts from Japanese eel *(Anguilla japonica)* against zinc-induced neuronal cell death: Carnosine and an unknown substance. *Trace Nutr. Res.* **2007**, *24*, 98–105.

92. Sadakane, Y.; Konoha, K.; Kawahara, M. Protective activity of mango *(Mangifera indica* L.) fruit against a zinc-induced neuronal cell death is independent of its antioxidant activity. *Trace Nutr. Res.* **2005**, *22*, 73–79.

93. Kawahara, M.; Sadakane, Y.; Koyama, H.; Konoha, K.; Ohkawara, S. D-histidine and L-histidine attenuate zinc-induced neuronal death in GT1-7 cells. *Metallomics* **2013**, *5*, 453–460. [CrossRef] [PubMed]

94. Mizuno, D.; Konoha-Mizuno, D.; Mori, M.; Sadakane, Y.; Koyama, H.; Ohkawara, S.; Kawahara, M. Protective activity of carnosine and anserine against zinc-induced neurotoxicity: A possible treatment for vascular dementia. *Metallomics* **2015**, *7*, 1233–1239. [CrossRef] [PubMed]

95. Tanaka, K.; Kawahara, M. Copper enhances zinc-induced neurotoxicity and the endoplasmic reticulum stress response in a neuronal model of vascular dementia. *Front. Neurosci.* **2017**, *11*, 58. [CrossRef] [PubMed]

96. Tanaka, K.; Shimoda, M.; Kawahara, M. Pyruvic acid prevents Cu^{2+}/Zn^{2+}-induced neurotoxicity by suppressing mitochondrial injury. *Biochem. Biophys. Res. Commun.* **2018**, *495*, 1335–1341. [CrossRef] [PubMed]

97. Tanaka, K.; Shimoda, M.; Chuang, V.T.G.; Nishida, K.; Kawahara, M.; Ishida, T.; Otagiri, M.; Maruyama, T.; Ishima, Y. Thioredoxin-albumin fusion protein prevents copper enhanced zinc-induced neurotoxicity via its antioxidative activity. *Int. J. Pharm.* **2018**, *535*, 140–147. [CrossRef] [PubMed]

98. Rajanikant, G.K.; Zemke, D.; Senut, M.C.; Frenkel, M.B.; Chen, A.F.; Gupta, R.; Majid, A. Carnosine is neuroprotective against permanent focal cerebral ischemia in mice. *Stroke* **2007**, *38*, 3023–3031. [CrossRef] [PubMed]

99. Zhang, X.; Song, L.; Cheng, X.; Yang, Y.; Luan, B.; Jia, L.; Xu, F.; Zhang, Z. Carnosine pretreatment protects against hypoxia-ischemia brain damage in the neonatal rat model. *Eur. J. Pharmacol.* **2011**, *667*, 202–207. [CrossRef] [PubMed]

100. Davis, C.K.; Laud, P.J.; Bahor, Z.; Rajanikant, G.K.; Majid, A. Systematic review and stratified meta-analysis of the efficacy of carnosine in animal models of ischemic stroke. *J. Cereb. Blood Flow Metab.* **2016**, *36*, 1686–1694. [CrossRef] [PubMed]

101. Kawahara, M.; Konoha, K.; Nagata, T.; Sadakane, Y. A Drug for Prevention or Treatment for Vascular Dementia. JP5382633, 11 October 2013.

102. Prusiner, S.B. Prion diseases and the BSE crisis. *Science* **1997**, *278*, 245–251. [CrossRef] [PubMed]

103. Carrell, R.W.; Lomas, D.A. Conformational disease. *Lancet* **1997**, *350*, 134–138. [CrossRef]

104. Jackson, G.S.; Murray, I.; Hosszu, L.L.; Gibbs, N.; Waltho, J.P.; Clarke, A.R.; Collinge, J. Location and properties of metal-binding sites on the human prion protein. *Proc. Natl. Acad. Sci. USA* **2001**, *98*, 8531–8535. [CrossRef] [PubMed]

105. Brown, D.R.; Qin, K.; Herms, J.W.; Madlung, A.; Manson, J.; Strome, R.; Fraser, P.E.; Kruck, T.; von Bohlen, A.; Schulz-Schaeffer, W.; et al. The cellular prion protein binds copper in vivo. *Nature* **1997**, *390*, 684–687. [CrossRef] [PubMed]

106. Brown, D.R. Brain proteins that mind metals: A neurodegenerative perspective. *Dalton Trans.* **2009**, *21*, 4069–4076. [CrossRef] [PubMed]

107. Schmitt-Ulms, G.; Ehsani, S.; Watts, J.C.; Westaway, D.; Wille, H. Evolutionary descent of prion genes from the ZIP family of metal ion transporters. *PLoS ONE* **2009**, *4*, e7208. [CrossRef] [PubMed]

108. Watt, N.T.; Griffiths, H.H.; Hooper, N.M. Neuronal zinc regulation and the prion protein. *Prion* **2013**, *7*, 203–208. [CrossRef] [PubMed]

109. Bonetto, V.; Massignan, T.; Chiesa, R.; Morbin, M.; Mazzoleni, G.; Diomede, L.; Angeretti, N.; Colombo, L.; Forloni, G.; Tagliavini, F.; et al. Synthetic miniprion PrP106. *J. Biol. Chem.* **2002**, *277*, 31327–31334. [CrossRef] [PubMed]

110. Kang, J.H.; Kim, K.S. Enhanced oligomerization of the alpha-synuclein mutant by the Cu, Zn-superoxide dismutase and hydrogen peroxide system. *Mol. Cells* **2003**, *15*, 87–93. [PubMed]

111. Villari, V.; Attanasio, F.; Micali, N. Control of the structural stability of α-crystallin under thermal and chemical stress: The role of carnosine. *J. Phys. Chem. B* **2014**, *118*, 13770–13776. [CrossRef] [PubMed]

112. Del Prete, D.; Lombino, F.; Liu, X.; D'Adamio, L. APP is cleaved by Bace1 in pre-synaptic vesicles and establishes a pre-synaptic interactome, via its intracellular domain, with molecular complexes that regulate pre-synaptic vesicles functions. *PLoS ONE* **2014**, *9*, e108576. [CrossRef] [PubMed]

113. Stys, P.K.; You, H.; Zamponi, G.W. Copper-dependent regulation of NMDA receptors by cellular prion protein: Implications for neurodegenerative disorders. *J. Physiol.* **2012**, *590*, 1357–1368. [CrossRef] [PubMed]

114. Mellone, M.; Pelucchi, S.; Alberti, L.; Genazzani, A.A.; Di Luca, M.; Gardoni, F. Zinc transporter-1: A novel NMDA receptor-binding protein at the postsynaptic density. *J. Neurochem.* **2015**, *132*, 159–168. [CrossRef] [PubMed]

115. Howells, C.; West, A.K.; Chung, R.S. Neuronal growth-inhibitory factor (metallothionein-3): Evaluation of the biological function of growth-inhibitory factor in the injured and neurodegenerative brain. *FEBS J.* **2010**, *277*, 2931–2939. [CrossRef] [PubMed]

116. Uchida, Y.; Takio, K.; Titani, K.; Ihara, Y.; Tomonaga, M. The growth inhibitory factor that is deficient in the Alzheimer's disease brain is a 68 amino acid metallothionein-like protein. *Neuron* **1991**, *7*, 337–347. [CrossRef]

117. De Marchis, S.; Modena, C.; Peretto, P.; Migheli, A.; Margolis, F.L.; Fasolo, A. Carnosine-related dipeptides in neurons and glia. *Biochemistry* **2000**, *65*, 824–833. [PubMed]
118. Bakardjiev, A. Carnosine and β-alanine release is stimulated by glutamatergic receptors in cultured rat oligodendrocytes. *Glia* **1998**, *24*, 346–351. [CrossRef]
119. Kaneko, J.; Enya, A.; Enomoto, K.; Ding, Q.; Hisatsune, T. Anserine (beta-alanyl-3-methyl-L-histidine) improves neurovascular-unit dysfunction and spatial memory in aged AβPPswe/PSEN1dE9 Alzheimer's-model mice. *Sci. Rep.* **2017**, *7*, 12571. [CrossRef] [PubMed]
120. Hisatsune, T.; Kaneko, J.; Kurashige, H.; Cao, Y.; Satsu, H.; Totsuka, M.; Katakura, Y.; Imabayashi, E.; Matsuda, H. Effect of anserine/carnosine supplementation on verbal episodic memory in elderly people. *J. Alzheimers Dis.* **2016**, *50*, 149–159. [CrossRef] [PubMed]
121. Tomonaga, S.; Hayakawa, T.; Yamane, H.; Maemura, H.; Sato, M.; Takahata, Y.; Morimatsu, F.; Furuse, M. Oral administration of chicken breast extract increases brain carnosine and anserine concentrations in rats. *Nutr. Neurosci.* **2007**, *10*, 181–186. [CrossRef] [PubMed]
122. Stuerenburg, H.J. The roles of carnosine in aging of skeletal muscle and in neuromuscular diseases. *Biochemistry* **2000**, *65*, 862–865. [PubMed]
123. Mori, M.; Mizuno, D.; Konoha-Mizuno, K.; Sadakane, Y.; Kawahara, M. Quantitative analysis of carnosine and anserine in foods by performing high performance liquid chromatography. *Biomed. Res. Trace Elem.* **2015**, *26*, 147–152.
124. Mori, M.; Mizuno, D.; Konoha-Mizuno, K.; Sadakane, Y.; Kawahara, M. Carnosine concentration in the muscle of thoroughbred horses and its implications in exercise performance. *Trace Nutr. Res.* **2015**, *32*, 49–53.
125. Trexler, E.T.; Smith-Ryan, A.E.; Stout, J.R.; Hoffman, J.R.; Wilborn, C.D.; Sale, C.; Kreider, R.B.; Jäger, R.; Earnest, C.P.; Bannock, L.; et al. International society of sports nutrition position stand: Beta-Alanine. *J. Int. Soc. Sports Nutr.* **2015**, *12*, 30. [CrossRef] [PubMed]

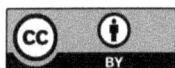

nutrients

MDPI

Review

Zinc and Skin Disorders

Youichi Ogawa *, Manao Kinoshita, Shinji Shimada and Tatsuyoshi Kawamura

Department of Dermatology, Faculty of Medicine, University of Yamanashi, Yamanashi 409-3898, Japan;
mkinoshita@yamanashi.ac.jp (M.K.); sshimada@yamanashi.ac.jp (S.S.); tkawa@yamanashi.ac.jp (T.K.)
* Correspondence: yogawa@yamanashi.ac.jp; Tel./Fax: +81-155-273-6766

Received: 7 December 2017; Accepted: 9 February 2018; Published: 11 February 2018

Abstract: The skin is the third most zinc (Zn)-abundant tissue in the body. The skin consists of the epidermis, dermis, and subcutaneous tissue, and each fraction is composed of various types of cells. Firstly, we review the physiological functions of Zn and Zn transporters in these cells. Several human disorders accompanied with skin manifestations are caused by mutations or dysregulation in Zn transporters; acrodermatitis enteropathica (Zrt-, Irt-like protein (ZIP)4 in the intestinal epithelium and possibly epidermal basal keratinocytes), the spondylocheiro dysplastic form of Ehlers-Danlos syndrome (ZIP13 in the dermal fibroblasts), transient neonatal Zn deficiency (Zn transporter (ZnT)2 in the secretory vesicles of mammary glands), and epidermodysplasia verruciformis (ZnT1 in the epidermal keratinocytes). Additionally, acquired Zn deficiency is deeply involved in the development of some diseases related to nutritional deficiencies (acquired acrodermatitis enteropathica, necrolytic migratory erythema, pellagra, and biotin deficiency), alopecia, and delayed wound healing. Therefore, it is important to associate the existence of mutations or dysregulation in Zn transporters and Zn deficiency with skin manifestations.

Keywords: zinc; skin; acrodermatitis enteropathica; Langerhans cells; ATP; nutrition

1. Introduction

In the human body, zinc (Zn) is stably maintained in the weight of 2–3 g [1]. Skin is the third most Zn-abundant tissue in the body (skeletal muscle 60%, bones 30%, liver 5%, and skin 5%) [1]. The epidermis contains more Zn compared with the dermis [2]. In the epidermis, Zn is more abundantly distributed throughout the stratum spinosum than the other three layers of keratinocytes (KCs) [3]. In the dermis, Zn concentration in the upper dermis is higher than it in the lower dermis [2]. Zn is enriched in the granules of mast cells (MCs) [4] and MCs are more abundant in the upper dermis than in the lower dermis [5,6]. Therefore, the difference in dermal MC distributions may explain the difference of Zn distributions within the dermis.

Zn is present as a divalent ion (Zn^{2+}) in cells and does not need a redox reaction upon crossing the cellular membrane. Thus, the tight regulation needed to maintain Zn homeostasis in cells is assumed by two solute-linked carrier (SLC) gene families: Zn transporter (ZnT; SLC30A) and Zrt-, Irt-like protein (ZIP; SLC39A) (reviewed in [7–10]). ZnTs and ZIPs are involved in Zn efflux and uptake, respectively. 10 ZnT and 14 ZIP were identified in humans so far [7]. Besides ZnTs and ZIPs, metallothioneins (MTs) also assume Zn regulation. MTs that ubiquitously distribute in the cytoplasm contain a unique cysteine-rich amino acid sequence. This allows MTs to bind to Zn, copper, and cadmium. An excess cytosolic Zn binds to MTs, whereas Zn is released from MTs in the condition of Zn deficiency or Zn required. Consequently, MTs function as a regulator of Zn homeostasis [11].

In this review, we review the relationship between Zn and the skin, including the function and distribution of Zn, ZnTs, ZIPs, and MTs in the skin with adding new recent findings in our recent review [12] by introducing the function of Zn and Zn transporters in various types of skin cells. Additionally, we expanded the description of Zn deficiency-related human disorders accompanied with skin manifestations. We started this review by describing the physiological functions of Zn and Zn transporters in various types of cells of skin (Section 2), followed by human skin disorders caused by mutations of Zn transporters (Section 3), human skin disorders caused by dysregulation of Zn transporters (Section 4), and human skin disorders associated with Zn deficiency (Section 5).

2. Physiological Functions of Zn and Zn Transporters in the Skin

Zn is a cofactor for over 1000 enzymatic reactions [13,14] and is necessary for over 2000 transcription factors [15]. Zn-finger proteins function for DNA interaction, RNA packaging, activation of transcription, regulation of apoptosis, folding and assembly of protein, and lipid binding [16–18]. Additionally, about 10% of human proteins binds to Zn [19]. Therefore, Zn is associated with a wide variety of organic activities such as development, differentiation, and cell growth.

The skin consists of the epidermis, dermis, and subcutaneous tissue. Each skin region contains the following cells: epidermis; KCs, Langerhans cells (LCs), and melanocytes, dermis; antigen-presenting cells (dendritic cells (DCs), macrophages, and monocytes), T cells, MCs, fibroblasts, endothelial cells, etc., subcutaneous tissue; adipocytes. A review of the reported function of Zn and Zn transporters in these cells follows below (Figure 1).

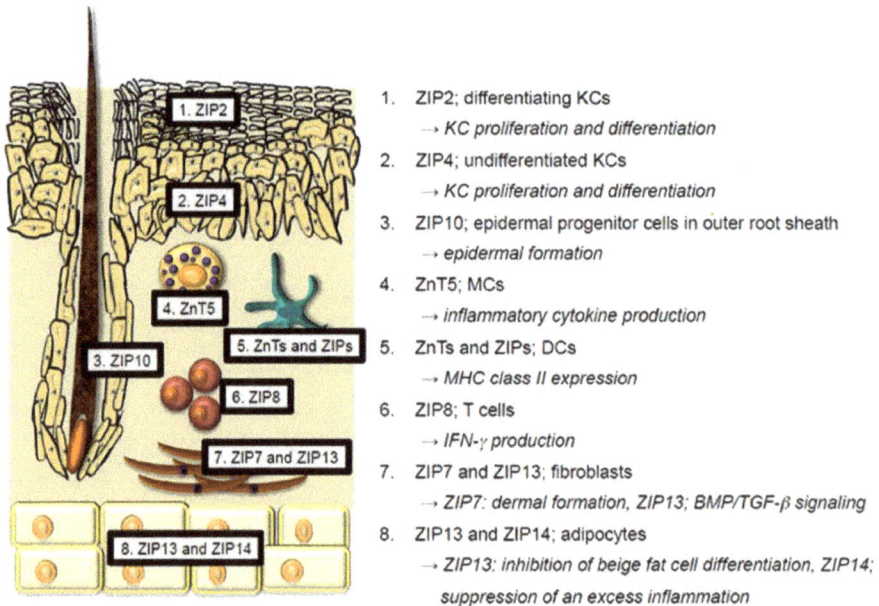

1. ZIP2; differentiating KCs
   → *KC proliferation and differentiation*
2. ZIP4; undifferentiated KCs
   → *KC proliferation and differentiation*
3. ZIP10; epidermal progenitor cells in outer root sheath
   → *epidermal formation*
4. ZnT5; MCs
   → *inflammatory cytokine production*
5. ZnTs and ZIPs; DCs
   → *MHC class II expression*
6. ZIP8; T cells
   → *IFN-γ production*
7. ZIP7 and ZIP13; fibroblasts
   → *ZIP7: dermal formation, ZIP13; BMP/TGF-β signaling*
8. ZIP13 and ZIP14; adipocytes
   → *ZIP13: inhibition of beige fat cell differentiation, ZIP14; suppression of an excess inflammation*

Figure 1. Reported distribution and function of Zn transporters in the skin. Every skin cell expresses many different Zn transporters. However, the expression and role of Zn transporters in skin cells are less understood. This figure shows the reported distribution and representative function of Zn transporters in the skin. 1 and 2. ZIP2 and ZIP4 in KCs facilitate KC proliferation and differentiation. 3. ZIP10 expressed in the epidermal progenitor cells in outer root sheath is crucial for the proper epidermal formation. 4. ZnT5 in MCs is involved in inflammatory cytokine production. 5. Many ZnTs and ZIPs regulate MHC class II expression in DCs. 6. ZIP8 in T cells is involved in interferon-γ (IFN-γ) production. 7. ZIP7 and ZIP13 in fibroblasts are required for the dermal formation and bone morphogenetic protein/transforming growth factor-β (BMP/TGF-β) signaling, respectively. 8. ZIP13 in adipocytes inhibits beige fat cell differentiation. ZIP14 in adipocytes suppresses an excess inflammation.

2.1. Keratinocytes

Keratinocytes (KCs) occupy approximately 97% of epidermis and are categorized into four layers according to the degree of differentiation and keratinization. These layers include the basal layer, stratum spinosum, stratum granulosum, and stratum corneum. As described, Zn concentrations are most abundant in the stratum spinosum, more so than in the other three KC layers [3]. However, the physiological reason for this is not known. An in vitro experiment demonstrated that exposing HaCaT KCs (human immortalized KCs) to a nontoxic concentration of Zn facilitates survival and proliferation [20]. In contrast, a chelation of intracellular Zn by N,N,N',N'-tetrakis (2-pyridylmethyl) ethylenediamine (TPEN) activates caspase-3 and DNA fragmentation, resulting in the apoptosis of KCs [21,22]. Further, a Zn-deficient diet alters the expression of keratin polypeptides in rats because of impaired keratinolytic enzyme activity [23]. In an in vitro experiment using normal human epidermal KCs, Zn suppressed IFN-γ-induced KC activation and tumor necrosis factor-α (TNF-α) production via unknown underlying mechanisms [24]. Zn also diminishes inducible nitric oxide synthase (iNOS) induction and subsequent nitric oxide (NO) production in Pam212 KCs (murine immortalized KCs) [25]. These data suggest that Zn is required for the proliferation of KCs and the suppression of inflammation in KCs (reviewed in [26]). These effects of Zn on KCs account for the clinical effects of Zn oxide ointment on skin inflammation and ulcers.

Recent research elucidated the functions of some ZIP proteins that are expressed in KCs. In mice, ZIP2 is almost exclusively expressed in the epidermis, but not in the dermis. ZIP2 is expressed in differentiating KCs. Knockdown (KD) of ZIP2 in KCs interferes with KC differentiation and proliferation. Thus, Zn uptake through ZIP2 is essential for terminal differentiation of KCs [3]. ZIP4 is associated with the development of acrodermatitis enteropathica (AE; OMIM 201100). Although ZIP4 is highly expressed in the apical side of the intestinal epithelium, human epidermal KCs also express ZIP4, particularly in undifferentitated KCs. In human epidermal KCs, ZIP4 KD reduces intracellular Zn levels up to half, interferes with normal KC differentiation, and promotes KC proliferation, thereby leading to the parakeratosis [27]. Although these histological changes by ZIP4 KD in KCs are not identical to the histological changes in AE, ZIP4, and ZIP2 are involved in the normal KC differentiation and proliferation. Zn is deeply involved in hair biology. For example, Zn deficiency (ZnD) induces telogen effluvium and abnormal hair keratinization (reviewed in [12]). Murine ZIP10 is highly expressed in the epidermal progenitor cells located in the outer root sheath of hair follicles. Thus, depletion of ZIP10 in keratin14-expressing cells results in a thin epidermis and hair follicle hypoplasia because of downregulation of the transcriptional activity of p63, a critical regulator of epidermal formation [28]. MTs are proteins that are ubiquitously expressed throughout various types of cells and predominantly distribute in the cytoplasm, and to a lesser extent in the nuclei and lysosomes [29]. MTs are comprised of four isoforms; MT-1, MT-2, MT-3, and MT-4 [30]. In the human skin, MT-1 and MT-2 are expressed in actively proliferating cells such as hair matrix, outer hair roots, and basal layer KCs [31]. These MT expressions are further upregulated in the hyperplastic KCs of inflamed skin lesions and skin cancers in conditions such as actinic keratosis, squamous cell carcinoma, and basal cell carcinoma [32]. Knock out (KO) of both MT-1 and MT-2 in mice impairs KC proliferation [33]. Thus, MT-1 and MT-2 regulate KC proliferation, likely cooperating with ZIP2 and ZIP4 in the epidermis. Similarly, MT-3 is expressed in human epidermal KCs, and its expression appears to be upregulated in skin cancers [34,35]. MT-4 expression in murine neonatal skin is reported [36]. However, the expression and function in human skin are not understood. In summary, ZIP2 and ZIP4 in KCs facilitate KC proliferation and differentiation. ZIP10 expressed in the epidermal progenitor cells in outer root sheath is crucial for the proper epidermal formation. MTs in KCs also facilitate KC proliferation.

2.2. Langerhans Cells

Langerhans cells (LCs) are one subset of antigen-presenting cells that distribute in the epidermis [37]. LCs are involved in the development of cutaneous manifestations of acrodermatitis enteropathica (AE), a rare autosomal recessive disease. AE is caused by a mutation in the SLC39A4 gene that encodes ZIP4 followed by Zn deficiency (ZnD) because of a disability of Zn absorption within the intestines (reviewed in [38] and [39]). We found that epidermal LCs were absent in AE skin lesions. Additionally, LC loss in the epidermis was reproducible using mice with Zn-deficient diets (ZD mice) [40] (Figure 2).

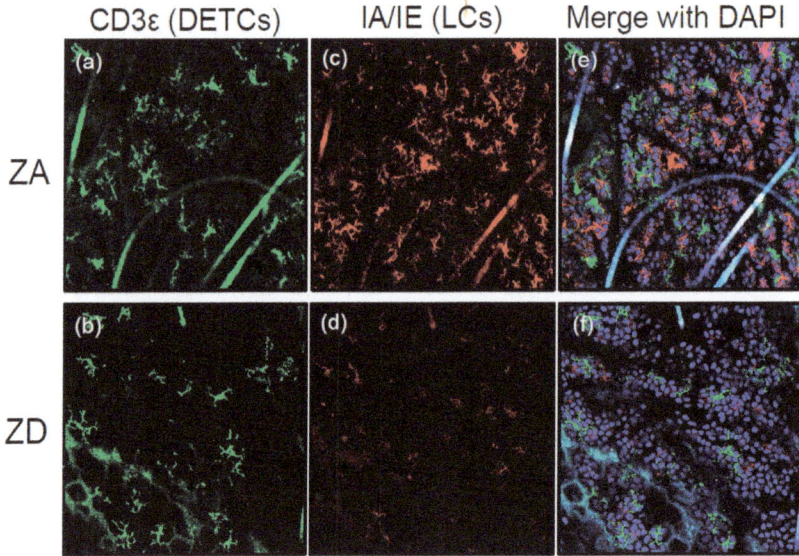

Figure 2. LC loss in ZD ear epidermis. Immunofluorescence of epidermal whole mounts stained for IA/IE (red) and CD3ε (green) from mice fed ZA or ZD diets for seven weeks. Original magnification, ×100. IA/IE-positive LCs are absent in ZD ear epidermis (**c**) and (**d**); whereas the distribution of CD3ε-positive dendritic epidermal T cells are unaffected (**a**) and (**b**). (**a**) and (**c**) merge with DAPI is (**e**); (**b**) and (**d**) merge with DAPI is (**f**).

In patients with AE and ZD mice, transforming growth factor-β1 (TGF-β1) expression in the epidermis was impaired compared with healthy people and mice with Zn-adequate (ZA) diets (ZA mice). TGF-β1 is essential for LC homeostasis [41]. Because several Zn finger transcription factors (e.g., ZNF580) are involved in TGF-β signaling [42], ZnD might decrease TGF-β1 production in LCs and KCs by influencing the activity of those transcription factors. Therefore, impaired TGF-β1 expression in the epidermis is, at least in part, responsible for LC loss (Figure 3). Another possibility for LC loss is apoptosis. In the steady state, epidermal LCs of ZD mice exhibited an increased apoptosis rate. Murine and human LCs underwent apoptosis when cultured with TPEN, whereas the culture condition did not induce apoptosis of KCs. This suggests that LCs are prone to apoptosis in the condition of ZnD. It is worth noting that LCs were replenished in the epidermis after Zn supplementation in patients with AE and ZD mice. Considered with these findings, severe ZnD induces LC apoptosis through a synergy of its direct effect and impaired TGF-β1 expression, leading to a disappearance of epidermal LC [40] (Figures 2 and 3). In summary, Zn is critical for LC homeostasis. Despite the importance of Zn in LCs, the expression and function of ZnTs, ZIPs, and MTs in LCs are poorly understood.

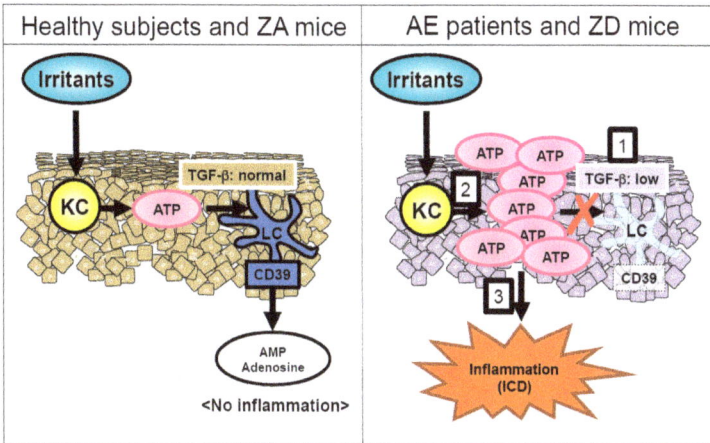

Figure 3. An underlying mechanism of development of acrodermatitis. Right panel: 1. In patients with AE and ZD mice, TGF-β1 expression in the epidermis is impaired compared with healthy subjects and ZA mice. Subsequently, LCs disappear from the epidermis. LCs are the sole CD39 (ecto-NTPDase1)-expressing cells in the epidermis. 2. Ear epidermis from ZD mice produces much more ATP upon the exposure of irritants than it from ZA mice. Additionally, this ATP is not hydrolyzed because of the absence of CD39-expressing LCs. 3. ATP in the epidermis elicits ICD, followed by the formation of acrodermatitis in AE.

2.3. Melanocytes

In an in vitro experiment, exposure of human melanocytes recovered from healthy skin to exogenous and nontoxic levels of Zn increases intracellular Zn levels, particularly in lysosomes and melanosomes. This enhances proliferation of human melanocytes with upregulated expression of AKT3, extracellular signal–regulated kinase1/2 (ERK1/2), c-MYC, and CYCD and enhances mitochondrial biosynthesis, followed by the upregulated process of autophagy [43]. In summary, Zn facilitates the melanocyte proliferation and the autophagy. The expression and function of ZnTs, ZIPs, and MTs in melanocytes are poorly understood. However, MT expression in melanoma may correlate with an increased risk of its progression and metastasis [44,45].

2.4. Mast Cells and Dendritic Cells

Besides the proliferative effect of Zn on various types of cells, Zn also functions as an intracellular signaling molecule, like calcium, by transducing extracellular stimuli into intracellular signaling (reviewed in [16,46]).

In mast cells (MCs), cytosolic Zn promotes FcεRI-induced granule translocation and subsequent degranulation. ZnT5 mRNA is abundant in MCs and its expression is upregulated by FcεRI stimulation. Zn and ZnT5 cooperatively translocate protein kinase C (PKC) to the plasma membrane, and the subsequent nuclear translocation of nuclear factor kappa-light-chain-enhancer of activated B cells (NF-κB), thereby promoting the production of inflammatory cytokines like IL-6 and TNF-α [47,48]. In summary, Zn and ZnT5 in MCs are involved in inflammatory cytokine production.

In dendritic cells (DCs), Zn is involved in its maturation. Upon lipopolysaccharides (LPS) stimulation of murine DCs, ZIP6 and ZIP10 are downregulated, whereas ZnT1, ZnT4, and ZnT6 are upregulated. This decreases intracellular free Zn. Because Zn promotes the endocytosis of major histocompatibility complex (MHC) class II and inhibits its trafficking from the lysosome/endosome to the plasma membrane. Decreased intracellular free Zn facilitates upregulation of surface MHC class II expression [49]. In summary, Zn and Zn transporters regulate MHC class II expression in DCs.

2.5. T cells

ZnD induces atrophy of the thymus accompanied by reduced double-positive thymocytes, decreasing the number of mature single positive T cells [50–52]. This is mediated by elevated glucocorticoids from adrenal glands and subsequent enhancement of apoptosis rate within double-positive thymocytes [53]. This suggests that Zn is required for the normal T cell generation [26].

Although the expressions and functions of ZnTs, ZIPs, and MTs in T cells are less understood, ZIP8 is enriched in human T cells, and its expression is markedly upregulated by in vitro activation with T cell receptor (TCR) engagement [54]. Although ZIP8 is localized to both the plasma membrane and lysosomes, ZIP8 in T cells is primarily localized to lysosomes. ZIP8 KD in T cells reduces IFN-γ production, whereas overexpression of ZIP8 in T cells enhances it [54], suggesting that Zn transport from lysosomes to the cytoplasm facilitates IFN-γ production in T cells. In summary, ZIP8 in T cells is involved in IFN-γ production.

2.6. Endothelial Cells

Zn chelation leads to death of endothelial cells (ECs). On the other hand, chronic exposure to Zn accelerates senescence of ECs in an in vitro experiment [55]. An exposure to 25 μM Zn^{2+} impedes the migration of human ECs [56]. Similarly, Zn oxide nanoparticles inhibit angiogenesis [57]. These data suggest that Zn is involved in the cell viability of ECs and angiogenesis.

Chronic exposure to Zn upregulates the mRNA expression of ZnT1 and ZIP6, downregulates the mRNA expression of ZnT5 and ZIP10, and does not alter the mRNA expression of ZIP1, ZIP2, and ZIP3 [55]. As for MTs in ECs, human ECs express MT-1E, MT-1X, MT-2A, and MT-3. An exposure to Zn induces the expression of most MT-1 isoforms. MT-2A KD leads to the decreased proliferation and the increased migration of ECs [58]. Collectively, Zn alters the expression of ZnTs, ZIPs, and MTs in ECs. However, the function of ZnTs and ZIPs in ECs remains to be identified.

2.7. Fibroblasts

It is known that Zn promotes lipogenesis and glucose transport via its insulin-like effects on 3T3-L1 fibroblasts and adipocytes [59]. Recent research elucidated the critical roles of ZIP7 and ZIP13 in connective tissue homeostasis. Both are intracellular Zn transporters, have quite similar amino acid sequences, and share various functional characteristics [60]. However, there are some differences. (1) ZIP7 is predominantly localized in the endoplasmic reticulum (ER), whereas ZIP13 is predominantly localized in the Golgi apparatus [60]. (2) ZIP7 is distributed throughout various types of cells, whereas ZIP13 is primarily localized in connective tissues [61,62]. ZIP7 KO mice in collagen1-expressing cells exhibit thin dermis with reduced collagen1 deposition, thin subcutaneous tissues, and a reduced number of hair follicles. Additionally, ZIP7 KD in human mesenchymal stem cells inhibits proliferation and differentiation into fibroblasts, osteoblasts, and chondrocytes [63]. As described, ZIP7 is localized in ER and transports Zn from the ER lumen to the cytoplasm. ZIP7 KD increases Zn levels in the ER, resulting in Zn-dependent aggregation and inactivation of protein disulfide isomerase, which controls proper protein folding. Thus, ER stress is overwhelming in ZIP7 KD cells, and these cells undergo apoptosis [63]. These data suggest that Zn regulation by ZIP7 in the ER is critical for the proper ER function and prevention of ER stress-induced cell death. Accordingly, the third difference between ZIP7 and ZIP13 is that ZIP7 KD induces ER stress, whereas ZIP13 KD does not induce it [64]. In conclusion, ZIP7 in fibroblasts is required for the proper dermal formation. The role of ZIP13 in fibroblasts is described later.

2.8. Adipocytes

ZIP13 is also involved in adipocyte biology. Adipocytes are divided into white and brown adipocytes. The former stores energy, whereas the latter consumes it. Additionally, other brown adipocyte-like cells, named beige adipocytes, are recently found within white adipose tissue, which is developed by various stimuli such as chronic cold exposure and long-term peroxisome proliferator-activated receptor γ (PPARγ) agonist treatment [65–67]. CCAAT-enhancer-binding protein-β (C/EBP-β) is induced in the early phases of adipogenesis and is necessary to activate PPARγ [68]. As described, ZIP13 is localized in the Golgi apparatus and transports Zn from the Golgi lumen to the cytoplasm. This Zn inhibits C/EBP-β activation and subsequent PPARγ activation, leading to the inhibition of beige fat cell differentiation. Conversely, ZIP13 KD facilitates beige fat cell differentiation. This enhances energy consumption, leading to the inhibition of obesity [69].

Inflammatory cytokines proliferate adipocytes, expanding cell mass through both hypertrophy and hyperplasia [70]. ZIP14 is localized to the plasma membrane, and its expression is upregulated by inflammatory cytokines and/or LPS [71]. Adipocytes from ZIP14 KO mice increase cytokine production by activating the NF-κB and signal transducer and activator of transcription 3 (STAT3) pathways [72]. These data suggest that ZIP14, which is upregulated in adipocytes during inflammation, may suppress excess inflammation.

Besides the involvement of ZIP13 and ZIP14 in adipocyte biology, many Zn finger proteins, which are proteins containing the Zn finger domains, are involved in adipogenesis [73].

3. Human Skin Disorders Caused by Mutations of Zn Transporters

Some genetic disorders are caused by mutations of Zn transporter genes. Among these disorders, mutations of ZIP4, ZIP13, and ZnT2 accompany skin manifestations.

3.1. ZIP4 Mutation; Acrodermatitis Enteropathica (AE; OMIM 201100)

As described in Section 2.2, AE is caused by loss-of-function mutations in ZIP4 followed by ZnD because of a disability of Zn absorption in the intestines. Since this discovery, over 30 mutations are reported [74]. The clinical symptoms are skin manifestations, alopecia, and diarrhea. Skin manifestations that are characterized by ZnD are referred to as acrodermatitis, and occur on periorificial, anogenital, and acral regions, where frequent contact with external substances is expected. Therefore, we presumed that acrodermatitis occurs as a consequence of contact dermatitis (CD). We utilized skin specimens of patients with AE and ZD mice to examine this hypothesis [40].

ZD mice exhibited an impaired allergic CD in response to dinitrofluorobenzene (DNFB) compared with ZA mice, because of an immunodeficiency in the ZD mice. On the other hand, ZD mice exhibited a significantly increased and prolonged irritant CD (ICD) in response to croton oil (CrO) compared with ZA mice. Adenosine triphosphate (ATP) is released from KCs in response to various environmental stimuli through lytic and non-lytic mechanisms [75–77]. ATP released from chemically injured mouse KCs causes ICD [77]. In an ex vivo organ culture, the released ATP amount from skin upon CrO application was much greater in the skin of ZD mice than in the skin of ZA mice. Additionally, an injection of apyrase that hydrolyzes ATP into adenosine monophosphate (AMP) restored the increased and prolonged ICD upon CrO application in ZD mice. These results suggest that the prolonged ICD response in ZD mice was mediated via the excess ATP release by KCs in response to irritants (Figure 3). As described in Section 2.2, epidermal LCs were absent in the lesioned skin of AE and ZD mice (Figure 2). LCs but not KCs express CD39 (ecto-nucleoside triphosphate diphosphohydrolase 1 (ecto-NTPDase1)) that potently hydrolyzes ATP into AMP [77,78]. Thus, the impaired ATP hydrolysis because of the disappearance of LCs leads to ATP-mediated inflammation in the epidermis, followed by the development of ICD (Figure 3).

3.2. ZIP13 Mutation; Spondylocheiro Dysplastic Form of Ehlers–Danlos Syndrome (SCD-EDS; OMIM 612350)

As described in Section 2.7, ZIP13 is localized to connective tissue cells including fibroblasts. A study with ZIP13 KO mice revealed that ZIP13 is necessary for the nuclear translocation of Smads in BMP/TGF-β signaling [61]. Thus, ZIP13 is crucial for connective tissue formation. Homozygous loss-of-function mutations of the ZIP13 gene cause SCD-EDS [61,79], characterized by hyperelastic and thin skin and hypermobility of the small joints.

3.3. ZnT2 Mutation; Transient Neonatal Zn Deficiency (TNZD; OMIM 608118)

Zn concentration in milk is maintained at higher levels than in serum, because Zn in breast milk is critical for the growth and survival of neonates [80]. In mice, the ZnT2 mutation causes severe ZnD in pups because of low Zn concentrations in breast milk. Like ZnT2-mutated mice, the breast milk from mice with a loss-of-function mutation of ZnT4 (lethal milk mutant mice; OMIM 602095) is deficient in Zn. Nursing pups of lethal milk mutant mice die before weaning [81]. Both ZnT2 and ZnT4 are localized in cytoplasmic secretory vesicles and efflux Zn from the cytoplasm to cytoplasmic secretory vesicles [7]. In humans, ZnT2 is essential for maintaining proper Zn concentrations in breast milk. Because breast milk from ZnT2-mutated mothers contains lower Zn, breast-feeding neonates show similar symptoms with AE [39,82–85]. On the other hand, there are no reports of ZnT4 involvement in Zn transport into secretory vesicles in humans.

4. Human Skin Disorders Caused by Dysregulation of Zn Transporters

Epidermodysplasia verruciformis (EV; OMIM 226400), a rare autosomal-recessive skin disease, develops non-melanoma skin cancers because of a susceptibility to oncogenic human papillomaviruses (HPVs). ZnT1 associates with the development of EV [86,87]. Although oncogenic HPVs can be detected in the skin of healthy individuals, they are asymptomatic. EV patients have mutations in either the EVER1 or EVER2 genes [88,89]. In KCs, EVER1 and 2 form a complex with ZnT1 primarily in the ER and to a lesser extent in the nuclear membrane and Golgi apparatus. The free Zn concentration in the KC nucleus is increased in patients with EV compared with healthy individuals, suggesting that the complex of ZnT1 and EVERs regulates free Zn transport in the nucleus, potentially altering cell function. A complex of ZnT1 with 'intact' EVERs inhibits the activator protein 1 (AP-1) activation that promotes the replication of HPV [90]. Accordingly, a complex of ZnT1 with 'mutated' EVERs increases free Zn transport into KC nucleus and subsequent AP-1 activity. This results in the aberrant replication of EV-related oncogenic HPVs, thereby developing skin cancers [86,87].

5. Human Skin Disorders Associated with Zn Deficiency

At present, acquired Zn deficiency (ZnD) still affects 17% of the world's population who are in the condition of general malnutrition due to starvation, severe illness, alcohol addiction. Additionally, infants, the elderly, and pregnant women are also prone to fall into acquired ZnD [91–94]. Acquired ZnD could cause acquired AE. Additionally, ZnD is observed in diseases linked to nutritional deficiencies such as necrolytic migratory erythema (elevated serum glucagon), pellagra (niacin or tryptophan deficiency), and biotin deficiency. AE-like erythema is also observed in these diseases. Interestingly, loss or decrease of epidermal LCs that is seen in patients with AE is reported in some cases of diseases related to nutritional deficiencies. Loss of epidermal LCs and subsequent AE-like erythema are common phenomena in diseases related to nutritional deficiencies. Additionally, the nature of these abnormalities might be attributable to ZnD, because Zn supplementation restores these abnormalities. Besides these diseases related to nutritional deficiencies, ZnD is involved in other skin disorders.

5.1. Nutritional Deficiency Diseases

5.1.1. Necrolytic Migratory Erythema

Necrolytic migratory erythema (NME) has been considered as a dermadrome of pancreatic glucagonoma, because NME skin lesions could resolve if the tumor is removed [95–97]. Patients with glucagonoma exhibit increased serum levels of glucagon. Because glucagon is involved in the metabolism of amino acids [98], excess glucagon decreases amino acids in the serum and in the epidermis, leading to epidermal necrosis.

However, it is now clarified that NME can develop within the context of other conditions including excess inflammatory mediators, liver dysfunction, and metabolic or nutritional deficiencies, particularly of Zn, and essential amino and fatty acids [97]. Because serum glucagon levels are variable in these conditions, glucagon is not the sole causative substance of NME. Decreased serum levels of Zn are reported in patients with NME suffering from inflammatory bowel disease, celiac disease, liver dysfunction, and a malignancy other than glucagonoma [99–111]. Supplementation of Zn restores skin lesions of NME, implying that decreased serum levels of Zn associate with the pathogenesis of NME. As described, AE-like erythema in patients with NME and its histopathological findings—such as cytoplasmic pallor, parakeratosis, subcorneal vacuolization, and ballooning degeneration of KCs—are identical to AE. In addition, one report demonstrates that epidermal LC number is reduced in patients with NME whose serum levels of Zn are decreased [111]. This suggests that similar mechanisms may underlie the development of skin lesions in patients with AE (described in Sections 2.2 and 3.1) and NME.

5.1.2. Pellagra

The compounds that have anti-pellagra activity are called niacin, and the major compound of niacin is nicotinamide and nicotinic acid. Nicotinamide is generated by two pathways. (1) Dietary nicotinic acid is promptly incorporated into the liver and is converted to nicotinamide; (2) Nicotinamide is synthesized from tryptophan, an essential amino acid, by the tryptophan–nicotinamide conversion pathway [112].

Deficiency of niacin and/or tryptophan contributes to pellagra. Diets rich in corn contain less niacin and tryptophan, contributing to the development of pellagra [113]. Patients with pellagra show AE-like erythema, diarrhea, and dementia [114]. Photosensitivity is a unique phenomenon in patients with pellagra and is not seen in other diseases associated with nutritional deficiencies. Niacin deficiency induces reactive oxygen species in KCs, followed by the production of prostaglandin E2 (PGE2). This PGE2 mediates photosensitivity in patients with pellagra [115]. A study investigating serum Zn levels in 81 pellagra patients showed a significant reduction of serum Zn level in patients with pellagra (69.7 ± 16.8 µg/dL) compared with that in healthy subjects (82.3 ± 34.0 µg/dL) [116]. Although the average serum Zn levels in patients with pellagra are in the range of latent ZnD, ZnD may be involved in the development of pellagra. Like AE and NME, loss or decrease of epidermal LCs is reported in the lesional skin of pellagra, but not in non-lesional skin of pellagra [117].

5.1.3. Biotin Deficiency

Biotin is a water-soluble vitamin and serves as a co-enzyme for five carboxylases in humans. Biotin-dependent carboxylases are involved in various metabolic pathways such as gluconeogenesis, fatty acid synthesis, and amino acid synthesis. Mammals cannot synthesize biotin. However, because biotin is contained in a wide range of foods and some gut microbiota produce biotin, biotin deficiency (BnD) does not occur in people who consume a mixed general diet. On the other hand, genetic deficiency of holocarboxylase synthetase and biotinidase; continuous consumption of raw egg whites; parenteral nutrition; and modified milk without biotin supplementation can lead to the development of BnD [118]. BnD causes similar symptoms as AE including skin lesions, alopecia, and diarrhea [119]. As for the underlying mechanism of development of the skin lesions in BnD, BnD causes abnormalities in fatty acid composition such as accumulation of odd-chain fatty acids and abnormal metabolism of long-chain polyunsaturated fatty acids [120–123]. Besides fatty acid abnormalities, ZnD is reported in some patients with BnD [124–126]. Although the serum Zn levels in patients with BnD are inconsistent among reports [127–129], ZnD might contribute to the development of BnD when considering their similar symptom profiles.

5.2. Alopecia

Alopecia is roughly classified into non-scarring and scarring. The former includes telogen effluvium, alopecia areata, and androgenic alopecia [130]. ZnD is related to some non-scarring alopecia.

5.2.1. Alopecia in Acrodermatitis Enteropathica

Alopecia developed in patients with acrodermatitis enteropathica (AE) shows the characteristics of telogen effluvium (TE), which is a type of non-scarring alopecia and is defined by the premature transition of anagen to telogen phase [131,132]. Patients with TE without AE also exhibit decreased serum levels of Zn compared with healthy individuals [132,133]. TE can be restored by supplementation of Zn [132]. In patients with AE, hair contains less Zn [134] and hair shafts show a characteristic irregular pattern because of impaired incorporation of cystine, a major content of hair keratin amino acids that is required for normal hair keratinization [135,136]. This is evidenced by impaired incorporation of radiolabeled cystine into hair in ZD rats [137–139]. Although alopecia-like hair loss is reported in dietary ZD AE models using mice [140], rats [141,142], and rabbits [143], no studies have addressed the underlying mechanisms. In summary, ZnD induces TE and abnormal hair keratinization.

5.2.2. Alopecia Areata

Alopecia areata (AA) is an autoimmune disease mediated by cytotoxic T lymphocytes [144]. IFN-γ KO mice do not develop experimental AA [145,146]. The association between AA and lower serum levels of Zn is a subject of active inquiry. The results of multiple analyses of serum Zn levels and AA are contradictory (reviewed in [12]). However, evidence indicates that serum levels of Zn are certainly decreased in patients with severe AA whose alopecia is broad and prolonged and is resistant to conventional therapies [147–149]. This implies that the serum levels of Zn are a useful parameter to predict the severity and that supplementation of Zn can be a promising adjuvant therapy, along with standard therapy for severe AA.

5.3. Cutaneous Wounds and Ulcers

The process of wound healing is complex and involves various Zn-related molecules, such as MTs, matrix metalloproteinases, integrins, alkaline phosphatase, and Zn finger proteins [150,151]. Oral and/or topical Zn has been long used to treat ulcers and wounds. Unexpectedly, a systematic review using data from the Cochrane Wound Group failed to conclude that oral Zn supplementation improves wound healing [152]. However, studies show the efficacy of topical Zn oxide for improving rates of wound healing, regardless of serum Zn levels of patients [153,154].

As described in Section 2.4, Zn acts as an intracellular signaling molecule. G-protein coupled receptor 39 (GPR39) has been identified as a Zn-sensing receptor [155]. GPR39 is an orphan G protein-coupled receptor that is conserved in vertebrates and transduces autocrine and paracrine Zn signals [155]. In an in vitro experiment, Zn released from injured KCs stimulates GPR39, and this signaling promotes epithelial repair [156]. Stem cells in the skin are localized in various regions including the interfollicular epidermis, hair follicles, sweat glands, and sebaceous glands (SGs) [157]. These stem cells are critical for wound repair [157]. In murine skin, GPR39 is exclusively localized to SGs and is co-localized with stem cells in SGs that express Blimp1. GPR39 KO mice show delayed wound healing [158]. These data demonstrate that Zn signaling through GPR39 plays an important role in wound healing by stimulating stem cell activity in SGs.

5.4. Other Skin Disorders Associated with Zn Deficiency

Zn deficiency (ZnD) is reported in some skin disorders including inflammatory diseases (atopic dermatitis [159,160], oral lichen planus [161], and Behcet's disease [162,163]), autoimmune bullous diseases (pemphigus vulgaris [164] and bullous pemphigoid [165]), inherited bullous diseases (inherited epidermolysis bullosa [166,167]), and hyperpigmentation (melasma [168]). Because Zn is deeply involved in the regulation of immune systems, it is likely that ZnD leads to the development of these inflammatory and autoimmune disorders [26,169].

Accumulation of evidence is required to determine the relationship between Zn and these skin disorders.

6. Conclusions

The association of skin manifestations and ZnD is well known. AE is caused by the mutations of ZIP4 and subsequent ZnD. Substantial numbers of patients suffering from diseases related to nutritional deficiencies such as acquired AE, NME, pellagra, and BnD show low serum Zn levels. This suggests that ZnD affects any cell type. Additionally, many micronutrients are also deficient in the conditions that fall into nutritional ZnD. Patients with these disorders share common skin manifestations of acrodermatitis. Additionally, LC loss in the epidermis is reported in patients with AE, NME, and pellagra. LCs are the sole CD39 (ecto-NTPDase1)-expressing cells in the epidermis. Thus, the disappearance of LCs in the epidermis exacerbates skin inflammation after irritant exposure (Figures 2 and 3). In conclusion, acrodermatitis in diseases associated with nutritional deficiencies may be caused by ICD, secondary to LC loss.

Although every cell expresses many different Zn transporters, which all contribute to homeostatic control of the cells and tissues, the role of Zn transporters in skin homeostasis is less understood. However, recent studies add some important information to this field (Figure 1). For instance, ZIP2 and ZIP4 contribute to KC proliferation and differentiation. ZIP10 is critical for skin homeostasis and epidermal formation. ZIP7 is important for proper dermal formation. ZIP13 is involved in adipocyte biology.

ZnD is a current problem in both developing and developed countries. We have to pay attention to cutaneous symptoms in order not to miss the 'dermadrome' of ZnD.

Author Contributions: Y.O. and T.K. conceived and constructed this manuscript with the assistance of M.K. and S.S.

Conflicts of Interest: The authors declare no conflict of interest.

References

1. Jackson, M.J. Physiology of zinc: General aspects. In *Zinc in Human Biology*; Mills, C.F., Ed.; Springer: Berlin/Heidelberg, Germany; New York, NY, USA, 1989; pp. 1–14.
2. Michaelsson, G.; Ljunghall, K.; Danielson, B.G. Zinc in epidermis and dermis in healthy subjects. *Acta Derm. Venereol.* **1980**, *60*, 295–299. [PubMed]
3. Inoue, Y.; Hasegawa, S.; Ban, S.; Yamada, T.; Date, Y. ZIP2 protein, a zinc transporter, is associated with keratinocyte differentiation. *J. Biol. Chem.* **2014**, *289*, 21451–21462. [CrossRef] [PubMed]
4. Gustafson, G.T. Heavy metals in rat mast cell granules. *Lab. Investig.* **1967**, *17*, 588–598. [PubMed]
5. Cowen, T.; Trigg, P.; Eady, R.A. Distribution of mast cells in human dermis: Development of a mapping technique. *Br. J. Dermatol.* **1979**, *100*, 635–640. [CrossRef] [PubMed]
6. Weber, A.; Knop, J.; Maurer, M. Pattern analysis of human cutaneous mast cell populations by total body surface mapping. *Br. J. Dermatol.* **2003**, *148*, 224–228. [CrossRef] [PubMed]
7. Kambe, T.; Tsuji, T.; Hashimoto, A.; Itsumura, N. The physiological, biochemical, and molecular roles of zinc transporters in zinc homeostasis and metabolism. *Physiol. Rev.* **2015**, *95*, 749–784. [CrossRef] [PubMed]
8. Hediger, M.A.; Romero, M.F.; Peng, J.B.; Rolfs, A.; Takanaga, H.; Bruford, E.A. The ABCs of solute carriers: Physiological, pathological and therapeutic implications of human membrane transport proteins. *Pflugers Arch.* **2004**, *447*, 465–468. [CrossRef] [PubMed]
9. Eide, D.J. The SLC39 family of metal ion transporters. *Pflugers Arch.* **2004**, *447*, 796–800. [CrossRef] [PubMed]
10. Palmiter, R.D.; Huang, L. Efflux and compartmentalization of zinc by members of the SLC30 family of solute carriers. *Pflugers Arch.* **2004**, *447*, 744–751. [CrossRef] [PubMed]

11. Tapiero, H.; Tew, K.D. Trace elements in human physiology and pathology: Zinc and metallothioneins. *Biomed. Pharmacother.* **2003**, *57*, 399–411. [CrossRef]

12. Ogawa, Y.; Kawamura, T.; Shimada, S. Zinc and skin biology. *Arch. Biochem. Biophys.* **2016**, *611*, 113–119. [CrossRef] [PubMed]

13. Andreini, C.; Bertini, I.; Cavallaro, G. Minimal functional sites allow a classification of zinc sites in proteins. *PLoS ONE* **2011**, *6*, e26325. [CrossRef] [PubMed]

14. Andreini, C.; Bertini, I. A bioinformatics view of zinc enzymes. *J. Inorg. Biochem.* **2012**, *111*, 150–156. [CrossRef] [PubMed]

15. Berg, J.M.; Shi, Y. The galvanization of biology: A growing appreciation for the roles of zinc. *Science* **1996**, *271*, 1081–1085. [CrossRef] [PubMed]

16. Fukada, T.; Yamasaki, S.; Nishida, K.; Murakami, M.; Hirano, T. Zinc homeostasis and signaling in health and diseases: Zinc signaling. *J. Biol. Inorg. Chem.* **2011**, *16*, 1123–1134. [CrossRef] [PubMed]

17. Klug, A. The discovery of zinc fingers and their applications in gene regulation and genome manipulation. *Annu. Rev. Biochem.* **2010**, *79*, 213–231. [CrossRef] [PubMed]

18. Laity, J.H.; Lee, B.M.; Wright, P.E. Zinc finger proteins: New insights into structural and functional diversity. *Curr. Opin. Struct. Biol.* **2001**, *11*, 39–46. [CrossRef]

19. Andreini, C.; Banci, L.; Bertini, I.; Rosato, A. Counting the zinc-proteins encoded in the human genome. *J. Proteome Res.* **2006**, *5*, 196–201. [CrossRef] [PubMed]

20. Emri, E.; Miko, E.; Bai, P.; Boros, G.; Nagy, G.; Rózsa, D.; Juhász, T.; Hegedűs, C.; Horkay, I.; Remenyik, É.; et al. Effects of non-toxic zinc exposure on human epidermal keratinocytes. *Metallomics* **2015**, *7*, 499–507. [CrossRef] [PubMed]

21. Chai, F.; Truong-Tran, A.Q.; Evdokiou, A. Intracellular zinc depletion induces caspase activation and p21$^{Waf1/Cip1}$ cleavage in human epithelial cell lines. *J. Infect. Dis.* **2000**, *182* (Suppl. 1), S85–S92. [CrossRef] [PubMed]

22. Wilson, D.; Varigos, G.; Ackland, M.L. Apoptosis may underlie the pathology of zinc-deficient skin. *Immunol. Cell Biol.* **2006**, *84*, 28–37. [CrossRef] [PubMed]

23. Hsu, D.J.; Daniel, J.C.; Gerson, S.J. Effect of zinc deficiency on keratins in buccal epithelium of rats. *Arch. Oral Biol.* **1991**, *36*, 759–763. [CrossRef]

24. Gueniche, A.; Viac, J.; Lizard, G.; Charveron, M.; Schmitt, D. Protective effect of zinc on keratinocyte activation markers induced by interferon or nickel. *Acta Derm. Venereol.* **1995**, *75*, 19–23. [PubMed]

25. Yamaoka, J.; Kume, T.; Akaike, A.; Miyachi, Y. Suppressive effect of zinc ion on iNOS expression induced by interferon-γ or tumor necrosis factor-α in murine keratinocytes. *J. Dermatol. Sci.* **2000**, *23*, 27–35. [CrossRef]

26. Wessels, I.; Maywald, M.; Rink, L. Zinc as a gatekeeper of immune function. *Nutrients* **2017**, *9*, 1286. [CrossRef] [PubMed]

27. Bin, B.H.; Bhin, J.; Kim, N.H.; Lee, S.-H.; Jung, H.-S.; Seo, J.; Kim, D.-K.; Hwang, D.; Fukada, T.; Lee, A.-Y.; et al. An acrodermatitis enteropathica-associated Zn transporter, ZIP4, Regulates human epidermal homeostasis. *J. Investig. Dermatol.* **2017**, *137*, 874–883. [CrossRef] [PubMed]

28. Bin, B.H.; Bhin, J.; Takaishi, M.; Toyoshima, K.-E.; Kawamata, S.; Ito, K.; Hara, T.; Watanabe, T.; Irié, T.; Takagishi, T.; et al. Requirement of zinc transporter ZIP10 for epidermal development: Implication of the ZIP10-p63 axis in epithelial homeostasis. *Proc. Natl. Acad. Sci. USA* **2017**, *114*, 12243–12248. [CrossRef] [PubMed]

29. Nartey, N.O.; Banerjee, D.; Cherian, M.G. Immunohistochemical localization of metallothionein in cell nucleus and cytoplasm of fetal human liver and kidney and its changes during development. *Pathology* **1987**, *19*, 233–238. [CrossRef] [PubMed]

30. Thirumoorthy, N.; Shyam Sunder, A.; Manisenthil Kumar, K.; Senthil kumar, M.; Ganesh, G.N.K.; Chatterjee, M. A review of metallothionein isoforms and their role in pathophysiology. *World J. Surg. Oncol.* **2011**, *9*, 54. [CrossRef] [PubMed]

31. Van den Oord, J.J.; De Ley, M. Distribution of metallothionein in normal and pathological human skin. *Arch. Dermatol. Res.* **1994**, *286*, 62–68. [CrossRef] [PubMed]

32. Zamirska, A.; Matusiak, L.; Dziegiel, P.; Szybejko-Machaj, G.; Szepietowski, J.C. Expression of metallothioneins in cutaneous squamous cell carcinoma and actinic keratosis. *Pathol. Oncol. Res.* **2012**, *18*, 849–855. [CrossRef] [PubMed]

33. Hanada, K.; Sawamura, D.; Hashimoto, I.; Kida, K.; Naganuma, A. Epidermal proliferation of the skin in metallothionein-null mice. *J. Investig. Dermatol.* **1998**, *110*, 259–262. [CrossRef] [PubMed]

34. Slusser, A.; Zheng, Y.; Zhou, X.D.; Somji, S.; Sens, D.A.; Sens, M.A.; Garrett, S.H. Metallothionein isoform 3 expression in human skin, related cancers and human skin derived cell cultures. *Toxicol. Lett.* **2015**, *232*, 141–148. [CrossRef] [PubMed]

35. Pula, B.; Tazbierski, T.; Zamirska, A.; Werynska, B.; Bieniek, A.; Szepietowski, J.; Rys, J.; Dziegiel, P.; Podhorska-Okolow, M. Metallothionein 3 expression in normal skin and malignant skin lesions. *Pathol. Oncol. Res.* **2015**, *21*, 187–193. [CrossRef] [PubMed]

36. Quaife, C.J.; Findley, S.D.; Erickson, J.C.; Froelick, G.J.; Kelly, E.J.; Zambrowicz, B.P.; Palmiter, R.D. Induction of a new metallothionein isoform (MT-IV) occurs during differentiation of stratified squamous epithelia. *Biochemistry* **1994**, *33*, 7250–7259. [CrossRef] [PubMed]

37. Merad, M.; Ginhoux, F.; Collin, M. Origin, homeostasis and function of Langerhans cells and other langerin-expressing dendritic cells. *Nat. Rev. Immunol.* **2008**, *8*, 935–947. [CrossRef] [PubMed]

38. Maverakis, E.; Fung, M.A.; Lynch, P.J.; Draznin, M.; Michael, D.J.; Ruben, B.; Fazel, N. Acrodermatitis enteropathica and an overview of zinc metabolism. *J. Am. Acad. Dermatol.* **2007**, *56*, 116–124. [CrossRef] [PubMed]

39. Kasana, S.; Din, J.; Maret, W. Genetic causes and gene-nutrient interactions in mammalian zinc deficiencies: Acrodermatitis enteropathica and transient neonatal zinc deficiency as examples. *J. Trace Elem. Med. Biol.* **2015**, *29*, 47–62. [CrossRef] [PubMed]

40. Kawamura, T.; Ogawa, Y.; Nakamura, Y.; Nakamizo, S.; Ohta, Y.; Nakano, H.; Kabashima, K.; Katayama, I.; Koizumi, S.; Kodama, T.; et al. Severe dermatitis with loss of epidermal Langerhans cells in human and mouse zinc deficiency. *J. Clin. Investig.* **2012**, *122*, 722–732. [CrossRef] [PubMed]

41. Borkowski, T.A.; Letterio, J.J.; Farr, A.G.; Udey, M.C. A role for endogenous transforming growth factor β1 in Langerhans cell biology: The skin of transforming growth factor β1 null mice is devoid of epidermal Langerhans cells. *J. Exp. Med.* **1996**, *184*, 2417–2422. [CrossRef] [PubMed]

42. Luo, Y.; Hu, W.; Xu, R.; Hou, B.; Zhang, L.; Zhang, W. ZNF580, a novel C2H2 zinc-finger transcription factor, interacts with the TGF-β signal molecule Smad2. *Cell Biol. Int.* **2011**, *35*, 1153–1157. [CrossRef] [PubMed]

43. Rudolf, E.; Rudolf, K. Increases in intracellular zinc enhance proliferative signaling as well as mitochondrial and endolysosomal activity in human melanocytes. *Cell. Physiol. Biochem.* **2017**, *43*, 1–16. [CrossRef] [PubMed]

44. Weinlich, G.; Bitterlich, W.; Mayr, V.; Fritsch, P.O.; Zelger, B. Metallothionein-overexpression as a prognostic factor for progression and survival in melanoma. A prospective study on 520 patients. *Br. J. Dermatol.* **2003**, *149*, 535–541. [CrossRef] [PubMed]

45. Emri, E.; Egervari, K.; Varvolgyi, T.; Rozsa, D.; Miko, E.; Dezso, B.; Veres, I.; Mehes, G.; Emri, G.; Remenyik, E. Correlation among metallothionein expression, intratumoural macrophage infiltration and the risk of metastasis in human cutaneous malignant melanoma. *J. Eur. Acad. Dermatol. Venereol.* **2013**, *27*, e320–e327. [CrossRef] [PubMed]

46. Hojyo, S.; Fukada, T. Roles of zinc signaling in the immune system. *J. Immunol. Res.* **2016**, *2016*, 6762343. [CrossRef] [PubMed]

47. Nishida, K.; Hasegawa, A.; Nakae, S.; Oboki, K.; Saito, H.; Yamasaki, S.; Hirano, T. Zinc transporter Znt5/Slc30a5 is required for the mast cell-mediated delayed-type allergic reaction but not the immediate-type reaction. *J. Exp. Med.* **2009**, *206*, 1351–1364. [CrossRef] [PubMed]

48. Kabu, K.; Yamasaki, S.; Kamimura, D.; Ito, Y.; Hasegawa, A.; Sato, E.; Kitamura, H.; Nishida, K.; Hirano, T. Zinc is required for FcεRI-mediated mast cell activation. *J. Immunol.* **2006**, *177*, 1296–1305. [CrossRef] [PubMed]

49. Kitamura, H.; Morikawa, H.; Kamon, H.; Iguchi, M.; Hojyo, S.; Fukada, T.; Yamashita, S.; Kaisho, T.; Akira, S.; Murakami, M.; et al. Toll-like receptor-mediated regulation of zinc homeostasis influences dendritic cell function. *Nat. Immunol.* **2006**, *7*, 971–977. [CrossRef] [PubMed]

50. Dowd, P.S.; Kelleher, J.; Guillou, P.J. T-lymphocyte subsets and interleukin-2 production in zinc-deficient rats. *Br. J. Nutr.* **1986**, *55*, 59–69. [CrossRef] [PubMed]

51. Fernandes, G.; Nair, M.; Onoe, K.; Tanaka, T.; Floyd, R.; Good, R.A. Impairment of cell-mediated immunity functions by dietary zinc deficiency in mice. *Proc. Natl. Acad. Sci. USA* **1979**, *76*, 457–461. [CrossRef] [PubMed]

52. Golden, M.H.; Jackson, A.A.; Golden, B.E. Effect of zinc on thymus of recently malnourished children. *Lancet* **1977**, *2*, 1057–1059. [CrossRef]
53. DePasquale-Jardieu, P.; Fraker, P.J. The role of corticosterone in the loss in immune function in the zinc-deficient A/J mouse. *J. Nutr.* **1979**, *109*, 1847–1855. [CrossRef] [PubMed]
54. Aydemir, T.B.; Liuzzi, J.P.; McClellan, S.; Cousins, R.J. Zinc transporter ZIP8 (SLC39A8) and zinc influence IFN-γ expression in activated human T cells. *J. Leukoc. Biol.* **2009**, *86*, 337–348. [CrossRef] [PubMed]
55. Malavolta, M.; Costarelli, L.; Giacconi, R.; Basso, A.; Piacenza, F.; Pierpaoli, E.; Provinciali, M.; Ogo, O.A.; Ford, D. Changes in Zn homeostasis during long term culture of primary endothelial cells and effects of Zn on endothelial cell senescence. *Exp. Gerontol.* **2017**, *99*, 35–45. [CrossRef] [PubMed]
56. Shearier, E.R.; Bowen, P.K.; He, W.; Drelich, A.; Drelich, J.; Goldman, J.; Zhao, F. In vitro cytotoxicity, adhesion, and proliferation of human vascular cells exposed to zinc. *ACS Biomater. Sci. Eng.* **2016**, *2*, 634–642. [CrossRef] [PubMed]
57. Tada-Oikawa, S.; Ichihara, G.; Suzuki, Y.; Izuoka, K.; Wu, W.; Yamada, Y.; Mishima, T.; Ichihara, S. Zn(II) released from zinc oxide nano/micro particles suppresses vasculogenesis in human endothelial colony-forming cells. *Toxicol. Rep.* **2015**, *2*, 692–701. [CrossRef] [PubMed]
58. Schulkens, I.A.; Castricum, K.C.; Weijers, E.M.; Koolwijk, P.; Griffioen, A.W.; Thijssen, V.L. Expression, regulation and function of human metallothioneins in endothelial cells. *J. Vasc. Res.* **2014**, *51*, 231–238. [CrossRef] [PubMed]
59. Tang, X.; Shay, N.F. Zinc has an insulin-like effect on glucose transport mediated by phosphoinositol-3-kinase and Akt in 3T3-L1 fibroblasts and adipocytes. *J. Nutr.* **2001**, *131*, 1414–1420. [CrossRef] [PubMed]
60. Bin, B.H.; Fukada, T.; Hosaka, T.; Yamasaki, S.; Ohashi, W.; Hojyo, S.; Miyai, T.; Nishida, K.; Yokoyama, S.; Hirano, T. Biochemical characterization of human ZIP13 protein: A homo-dimerized zinc transporter involved in the spondylocheiro dysplastic Ehlers-Danlos syndrome. *J. Biol. Chem.* **2011**, *286*, 40255–40265. [CrossRef] [PubMed]
61. Fukada, T.; Civic, N.; Furuichi, T.; Shimoda, S.; Mishima, K.; Higashiyama, H.; Idaira, Y.; Asada, Y.; Kitamura, H.; Yamasaki, S.; et al. The zinc transporter SLC39A13/ZIP13 is required for connective tissue development; its involvement in BMP/TGF-β signaling pathways. *PLoS ONE* **2008**, *3*, e3642. [CrossRef]
62. Taylor, K.M.; Morgan, H.E.; Johnson, A.; Nicholson, R.I. Structure-function analysis of HKE4, A member of the new LIV-1 subfamily of zinc transporters. *Biochem. J.* **2004**, *377*, 131–139. [CrossRef] [PubMed]
63. Bin, B.H.; Bhin, J.; Seo, J.; Kim, S.Y.; Lee, E.; Park, K.; Choi, D.H.; Takagishi, T.; Hara, T.; Hwang, D.; et al. Requirement of zinc transporter SLC39A7/ZIP7 for dermal development to fine-tune endoplasmic reticulum function by regulating protein disulfide isomerase. *J. Investig. Dermatol.* **2017**, *137*, 1682–1691. [CrossRef] [PubMed]
64. Bin, B.H.; Hojyo, S.; Hosaka, T.; Shimoda, S.; Mishima, K.; Higashiyama, H.; Idaira, Y.; Asada, Y.; Kitamura, H.; Yamasaki, S.; et al. Molecular pathogenesis of spondylocheirodysplastic Ehlers-Danlos syndrome caused by mutant ZIP13 proteins. *EMBO Mol. Med.* **2014**, *6*, 1028–1042. [CrossRef] [PubMed]
65. Kajimura, S.; Spiegelman, B.M.; Seale, P. Brown and beige fat: Physiological roles beyond heat generation. *Cell Metab.* **2015**, *22*, 546–559. [CrossRef] [PubMed]
66. Harms, M.; Seale, P. Brown and beige fat: Development, function and therapeutic potential. *Nat. Med.* **2013**, *19*, 1252–1263. [CrossRef] [PubMed]
67. Ohno, H.; Shinoda, K.; Spiegelman, B.M.; Kajimura, S. PPARγ agonists induce a white-to-brown fat conversion through stabilization of PRDM16 protein. *Cell Metab.* **2012**, *15*, 395–404. [CrossRef] [PubMed]
68. Tang, Q.Q.; Lane, M.D. Adipogenesis: From stem cell to adipocyte. *Annu. Rev. Biochem.* **2012**, *81*, 715–736. [CrossRef] [PubMed]
69. Fukunaka, A.; Fukada, T.; Bhin, J.; Suzuki, L.; Tsuzuki, T.; Takamine, Y.; Bin, B.H.; Yoshihara, T.; Ichinoseki-Sekine, N.; Naito, H.; et al. Zinc transporter ZIP13 suppresses beige adipocyte biogenesis and energy expenditure by regulating C/EBP-β expression. *PLoS Genet.* **2017**, *13*, e1006950. [CrossRef] [PubMed]
70. Chung, S.; Lapoint, K.; Martinez, K.; Kennedy, A.; Boysen Sandberg, M.; McIntosh, M.K. Preadipocytes mediate lipopolysaccharide-induced inflammation and insulin resistance in primary cultures of newly differentiated human adipocytes. *Endocrinology* **2006**, *147*, 5340–5351. [CrossRef] [PubMed]

71. Liuzzi, J.P.; Lichten, L.A.; Rivera, S.; Blanchard, R.K.; Aydemir, T.B.; Knutson, M.D.; Ganz, T.; Cousins, R.J. Interleukin-6 regulates the zinc transporter Zip14 in liver and contributes to the hypozincemia of the acute-phase response. *Proc. Natl. Acad. Sci. USA* **2005**, *102*, 6843–6848. [CrossRef] [PubMed]

72. Troche, C.; Aydemir, T.B.; Cousins, R.J. Zinc transporter Slc39a14 regulates inflammatory signaling associated with hypertrophic adiposity. *Am. J. Physiol. Endocrinol. Metab.* **2016**, *310*, E258–E268. [CrossRef] [PubMed]

73. Wei, S.; Zhang, L.; Zhou, X.; Du, M.; Jiang, Z.; Hausman, G.J.; Bergen, W.G.; Zan, L.; Dodson, M.V. Emerging roles of zinc finger proteins in regulating adipogenesis. *Cell. Mol. Life Sci.* **2013**, *70*, 4569–4584. [CrossRef] [PubMed]

74. Schmitt, S.; Kury, S.; Giraud, M.; Dreno, B.; Kharfi, M.; Bezieau, S. An update on mutations of the SLC39A4 gene in acrodermatitis enteropathica. *Hum. Mutat.* **2009**, *30*, 926–933. [CrossRef] [PubMed]

75. Lazarowski, E.R.; Boucher, R.C.; Harden, T.K. Mechanisms of release of nucleotides and integration of their action as P2X- and P2Y-receptor activating molecules. *Mol. Pharmacol.* **2003**, *64*, 785–795. [CrossRef] [PubMed]

76. Koizumi, S.; Fujishita, K.; Inoue, K.; Shigemoto-Mogami, Y.; Tsuda, M.; Inoue, K. Ca^{2+} waves in keratinocytes are transmitted to sensory neurons: The involvement of extracellular ATP and P2Y2 receptor activation. *Biochem. J.* **2004**, *380*, 329–338. [CrossRef] [PubMed]

77. Mizumoto, N.; Kumamoto, T.; Robson, S.C.; Sevigny, J.; Matsue, H.; Enjyoji, K.; Takashima, A. CD39 is the dominant Langerhans cell-associated ecto-NTPDase: Modulatory roles in inflammation and immune responsiveness. *Nat. Med.* **2002**, *8*, 358–365. [CrossRef] [PubMed]

78. Ho, C.L.; Yang, C.Y.; Lin, W.J.; Lin, C.H. Ecto-nucleoside triphosphate diphosphohydrolase 2 modulates local ATP-induced calcium signaling in human HaCaT keratinocytes. *PLoS ONE* **2013**, *8*, e57666. [CrossRef] [PubMed]

79. Giunta, C.; Elcioglu, N.H.; Albrecht, B.; Eich, G.; Chambaz, C.; Janecke, A.R.; Yeowell, H.; Weis, M.; Eyre, D.R.; Kraenzlin, M.; et al. Spondylocheiro dysplastic form of the Ehlers-Danlos syndrome—An autosomal-recessive entity caused by mutations in the zinc transporter gene SLC39A13. *Am. J. Hum. Genet.* **2008**, *82*, 1290–1305. [CrossRef] [PubMed]

80. Yamawaki, N.; Yamada, M.; Kan-no, T.; Kojima, T.; Kaneko, T.; Yonekubo, A. Macronutrient, mineral and trace element composition of breast milk from Japanese women. *J. Trace Elem. Med. Biol.* **2005**, *19*, 171–181. [CrossRef] [PubMed]

81. Huang, L.; Gitschier, J. A novel gene involved in zinc transport is deficient in the lethal milk mouse. *Nat. Genet.* **1997**, *17*, 292–297. [CrossRef] [PubMed]

82. Chowanadisai, W.; Lonnerdal, B.; Kelleher, S.L. Identification of a mutation in SLC30A2 (ZnT-2) in women with low milk zinc concentration that results in transient neonatal zinc deficiency. *J. Biol. Chem.* **2006**, *281*, 39699–39707. [CrossRef] [PubMed]

83. Lasry, I.; Seo, Y.A.; Ityel, H.; Shalva, N.; Pode-Shakked, B.; Glaser, F.; Berman, B.; Berezovsky, I.; Goncearenco, A.; Klar, A.; et al. A dominant negative heterozygous G87R mutation in the zinc transporter, ZnT-2 (SLC30A2), results in transient neonatal zinc deficiency. *J. Biol. Chem.* **2012**, *287*, 29348–29361. [CrossRef] [PubMed]

84. Itsumura, N.; Inamo, Y.; Okazaki, F.; Teranishi, F.; Narita, H.; Kambe, T.; Kodama, H. Compound heterozygous mutations in SLC30A2/ZnT2 results in low milk zinc concentrations: A novel mechanism for zinc deficiency in a breast-fed infant. *PLoS ONE* **2013**, *8*, e64045. [CrossRef] [PubMed]

85. Miletta, M.C.; Bieri, A.; Kernland, K.; Schoni, M.H.; Petkovic, V.; Fluck, C.E.; Eble, A.; Mullis, P.E. Transient neonatal zinc deficiency caused by a heterozygous G87R mutation in the *Zinc transporter ZnT-2* (*SLC30A2*) Gene in the mother highlighting the importance of Zn^{2+} for normal growth and development. *Int. J. Endocrinol.* **2013**, *2013*, 259189. [CrossRef] [PubMed]

86. Lazarczyk, M.; Pons, C.; Mendoza, J.A.; Cassonnet, P.; Jacob, Y.; Favre, M. Regulation of cellular zinc balance as a potential mechanism of EVER-mediated protection against pathogenesis by cutaneous oncogenic human papillomaviruses. *J. Exp. Med.* **2008**, *205*, 35–42. [CrossRef] [PubMed]

87. Orth, G. Host defenses against human papillomaviruses: Lessons from epidermodysplasia verruciformis. *Curr. Top. Microbiol. Immunol.* **2008**, *321*, 59–83. [PubMed]

88. Ramoz, N.; Taieb, A.; Rueda, L.A.; Montoya, L.S.; Bouadjar, B.; Favre, M.; Orth, G. Evidence for a nonallelic heterogeneity of epidermodysplasia verruciformis with two susceptibility loci mapped to chromosome regions 2p21-p24 and 17q25. *J. Investig. Dermatol.* **2000**, *114*, 1148–1153. [CrossRef] [PubMed]

89. Ramoz, N.; Rueda, L.A.; Bouadjar, B.; Montoya, L.S.; Orth, G.; Favre, M. Mutations in two adjacent novel genes are associated with epidermodysplasia verruciformis. *Nat. Genet.* **2002**, *32*, 579–581. [CrossRef] [PubMed]

90. Offord, E.A.; Beard, P. A member of the activator protein 1 family found in keratinocytes but not in fibroblasts required for transcription from a human papillomavirus type 18 promoter. *J. Virol.* **1990**, *64*, 4792–4798. [PubMed]

91. Stammers, A.L.; Lowe, N.M.; Medina, M.W.; Patel, S.; Dykes, F.; Perez-Rodrigo, C.; Serra-Majam, L.; Nissensohn, M.; Moran, V.H. The relationship between zinc intake and growth in children aged 1–8 years: A systematic review and meta-analysis. *Eur. J. Clin. Nutr.* **2015**, *69*, 147–153. [CrossRef] [PubMed]

92. Krebs, N.F.; Miller, L.V.; Hambidge, K.M. Zinc deficiency in infants and children: A review of its complex and synergistic interactions. *Paediatr. Int. Child Health* **2014**, *34*, 279–288. [CrossRef] [PubMed]

93. Penny, M.E. Zinc supplementation in public health. *Ann. Nutr. Metab.* **2013**, *62* (Suppl. 1), 31–42. [CrossRef] [PubMed]

94. Wang, H.; Hu, Y.F.; Hao, J.H.; Chen, Y.H.; Su, P.Y.; Wang, Y.; Yu, Z.; Fu, L.; Xu, Y.Y.; Zhang, C.; et al. Maternal zinc deficiency during pregnancy elevates the risks of fetal growth restriction: A population-based birth cohort study. *Sci. Rep.* **2015**, *5*, 11262. [CrossRef] [PubMed]

95. Mullans, E.A.; Cohen, P.R. Iatrogenic necrolytic migratory erythema: A case report and review of nonglucagonoma-associated necrolytic migratory erythema. *J. Am. Acad. Dermatol.* **1998**, *38*, 866–873. [CrossRef]

96. Alexander, E.K.; Robinson, M.; Staniec, M.; Dluhy, R.G. Peripheral amino acid and fatty acid infusion for the treatment of necrolytic migratory erythema in the glucagonoma syndrome. *Clin. Endocrinol.* **2002**, *57*, 827–831. [CrossRef]

97. Tierney, E.P.; Badger, J. Etiology and pathogenesis of necrolytic migratory erythema: Review of the literature. *MedGenMed* **2004**, *6*, 4. [PubMed]

98. Van Beek, A.P.; de Haas, E.R.; van Vloten, W.A.; Lips, C.J.; Roijers, J.F.; Canninga-van Dijk, M.R. The glucagonoma syndrome and necrolytic migratory erythema: A clinical review. *Eur. J. Endocrinol.* **2004**, *151*, 531–537. [CrossRef] [PubMed]

99. Walker, N.P. Atypical necrolytic migratory erythema in association with a jejunal adenocarcinoma. *J. R. Soc. Med.* **1982**, *75*, 134–135. [PubMed]

100. Kelly, C.P.; Johnston, C.F.; Nolan, N.; Keeling, P.W.; Weir, D.G. Necrolytic migratory erythema with elevated plasma enteroglucagon in celiac disease. *Gastroenterology* **1989**, *96*, 1350–1353. [CrossRef]

101. Blackford, S.; Wright, S.; Roberts, D.L. Necrolytic migratory erythema without glucagonoma: The role of dietary essential fatty acids. *Br. J. Dermatol.* **1991**, *125*, 460–462. [CrossRef] [PubMed]

102. Kerleau, J.M.; Levesque, H.; Cailleux, N.; Gancel, A.; Boullie, M.C.; Courtois, H. Isolated zinc deficiency and necrolytic migratory erythema. Apropos of a case. *Rev. Med. Interne* **1993**, *14*, 784–787. [CrossRef]

103. Thorisdottir, K.; Camisa, C.; Tomecki, K.J.; Bergfeld, W.F. Necrolytic migratory erythema: A report of three cases. *J. Am. Acad. Dermatol.* **1994**, *30*, 324–329. [CrossRef]

104. Marinkovich, M.P.; Botella, R.; Datloff, J.; Sangueza, O.P. Necrolytic migratory erythema without glucagonoma in patients with liver disease. *J. Am. Acad. Dermatol.* **1995**, *32*, 604–609. [CrossRef]

105. Delaporte, E.; Catteau, B.; Piette, F. Necrolytic migratory erythema-like eruption in zinc deficiency associated with alcoholic liver disease. *Br. J. Dermatol.* **1997**, *137*, 1027–1028. [CrossRef] [PubMed]

106. Sinclair, S.A.; Reynolds, N.J. Necrolytic migratory erythema and zinc deficiency. *Br. J. Dermatol.* **1997**, *136*, 783–785. [CrossRef] [PubMed]

107. Al-Rikabi, A.C.; Al-Homsi, H.I. Propionic acidemia and zinc deficiency presenting as necrolytic migratory erythema. *Saudi Med. J.* **2004**, *25*, 660–662. [PubMed]

108. Topham, E.J.; Child, F.J. Exfoliative erythema of malnutrition with zinc and essential amino acid deficiency. *Clin. Exp. Dermatol.* **2005**, *30*, 235–237. [CrossRef] [PubMed]

109. Nakashima, H.; Komine, M.; Sasaki, K.; Mitsui, H.; Fujimoto, M.; Ihn, H.; Asahina, A.; Kikuchi, K.; Tamaki, K. Necrolytic migratory erythema without glucagonoma in a patient with short bowel syndrome. *J. Dermatol.* **2006**, *33*, 557–562. [CrossRef] [PubMed]

110. Healy, E.; Scanlain, N.I.; Barnes, L. Necrolytic migratory erythema due to zinc deficiency. *Br. J. Dermatol.* **1992**, *127*, 57–58. [CrossRef]

111. Rokunohe, D.; Nakano, H.; Ikenaga, S.; Umegaki, N.; Kaneko, T.; Matsuhashi, Y.; Tando, Y.; Toyoki, Y.; Hakamada, K.; Kusumi, T.; et al. Reduction in epidermal Langerhans cells in patients with necrolytic migratory erythema. *J. Dermatol. Sci.* **2008**, *50*, 76–80. [CrossRef] [PubMed]

112. Bogan, K.L.; Brenner, C. Nicotinic acid, nicotinamide, and nicotinamide riboside: A molecular evaluation of NAD+ precursor vitamins in human nutrition. *Annu. Rev. Nutr.* **2008**, *28*, 115–130. [CrossRef] [PubMed]

113. Rajakumar, K. Pellagra in the United States: A historical perspective. *South. Med. J.* **2000**, *93*, 272–277. [CrossRef] [PubMed]

114. Chick, H. The aetiology of pellagra: A review of current theories. *J. Trop. Med. Hyg.* **1951**, *54*, 207–213. [CrossRef]

115. Sugita, K.; Ikenouchi-Sugita, A.; Nakayama, Y.; Yoshioka, H.; Nomura, T.; Sakabe, J.; Nakahigashi, K.; Kuroda, E.; Uematsu, S.; Nakamura, J.; et al. Prostaglandin E_2 is critical for the development of niacin-deficiency-induced photosensitivity via ROS production. *Sci. Rep.* **2013**, *3*, 2973. [CrossRef] [PubMed]

116. Vannucchi, H.; Favaro, R.M.; Cunha, D.F.; Marchini, J.S. Assessment of zinc nutritional status of pellagra patients. *Alcohol Alcohol.* **1995**, *30*, 297–302. [PubMed]

117. Yamaguchi, S.; Miyagi, T.; Sogabe, Y.; Yasuda, M.; Kanazawa, N.; Utani, A.; Izaki, S.; Uezato, H.; Takahashi, K. Depletion of Epidermal Langerhans Cells in the Skin Lesions of Pellagra Patients. *Am. J. Dermatopathol.* **2017**, *39*, 428–432. [CrossRef] [PubMed]

118. Zempleni, J.; Wijeratne, S.S.; Hassan, Y.I. Biotin. *Biofactors* **2009**, *35*, 36–46. [CrossRef] [PubMed]

119. Mock, D.M. Skin manifestations of biotin deficiency. *Semin. Dermatol.* **1991**, *10*, 296–302. [PubMed]

120. Mock, D.M.; Johnson, S.B.; Holman, R.T. Effects of biotin deficiency on serum fatty acid composition: Evidence for abnormalities in humans. *J. Nutr.* **1988**, *118*, 342–348. [CrossRef] [PubMed]

121. Mock, D.M.; Mock, N.I.; Johnson, S.B.; Holman, R.T. Effects of biotin deficiency on plasma and tissue fatty acid composition: Evidence for abnormalities in rats. *Pediatr. Res.* **1988**, *24*, 396–403. [CrossRef] [PubMed]

122. Kramer, T.R.; Briske-Anderson, M.; Johnson, S.B.; Holman, R.T. Effects of biotin deficiency on polyunsaturated fatty acid metabolism in rats. *J. Nutr.* **1984**, *114*, 2047–2052. [CrossRef] [PubMed]

123. Suchy, S.F.; Rizzo, W.B.; Wolf, B. Effect of biotin deficiency and supplementation on lipid metabolism in rats: Saturated fatty acids. *Am. J. Clin. Nutr.* **1986**, *44*, 475–480. [CrossRef] [PubMed]

124. Matsusue, S.; Kashihara, S.; Takeda, H.; Koizumi, S. Biotin deficiency during total parenteral nutrition: Its clinical manifestation and plasma nonesterified fatty acid level. *JPEN J. Parenter. Enter. Nutr.* **1985**, *9*, 760–763. [CrossRef] [PubMed]

125. Higuchi, R.; Mizukoshi, M.; Koyama, H.; Kitano, N.; Koike, M. Intractable diaper dermatitis as an early sign of biotin deficiency. *Acta Paediatr.* **1998**, *87*, 228–229. [CrossRef] [PubMed]

126. Lagier, P.; Bimar, P.; Seriat-Gautier, S.; Dejode, J.M.; Brun, T.; Bimar, J. Zinc and biotin deficiency during prolonged parenteral nutrition in the infant. *Presse Med.* **1987**, *16*, 1795–1797. [PubMed]

127. Khalidi, N.; Wesley, J.R.; Thoene, J.G.; Whitehouse, W.M., Jr.; Baker, W.L. Biotin deficiency in a patient with short bowel syndrome during home parenteral nutrition. *JPEN J. Parenter. Enter. Nutr.* **1984**, *8*, 311–314. [CrossRef] [PubMed]

128. Higuchi, R.; Noda, E.; Koyama, Y.; Shirai, T.; Horino, A.; Juri, T.; Koike, M. Biotin deficiency in an infant fed with amino acid formula and hypoallergenic rice. *Acta Paediatr.* **1996**, *85*, 872–874. [CrossRef] [PubMed]

129. Fujimoto, W.; Inaoki, M.; Fukui, T.; Inoue, Y.; Kuhara, T. Biotin deficiency in an infant fed with amino acid formula. *J. Dermatol.* **2005**, *32*, 256–261. [CrossRef] [PubMed]

130. Sullivan, J.R.; Kossard, S. Acquired scalp alopecia. Part I: A review. *Australas. J. Dermatol.* **1998**, *39*, 207–219. [CrossRef] [PubMed]

131. Finner, A.M. Nutrition and hair: Deficiencies and supplements. *Dermatol. Clin.* **2013**, *31*, 167–172. [CrossRef] [PubMed]

132. Karashima, T.; Tsuruta, D.; Hamada, T.; Ono, F.; Ishii, N.; Abe, T.; Ohyama, B.; Nakama, T.; Dainichi, T.; Hashimoto, T. Oral zinc therapy for zinc deficiency-related telogen effluvium. *Dermatol. Ther.* **2012**, *25*, 210–213. [CrossRef] [PubMed]

133. Kil, M.S.; Kim, C.W.; Kim, S.S. Analysis of serum zinc and copper concentrations in hair loss. *Ann. Dermatol.* **2013**, *25*, 405–409. [CrossRef] [PubMed]

134. Amador, M.; Pena, M.; Garcia-Miranda, A.; Gonzalez, A.; Hermelo, M. Letter: Low hair-zinc concentrations in acrodermatitis enteropathica. *Lancet* **1975**, *1*, 1379. [CrossRef]

135. Traupe, H.; Happle, R.; Grobe, H.; Bertram, H.P. Polarization microscopy of hair in acrodermatitis enteropathica. *Pediatr. Dermatol.* **1986**, *3*, 300–303. [CrossRef] [PubMed]

136. Dupre, A.; Bonafe, J.L.; Carriere, J.P. The hair in acrodermatitis interopathica—A disease indicator? *Acta Derm. Venereol.* **1979**, *59*, 177–178. [PubMed]

137. Follis, R.H.; Day, H.G.; McCollum, E.V. Histological studies of the tissues of rats fed a diet extremely low in zinc. *J. Nutr.* **1941**, *22*, 223–237. [CrossRef]

138. Hsu, J.N. *Zinc as Related to Cystine Metabolism*; Academic Press: London, UK, 1976.

139. Wilson, R.H.; Lewis, H.B. The cystine content of hair and other epidermal tissues. *J. Biol. Chem.* **1927**, *73*, 543–553.

140. Day, H.G.; Skidmore, B.E. Some effects of dietary zinc deficiency in the mouse. *J. Nutr.* **1946**, *33*, 27–38. [CrossRef]

141. Swenerton, H.; Hurley, L.S. Severe zinc deficiency in male and female rats. *J. Nutr.* **1968**, *95*, 8–18. [CrossRef] [PubMed]

142. Todd, W.R.; Elvehjem, C.A.; Hart, E.B. Zinc in the nutrition of the rat. *Am. J. Physiol.* **1933**, *107*, 146–156. [CrossRef]

143. Shaw, N.A.; Dickey, H.C.; Brugman, H.H.; Blamberg, D.L.; Witter, J.F. Zinc deficiency in female rabbits. *Lab. Anim.* **1974**, *8*, 1–7. [CrossRef] [PubMed]

144. Xing, L.; Dai, Z.; Jabbari, A.; Cerise, J.E.; Higgins, C.A.; Gong, W.; de Jong, A.; Harel, S.; DeStefano, G.M.; Rothman, L.; et al. Alopecia areata is driven by cytotoxic T lymphocytes and is reversed by JAK inhibition. *Nat. Med.* **2014**, *20*, 1043–1049. [CrossRef] [PubMed]

145. Petukhova, L.; Duvic, M.; Hordinsky, M.; Norris, D.; Price, V.; Shimomura, Y.; Kim, H.; Singh, P.; Lee, A.; Chen, W.V.; et al. Genome-wide association study in alopecia areata implicates both innate and adaptive immunity. *Nature* **2010**, *466*, 113–117. [CrossRef] [PubMed]

146. Freyschmidt-Paul, P.; McElwee, K.J.; Hoffmann, R.; Sundberg, J.P.; Vitacolonna, M.; Kissling, S.; Zoller, M. Interferon-gamma-deficient mice are resistant to the development of alopecia areata. *Br. J. Dermatol.* **2006**, *155*, 515–521. [CrossRef] [PubMed]

147. Park, H.; Kim, C.W.; Kim, S.S.; Park, C.W. The therapeutic effect and the changed serum zinc level after zinc supplementation in alopecia areata patients who had a low serum zinc level. *Ann. Dermatol.* **2009**, *21*, 142–146. [CrossRef] [PubMed]

148. Bhat, Y.J.; Manzoor, S.; Khan, A.R.; Qayoom, S. Trace element levels in alopecia areata. *Indian J. Dermatol. Venereol. Leprol.* **2009**, *75*, 29–31. [CrossRef] [PubMed]

149. Abdel Fattah, N.S.; Atef, M.M.; Al-Qaradaghi, S.M. Evaluation of serum zinc level in patients with newly diagnosed and resistant alopecia areata. *Int. J. Dermatol.* **2016**, *55*, 24–29. [CrossRef] [PubMed]

150. Lansdown, A.B.; Mirastschijski, U.; Stubbs, N.; Scanlon, E.; Agren, M.S. Zinc in wound healing: Theoretical, experimental, and clinical aspects. *Wound Repair Regen.* **2007**, *15*, 2–16. [CrossRef] [PubMed]

151. Schwartz, J.R.; Marsh, R.G.; Draelos, Z.D. Zinc and skin health: Overview of physiology and pharmacology. *Dermatol. Surg.* **2005**, *31*, 837–847. [CrossRef] [PubMed]

152. Wilkinson, E.A.; Hawke, C.I. Does oral zinc aid the healing of chronic leg ulcers? A systematic literature review. *Arch. Dermatol.* **1998**, *134*, 1556–1560. [CrossRef] [PubMed]

153. Agren, M.S.; Stromberg, H.E. Topical treatment of pressure ulcers. A randomized comparative trial of Varidase and zinc oxide. *Scand. J. Plast. Reconstr. Surg.* **1985**, *19*, 97–100. [CrossRef] [PubMed]

154. Agren, M.S. Studies on zinc in wound healing. *Acta Derm. Venereol. Suppl.* **1990**, *154*, 1–36.

155. Popovics, P.; Stewart, A.J. GPR39, a Zn^{2+}-activated G protein-coupled receptor that regulates pancreatic, gastrointestinal and neuronal functions. *Cell. Mol. Life Sci.* **2011**, *68*, 85–95. [CrossRef] [PubMed]

156. Sharir, H.; Zinger, A.; Nevo, A.; Sekler, I.; Hershfinkel, M. Zinc released from injured cells is acting via the Zn2+-sensing receptor, ZnR, to trigger signaling leading to epithelial repair. *J. Biol. Chem.* **2010**, *285*, 26097–26106. [CrossRef] [PubMed]

157. Gonzales, K.A.U.; Fuchs, E. Skin and its regenerative powers: An alliance between stem cells and their niche. *Dev. Cell* **2017**, *43*, 387–401. [CrossRef] [PubMed]

158. Zhao, H.; Qiao, J.; Zhang, S.; Zhang, H.; Lei, X.; Wang, X.; Deng, Z.; Ning, L.; Cao, Y.; Guo, Y.; et al. GPR39 marks specific cells within the sebaceous gland and contributes to skin wound healing. *Sci. Rep.* **2015**, *5*, 7913. [CrossRef] [PubMed]

159. David, T.J.; Wells, F.E.; Sharpe, T.C.; Gibbs, A.C. Low serum zinc in children with atopic eczema. *Br. J. Dermatol.* **1984**, *111*, 597–601. [CrossRef] [PubMed]

160. Kim, J.E.; Yoo, S.R.; Jeong, M.G.; Ko, J.Y.; Ro, Y.S. Hair zinc levels and the efficacy of oral zinc supplementation in patients with atopic dermatitis. *Acta Derm. Venereol.* **2014**, *94*, 558–562. [CrossRef] [PubMed]

161. Gholizadeh, N.; Mehdipour, M.; Najafi, S.; Bahramian, A.; Garjani, S.; Khoeini Poorfar, H. Evaluation of the serum zinc level in erosive and non-erosive oral lichen planus. *J. Dent.* **2014**, *15*, 52–56.

162. Dogan, P.; Dogan, M.; Klockenkamper, R. Determination of trace elements in blood serum of patients with Behcet disease by total reflection X-ray fluorescence analysis. *Clin. Chem.* **1993**, *39*, 1037–1041. [PubMed]

163. Saglam, K.; Serce, A.F.; Yilmaz, M.I.; Bulucu, F.; Aydin, A.; Akay, C.; Sayal, A. Trace elements and antioxidant enzymes in Behcet's disease. *Rheumatol. Int.* **2002**, *22*, 93–96. [PubMed]

164. Yazdanpanah, M.J.; Ghayour-Mobarhan, M.; Taji, A.; Javidi, Z.; Pezeshkpoor, F.; Tavallaie, S.; Momenzadeh, A.; Esmaili, H.; Shojaie-Noori, S.; Khoddami, M.; et al. Serum zinc and copper status in Iranian patients with pemphigus vulgaris. *Int. J. Dermatol.* **2011**, *50*, 1343–1346. [CrossRef] [PubMed]

165. Tasaki, M.; Hanada, K.; Hashimoto, I. Analyses of serum copper and zinc levels and copper/zinc ratios in skin diseases. *J. Dermatol.* **1993**, *20*, 21–24. [CrossRef] [PubMed]

166. Ingen-Housz-Oro, S.; Blanchet-Bardon, C.; Vrillat, M.; Dubertret, L. Vitamin and trace metal levels in recessive dystrophic epidermolysis bullosa. *J. Eur. Acad. Dermatol. Venereol.* **2004**, *18*, 649–653. [CrossRef] [PubMed]

167. Fine, J.D.; Tamura, T.; Johnson, L. Blood vitamin and trace metal levels in epidermolysis bullosa. *Arch. Dermatol.* **1989**, *125*, 374–379. [CrossRef] [PubMed]

168. Rostami, M.M.; Safavi, A.N.; Iranparvar, A.M.; Maleki, N.; Aghabalaei, D.M. Evaluation of the serum zinc level in adult patients with melasma: Is there a relationship with serum zinc deficiency and melasma? *J. Cosmet. Dermatol.* **2017**. [CrossRef] [PubMed]

169. Fraker, P.J.; King, L.E. Reprogramming of the immune system during zinc deficiency. *Annu. Rev. Nutr.* **2004**, *24*, 277–298. [CrossRef] [PubMed]

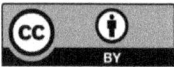

nutrients

MDPI

Review

The Role of the Slc39a Family of Zinc Transporters in Zinc Homeostasis in Skin

Bum-Ho Bin [1,†], Shintaro Hojyo [2,†], Juyeon Seo [3], Takafumi Hara [4], Teruhisa Takagishi [4], Kenji Mishima [1] and Toshiyuki Fukada [1,4,5,*]

[1] Division of Pathology, Department of Oral Diagnostic Sciences, School of Dentistry, Showa University, Tokyo 142-8555, Japan; bbh82429@gmail.com (B.-H.B); mishima-k@dent.showa-u.ac.jp (K.M.)
[2] Osteoimmunology, Deutsches Rheuma-Forschungszentrum, 10117 Berlin, Germany; Shintaro.Hojyo@drfz.de
[3] AmorePacific Corporation R&D Center, Yongin, Gyeonggi-do 446-729, Korea; yeon8687@amorepacific.com
[4] Faculty of Pharmaceutical Sciences, Tokushima Bunri University, Tokushima 770-8055, Japan; t-hara@ph.bunri-u.ac.jp (T.H.); t.takagishi@ph.bunri-u.ac.jp (T.T.)
[5] RIKEN Center for Integrative Medical Sciences, Yokohama 230-0042, Japan
* Correspondence: fukada@ph.bunri-u.ac.jp; Tel.: +81-88-602-8593
† These authors contributed equally to this work.

Received: 20 December 2017; Accepted: 11 February 2018; Published: 16 February 2018

Abstract: The first manifestations that appear under zinc deficiency are skin defects such as dermatitis, alopecia, acne, eczema, dry, and scaling skin. Several genetic disorders including acrodermatitis enteropathica (also known as Danbolt-Closs syndrome) and Brandt's syndrome are highly related to zinc deficiency. However, the zinc-related molecular mechanisms underlying normal skin development and homeostasis, as well as the mechanism by which disturbed zinc homeostasis causes such skin disorders, are unknown. Recent genomic approaches have revealed the physiological importance of zinc transporters in skin formation and clarified their functional impairment in cutaneous pathogenesis. In this review, we provide an overview of the relationships between zinc deficiency and skin disorders, focusing on the roles of zinc transporters in the skin. We also discuss therapeutic outlooks and advantages of controlling zinc levels via zinc transporters to prevent cutaneous disorganization.

Keywords: zinc; skin; homeostasis; transporter

1. Introduction

Zinc is an essential micronutrient obtained from food and drink [1]. Zinc is abundantly contained in mollusks such as oysters and in crustaceans such as crabs and crayfish [2]. The biological role of zinc was first revealed in 1869 by Raulin, who showed that zinc is essential for the growth of *Aspergillus niger* [1]. Subsequently, its importance for rodent growth was demonstrated using experimental rats in 1934 [1,3]. However, zinc's physiological role in humans was unknown until 1961 when zinc deficiency in humans was discovered [4]. Zinc is associated with growth, gonad development, immune function and pregnancy outcome improvement, and hair loss prevention [1,5,6]. In 1961, growth retardation and hypogonadism observed in Iranian and Egyptian adults were reported to be associated with zinc deficiency, which was closely related to dietary habits [4,7,8]. Middle Eastern diets typically include bread and beans, which contain large quantities of phytate [9]. Phytate has a negative effect on zinc absorption, thereby causing zinc deficiency. Zinc deficiency is also observed in vegetarians, single people, alcoholics, dieters, pregnant women, and the malnourished in developing and developed countries [4]. In this review, we outline the characteristics of zinc transporters and identify skin phenotypes of their knockout mouse models and human skin genetic diseases caused by mutations in zinc transporters. Furthermore, we discuss how zinc deficiency impacts normal skin development and homeostasis, based on the most recent research.

2. Zinc Homeostasis in Skin

2.1. Skin Structure

The skin largely consists of three layers [10,11]. The epidermis functions as a barrier to protect the interior from direct contact with the external environment. The dermis supports the epidermis by filling the skin volume with fibers. The hypodermis is present under the dermis and is composed of subcutaneous fat layers [10–12].

The epidermis is a cell layer composed of keratinocytes, the basal layer of which contains progenitor cells (called basal cells) at the interface with the dermal layer. These cells gradually proliferate perpendicularly to the basal layer. At the same time, they differentiate into spinous cells and induce keratinization while undergoing enucleation [10]. Spinous cells are first differentiated from the basal layer and produce keratin, which contributes to tight cell-to-cell adhesion [10,11]. These cells then differentiate into granular cells that are rich in keratohyalin and eject lipids and proteins, as well as connect keratin fibers with higher density [10–12]. Next, the granular cells immediately die after denucleation and form corneocytes that are eventually pushed up to the surface of the skin, resulting in a firm stratum corneum, the outermost layer of the dermal barrier.

Most of the dermis consists of collagen, elastin, and the polysaccharide hyaluronan, which is produced by fibroblasts [10–12]. There are various nerves, blood vessels, hair follicles, sweat glands, macrophages, and T-cells, which play important roles in the secondary function of skin sensation and immunity [4,13–15]. Upon aging or ultraviolet (UV) stimulation, the levels of these substances are decreased, leading to the production of matrix metalloproteinases (MMPs), which are degrading enzymes that reduce skin volume.

The hypodermis is a subcutaneous organization of adipocyte-derived lipids [4,13–15]. Fat tissue is important for maintaining body temperature in humans. Unlike reptiles, which change temperature depending on the environment, humans, with a thin epidermis, develop fat tissue in the hypodermis to maintain body temperature and protect the body organs. Therefore, surplus energy can be stored in the hypodermis, and nerves and blood vessels larger than the dermis are safely preserved from external impact, completing the complex human body as an organic and safe system.

2.2. Zinc Transporters

Intracellular zinc homeostasis is tightly regulated by zinc transporters and metal binding proteins, known as metallothioneins (MTs) (Figure 1) [16]. Because zinc is a metal ion that cannot pass through the cell wall, where lipid is abundant, cells must use carriers to maintain intracellular zinc homeostasis [16,17]. There are two types of zinc transporters: ZIP, which transports zinc into cells from extracellular regions or the luminal side of intracellular compartments and is dependent on zinc concentration, and ZnT, which transports zinc to the exterior of cells or the lumen side from cell cytoplasm. There are 14 ZIP and 10 ZnT family members in humans, and their expression patterns and intracellular locations vary depending on the cell type, developmental stage, and Zn status [18]. Currently, the structure of the ZIP family has not been clarified, but it is thought to possess a domain that penetrates the cell membranes approximately eight times and constitutes a homodimer or a heterodimer with other ZIP members [19,20]. Both ends of ZIP family member peptides face the extracellular or luminal side, with a variety of N-terminal domains, while the intracellular domain has two lengths [19]. In particular, the two domains contain a large number of histidine residues that can bind zinc. Proteoliposome studies using bacterial homologs have suggested that ZIP family members have transport mechanisms such as channels that are independent of other ionic concentrations or adenosine triphosphate (ATP) [21]. In some cases, the filter allowing the passage of zinc is thought to flexibly transport other metals with physicochemical properties similar to those of zinc such as cadmium. For instance, ZIP14 is responsible for transporting iron and manganese in the liver [22–24]. ZIP8 and ZIP14 are symporters that carry metal and biscarbonate ions [25].

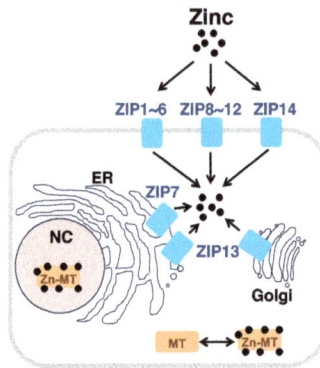

Figure 1. Zinc transporters and metallothionein (MT) are involved in intracellular zinc homeostasis. NC; nucleus, ER; endoplasmic reticulum, Zn; zinc.

ZIP4 is an intensively studied transporter expressed in enterocytes of the small intestine and plays a first gate role in absorbing zinc into the body [26,27]. When zinc is deficient, the N-terminus of ZIP4 is cleaved and the remaining truncated protein migrates to the cell surface to help absorb zinc [28–30]. ZIP4 is a causative gene for acrodermatitis enteropathica (AE), in which systemic zinc deficiency occurs because of impaired intestinal zinc transport [31]. Dozens of pathogenic mutations have been identified. Recent studies showed that single-nucleotide polymorphisms (SNPs) in *ZIP4* differ significantly among various regions of sub-Saharan Africa, where people exhibit high sensitivity to zinc deficiency [32]. Some people have a leucine-to-valine (Leu372Val) replacement in the ZIP4 protein that allows for the expression of small amounts of ZIP4 on cell surfaces and thus transport a low amount of zinc, whereas others show the pathogenic mutations Leu372Pro and Leu372Arg, which prevent ZIP4 from migrating to the cell surface. Homozygous knockout of *ZIP4* in an AE mouse model shows embryonic lethality [27], indicating that ZIP4 is essential for embryonic development in mice. A conditional *Zip4*-knockout mouse in which a *Zip4* allele is specifically deleted by Cre-Lox recombination controlled under the villin promoter has also been generated [33]. These mice show collapse of the stem cell niche and integrity of the small intestine, but do not present any skin abnormality.

ZIP10 is mainly localized to the cell surface and carries zinc in B-cells [34,35]. A conditional *Zip10*-knockout mouse in which a *Zip10* allele is specifically deleted by Cre-Lox recombination controlled under the keratin 14 promoter shows impaired skin barrier [36]. ZIP7 and ZIP13 are present in the endoplasmic reticulum (ER)/Golgi and play important roles in zinc homeostasis within these compartments [37,38]. A conditional *Zip7*-knockout mouse under the collagen 1 promoter results in a thin epidermis; thus, both ZIP7 and ZIP10 are essential for skin homeostasis [39]. In contrast to ZIPs, ZnTs are unique secondary transporters with Y-type and transport zinc using a concentration gradient of a partner transport substrate such as hydrogen ions [40,41]. As in the ZIP family, the ZnT group is present on the cell surface or within the cells depending on the cell type, and thus plays an indispensable role in zinc export [17].

As ZIPs and ZnTs, several transporters and channels were also found to mediate zinc influx. Although their main substrates do not appear to be zinc, transient receptor potential (TRP) channels, divalent metal transporter (DMT1), N-methyl-D-aspartate receptors (NMDA), amino-3-hydroxy-5-methyl-4-isoxazolepropionate receptors (AMPA-Rs), and voltage-dependent calcium channels (VDCCs), are reported to transport zinc [42,43]. However, their involvement in skin development and homeostasis is unknown.

2.3. MTs

MTs were first purified from the cortex of horse kidneys in 1957 [44]. MTs are small proteins (molecular weight less than 7 kDa) containing more than 33% cysteine residues and facilitate the storage of zinc, cadmium, and copper, etc. with high thermal stability [45,46]. MTs are important for acquiring resistance to epithelial apoptosis mediated by reactive oxygen species, possibly through their antioxidant activities [15,47]. Currently, more than 10 isoforms have been identified in humans, located in both the cytoplasm and nucleus [48–50]. Mice lacking *Mt1* or *Mt2* exhibit no specific skin abnormalities [51]. However, the epidermal swelling caused by cholera toxin or UV-B irradiation is not observed in *Mt1/2*-double knockout mice [52]. In a mouse wound healing model, zinc enrichment in hair follicles was found in parallel with increased MT1 and MT2 expression during the wound healing process [53], suggesting that MT1 and MT2 play important roles in epidermal proliferation in certain situations.

2.4. Zinc Levels in Skin

The expression of MTs is induced by metal-responsive transcription factor 1 (MTF1) in a zinc concentration-dependent manner. Therefore, many studies have indirectly monitored the quantity of zinc in cells and tissues by measuring MT expression levels [19,54,55]. MT in the skin is mainly accumulated in progenitor cells and initial spinous cells at the bottom of the epidermis near the basal layers [56]. MTs are also found in out-root sheath cells of hair follicles and epidermal stem cells [57], which are undifferentiated cells with common features and show strong proliferative capacity when necessary [11,12]. Given that zinc is required as a structural component or activating cofactor for over 300 enzymes and other proteins related to cell proliferation, survival, and differentiation, undifferentiated cells with proliferative capacity contain high amounts of zinc [17,46]. It is known that zinc has excellent efficacy for treating and regenerating skin wounds. Indeed, zinc deficiency causes delayed growth with skin anomalies [1,58]. Therefore, zinc is crucial for epidermal stem cells that regenerate inter-follicular epidermis, sebaceous gland, and hair follicle cells by rapidly migrating and dividing basal cells in the early stages of differentiation and scar tissue formation. Treatment with materials that thicken the epidermis have been shown to increase the amount of MT1 in such regions [52,57]. Fibroblasts are sparse in the dermis and do not undergo rapid cell division, suggesting that the dermis contains less zinc than the epidermis. In fact, zinc is present at 60 μg/g in the epidermis and 40 μg/g in the dermis [13,59]. Furthermore, it has been reported that the upper dermis contains higher zinc levels than the lower dermis [59]. This difference may be attributed, in part, to mast cells that contain a large quantity of zinc in the granules. Recently, the skin zinc concentration was measured by synchrotron radiation high energy X-ray fluorescence [60]. This study suggested that the greatest amount of dermal zinc exists in the stratum spinosum, a finding that somewhat differs from those of previous studies that showed a large quantity of zinc in spinous and granular cells compared to basal cells. Given that it is difficult to accurately measure the concentration of specific metals without interference from other metals, a new method for precise measurement of zinc concentration should be developed.

2.5. Zinc Deficiency in Skin

There are two major causes of zinc deficiency in humans. First, zinc deficiency is caused by a diet that is low in zinc content. Approximately 17% of the world's population is confronting health risks related to zinc deficiency, particularly in developing countries. However, in even developed countries, vegetarians, pregnant women, and singles also suffer from zinc deficiency. Second, zinc deficiency can be caused by genetic defects. In 1988, it was reported that babies with severe skin diseases and hair loss were diagnosed with transient neonatal zinc deficiency [61], but recovered by eating normal infant foods [62]. Their mothers have a variety of mutations in alleles of the zinc transporter ZnT2 [63].

When ZnT2 function is impaired, mammary epithelial cells do not release zinc into breast tissue [63]. Therefore, patients with transient neonatal zinc deficiency cannot expect to increase zinc concentrations in the breast milk unless zinc is prescribed. Mice carrying mutations involving ZnT4 exhibit lethal milk (*lm*) syndrome, causing dermatitis and alopecia, but this is irrelevant to humans. Thus, clinical features according to the zinc transport species involved differ among species [64]. Although zinc deficiency is diagnosed by direct measurement of zinc concentrations in the blood, accuracy can be low and perturbed even under healthy conditions. Therefore, the development of new zinc biomarkers has been widely pursued for more precise measurement of zinc levels (e.g., erythrocyte linoleic acid:dihomo-y-linolenic acid (LA:DGLA) [65].

Zinc deficiency initially causes skin problems such as dermatitis, alopecia (thin and sparse hair), acne, eczema, dry, scaling skin, delayed wound healing, and oral ulceration, as well as problems such as stomatitis. [1,17,58,66]. Dermatitis due to zinc deficiency is termed as AE. Brandt's syndrome also includes autosomal recessive metabolic disorders associated with AE, which is accompanied by inherited genetic abnormalities with low zinc distribution. In AE patients, personality disorders are observed, with blistering of the skin (dry skin), hair loss from the scalp, eyebrows, and eyelashes, glossitis, and pustules. Therefore, secondary infections can be easily caused by pathogens such as *Staphylococcus aureus* and fungi such as *Candida albicans* in the weakened epidermis due to zinc deficiency. Recent reports revealed that keratinocytes produce excess amounts of ATP, which induces inflammation upon contact with irritants in individuals with zinc-deficient skin [67]. In zinc-deficient mice, Langerhans cells (LCs), which can neutralize harmful ATP by surface CD39, are greatly reduced in the skin, resulting in augmented skin inflammation by ATP. In AE patients, the number of LCs is also decreased, and is recovered by zinc treatment. The effects of zinc deficiency have also been studied on a cellular basis. When keratinocytes in monolayer culture are scratched, zinc is released from these cells [68]. Subsequently, zinc binds to zinc-sensing receptors and induces cell proliferation in an autocrine/paracrine manner, suggesting that zinc is required for skin regeneration. In fact, the removal of zinc by *N,N,N,N* tetrakis (2-pyridylmethyl) ethylenediamine (TPEN) during keratinocyte culture induces caspase-3 activity and DNA fragmentation followed by apoptosis [69]. Zinc also has an anti-inflammatory effect and reduces tumor necrosis factor-α production by keratinocytes [59]. A recent study demonstrated that R1 and EVER2 proteins found in epidermodysplasia verruciformis (EV) patients with high susceptibility to papillomaviruses causing skin cancer interact with ZnT1 to control the zinc balance in keratinocytes, suggesting the importance of maintaining intracellular zinc homeostasis in skin cancer induced by viral infection [70].

3. Zinc Transporters and Skin Disorders

3.1. Epidermis

Zinc transporters known for their role in the epidermis are ZIP4 and ZIP10. *ZIP4* is actively expressed in human but not in mouse skin [33,71]. Recent skin equivalent experiments with human keratinocytes demonstrated the importance of ZIP4 in epidermis formation [56]. When *ZIP4* is knocked-down by siRNA, epidermal hypoplasia occurs, accompanied by decreased activity of p63, an master regulator with a zinc binding site that promotes the proliferation and differentiation of epidermal progenitor cells in epithelium formation (Figure 2) [56,72,73]. When zinc is deficient, nuclear translocation of p63 is disturbed, followed by abnormal epidermal formation (Figure 2) [56]. Detailed analysis revealed that the 205th Cys among the four Cys residues in the zinc binding site plays an important role in post-modification of p63, suggesting that zinc deficiency affects the DNA binding affinity of p63 involved in signal transduction. Since Zn affects the structure and functions of many proteins [17], ZIP4 may not only target the p63, but also influence the structure and activity of other zinc binding enzymes for epidermal growth. With regard to this issue, further studies are needed to clarify the relationship between ZIP4 and AE. Interestingly, it was recently found that natural products such as soybean extracts increase the expression of ZIP4 [74]. Therefore, this can be a starting point for controlling the rate of zinc absorption.

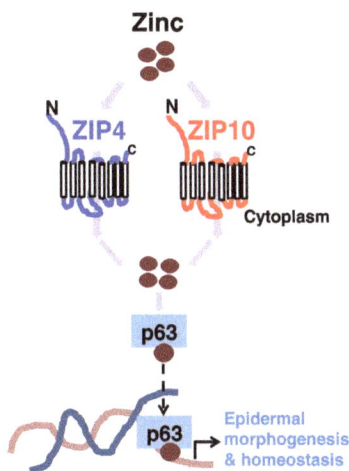

Figure 2. ZIP4 and ZIP10 support p63 activity for adult epidermal homeostasis. ZIP4 and ZIP10 supply zinc to epidermal master regulator p63 for their activity. Zinc deficiency leads to improper function of p63, resulting in epidermal hypoplasia. Zinc is depicted as a brown circle.

Of note, the murine and human epidermis have several different characteristics. Overall, the human epidermis is thicker than the mouse epidermis [11,12]. The stratum corneum shows a solid and thick-layered structure, and has a rete ridge structure because of the diversity of the number of spinous layers. The patterns of epidermal stem cells in the basal layer also differ between mouse and human. Therefore, the use of mouse models in human epidermal studies should be carefully assessed.

ZIP10 also plays important roles in epidermal development [36]. In situ hybridization analysis using mouse whole body sections showed that ZIP10 expression appears in hair follicles near embryonic day 14 (E14) during epidermal development, after which it gradually increases. In a postnatal phase after the completion of epidermis formation, ZIP10 expression is decreased. In the epidermis, ZIP10 accumulates in the outer root sheath region of the hair follicle, which is rich in various Lgr6-positive epidermal stem cells that migrate to the sebaceous glands, hair follicles, and wound space, when epidermis is regenerated upon injury. Consistent with this, next-generation sequencing analysis confirmed that *Zip10*-expressing cells co-express *Lgr6*. A conditional knockout mouse line in which *Zip10* was specifically deleted in Keratin14-expressing cells was born with severe epidermal hypoplasia (Figure 3a,b). In these mice, the p63-positive basal layer formed normally, and slight stratification of the dorsal part of the epidermis occurred by E14. However, such mice fail to form a thick and firm epidermis following rapid proliferation and differentiation of epidermal progenitor cells after E14 when the expression of both ZIP10 and p63 is increased in wild-type mice (Figure 3b,c). Further detailed analysis revealed that ZIP10 augments the activity of p63 by regulating its nuclear translocation (Figure 3c).

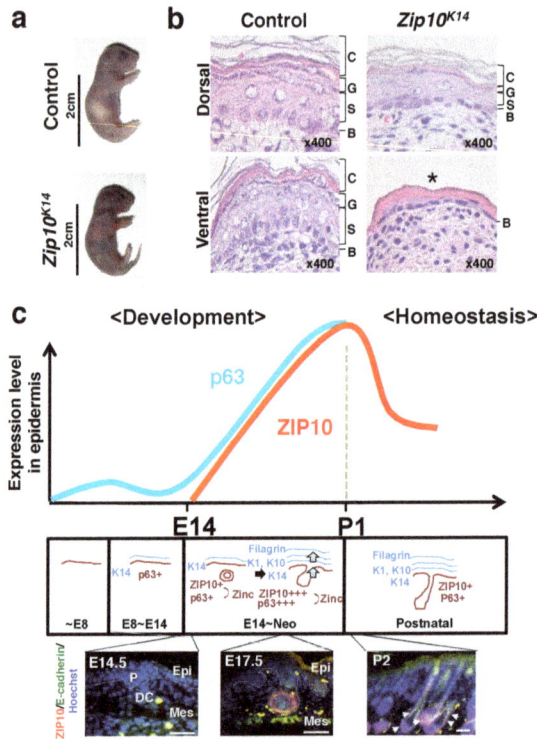

Figure 3. ZIP10 reinforces p63 function for epidermis development. (**a**) ZIP10 deficiency leads to epidermal hypoplasia in mice. (**b**) Hematoxylin and eosin staining revealed dorsal epidermal hypoplasia and ventral embryonic epidermis (asterisk) in P1 *Zip10^{K14}* mice. C, cornified layer; G, granular layer; S, spinous layer; B, basal layer. (**c**) Model for ZIP10's involvement in p63 function during epidermis development. ZIP10, whose expression is elevated from E14, contributes to the activities of increased p63 by supplying zinc. This allows p63 to properly bind to DNA for initiating gene expression for epidermis development, including cell proliferation and stratification. DC, dermal condensate; Epi, epithelium; Mes, mesenchyme; P, placode (Scale bar, 100 μm). Red (E17.5) and arrows (P2) indicate the ZIP10 protein expression. Modified from Bin et al. [36].

3.2. Dermis

Zinc transporters known to be important in the dermis are ZIP 7 and ZIP 13 [37,38]. Both ZIP7 and ZIP13 are present in skin cells and are mainly located in the ER and Golgi, respectively [19,37,38]. These two zinc transporters are closest to each other when a phylogenetic tree of ZIP family members is constructed. ZIP13 is also close to the zinc transporter of insects/bacteria [19]. ZIP13 is the smallest of the mammalian zinc transporters classified in the LIV-1 family, and thus has a shorter N-terminus and intracellular domain 2 than other transporters. The most abundant amino acid in ZIP7 is histidine, which is a characteristic of the LIV-1 family whose role is unknown; this is also the case for the methionine-rich motif that is largely conserved in copper transporters for copper binding and storage [19,75]. During functional analysis of zinc carriers, the first association of the zinc transporter with skin was found in *Zip13*-knockout mice [38]. The *Zip13*-knockout mice showed impaired collagen production with abnormal morphology of collagen-producing cells and shrunken cartilage with defective chondrocyte differentiation. The number of collagen fibers in *Zip13*-knockout mice was remarkably reduced as visualized under an electron microscope, and skin cracking and swelling phenomena were also remarkable because of severely decreased skin strength. This abnormal collagen production was reflected in the mouse face features with an enophthalmos-like appearance, eye blindness, and down-slanting palpebral fissures. The fibroblasts isolated from *Zip13*-knockout mice exhibited dysfunction in the BMP/TGF-β signaling pathway, which is essential for collagen formation. In *Zip13*-knockout mice, the nuclear translocation of SMAD transcription factors in the BMP/TGF-β signaling pathway was impaired, while remaining intact in terms of their phosphorylation status (Figure 4a). Examination of the zinc distribution in *Zip13*-deficient fibroblasts with an electron probe X-ray micro analyzer revealed that the nuclear zinc content was reduced, while that in the Golgi was increased [38,76].

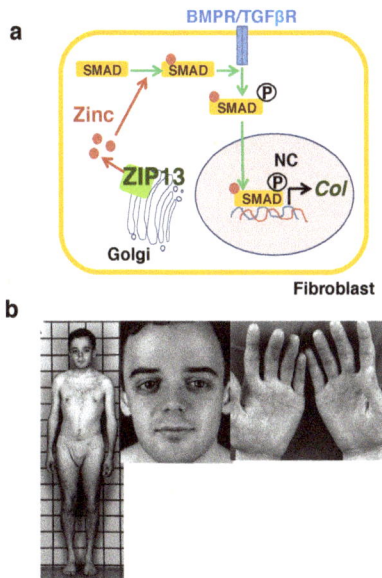

Figure 4. Ehlers–Danlos syndrome spondylodysplastic type 3 is caused by impaired collagen production due to ZIP13 dysfunction. (**a**) ZIP13 supplies zinc (brown circle) to SMAD proteins for their nuclear translocation. Phosphorylatoin is depicted as circled P. (**b**) The elder affected sib is shown at age 22 years. Patient exhibits short stature with mildly shortened trunk, antimongoloid eye slant with lack of periorbital tissue, thin and finely wrinkled skin on the palms of the hands. BMPR/TGFβR, BMP receptor/TGF-β receptor; *Col*, collagen. Modified from Fukada et al. [38].

The phenotypes of *Zip13*-knockout mice are similar to those of patients with spondylocheiro dysplastic form of Ehlers–Danlos syndrome (Ehlers–Danlos syndrome spondylodysplastic type 3, EDSSPD3), with an extremely thin layer of dermis and many wrinkles. EDSSPD3 patients have similar phenotypes such as sagging of the eyes, cracking of the skin, and prominent blood vessels (Figure 4b) [38,76,77]. To date, two mutated Gly64Asp and ΔPhe-Leu-Ala residues in ZIP13 protein have been identified in patients with EDSSPD3. Each of these mutations results in rapid clearance of ZIP13 protein due to ER-associated degradation via valprotein (VCP)/ubiquitination/proteasome machinery [78,79]. Thus, the compounds that increase the activity of ZIP13 or slow the degradation of ZIP13 are considered as therapeutic drugs that can increase collagen synthesis. Since ZIP13 is not only expressed in the Golgi, but also in putative zinc stores [80], another potential mechanism of EDSSPD3 development may be due to non-smooth zinc transport from zinc stores to the cytoplasm in the absence of ZIP13, resulting in low zinc levels in the cytoplasm. If this is the case, this condition also may induce ER stress, as the cytoplasm is a main zinc source for zinc homeostasis in the ER.

ZIP7 is ubiquitously expressed in the ER of nearly all mammalian tissues [17,18] and maintains zinc homeostasis in this intracellular organelle, and the ER acts as a zinc reservoir, although a study showed that ZIP7 also exists in the Golgi [81]. *Zip13*-knockout mice display specific abnormalities in connective tissues irrespective of ZIP7 expression [37], suggesting that ZIP13 and ZIP7 play distinct physiological roles in connective tissue development. Similar to in *Zip13*-knockout mice, *Zip7*-conditional knockout mice, in which Cre-Lox recombination is under the control of the collagen promoter, dysfunction of connective tissues including the dermis and cartilage is observed (Figure 5a,b) [37,38]. The width of the growth plate in *Zip7*-knockout mice is reduced with a normal columnar structure, while that of *Zip13*-knockout mice is disorganized. Unlike *Zip13*-knockdown cells, *Zip7*-knockdown cells show elevated ER stress with increased zinc concentrations in the ER and protein aggregation of protein disulfide isomerase (PDI) [37]. In a *Zip7*-deficient environment, PDI does not function properly because of persistent sticking of zinc on the protein. In fact, *Zip7*-deficient cells fail to achieve the classical protein folding function in the ER, leading to ER stress, unfolded protein response, cell growth inhibition, and apoptosis (Figure 5c). Taken together, this series of studies indicate that proper intracellular zinc distributions in the ER and Golgi by ZIP7 and ZIP13, respectively, are critical for collagen synthesis.

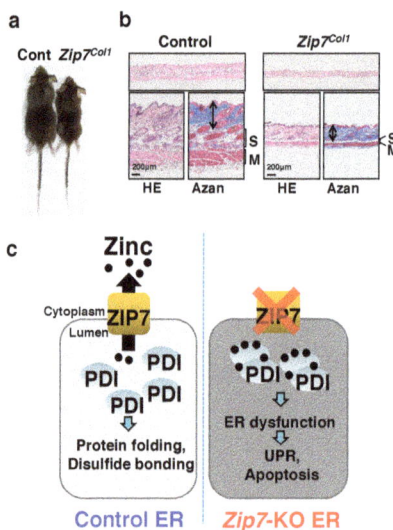

Figure 5. ZIP7 is essential for dermis formation. (**a**) Five-week-old female wild-type (WT) and *Zip7^{Col1}* mice. (**b**) The thickness of the Azan-stained *Zip7^{Col1}* dermis is reduced. M, muscle; S, Subcutis. (**c**) Models for the involvement of ZIP7 in ER function. When ZIP7 is dysregulated (right), the luminal zinc level is elevated, which would induce zinc-dependent aggregation of PDIs. Therefore, protein folding and disulfide bond formation would proceed aberrantly, leading to unfolded protein responses. ER, endoplasmic reticulum; KO, knockout; PDI, protein disulfide isomerase; UPR, unfolded protein response. Modified from Bin et al. [37].

3.3. Hypodermis

Zip7- and *Zip13*-knockout mice display reduced thickness of subcutaneous fat and dermal layers [37,38]. In EDSSPD3 patients, the subcutaneous fat layer is also significantly reduced in the aging skin [38]. Adipocytes play a major role in the formation of subcutaneous fat layers, and fibroblasts produce collagen for dermal formation. Thus, the abnormality of fat layers in *Zip7*- and *Zip13*-knockout mice may be attributed to impaired differentiation of mesenchymal stem cells and the generation of connective tissue cells. In fact, *Zip7*-deficiency in human mesenchymal stem cells leads to ER stress, resulting in defects in fibrogenic and chondrogenic lineage differentiation [37]. However, although *Zip13*-deficient mice show defective formation of connective tissue [38], the effect of mesenchymal stem cells on adipocyte differentiation has not been investigated. Recent research demonstrated that the inguinal white adipose tissue (iWAT) in *Zip13*-knockout mice shows a browning phenotype that reflects increased energy expenditure, thereby reducing iWAT mass. Further analysis revealed that *Zip13*-deficiency causes stabilization of C/EBP-β, an essential transcription factor for adipocyte browning, and thus promotes this process. These data suggest that the ZIP13-zinc axis plays a specific role in clearing C/EBP-β proteins to inhibit adipocyte browning [82].

4. Conclusions

Skin plays an important role as a primary defense line to protect the human body from the external environment. Healthy skin is an important factor that affects social activities and quality of life. It has long been known that zinc is important for maintaining healthy skin. Studies using knockout mouse models have demonstrated that specific zinc signaling axes mediated by individual zinc transporters play crucial roles in skin homeostasis and development. Aging is associated with reduced zinc levels in the human body. Therefore, the development of technology to control the versatile functions of zinc transporters in relation to anti-aging will contribute to regeneration of aged skin.

Acknowledgments: This study was supported by KAKENHI (17H04011) of the Ministry of Education, Culture, Sports, Science, and Technology (MEXT), the Vehicle Racing Commemorative Foundation, the Mitsubishi Foundation, and Takeda Science Foundation to Toshiyuki Fukada. Amorepacific Corporation R&D Center provided financial support to Juyeon Seo. We also thank Andrea Superti-Furga (University of Lausanne) for use of the human case images [30].

Author Contributions: Bum-Ho Bin, Shintaro Hojyo, Juyeon Seo, Takafumi Hara, Teruhisa Takagishi, Kenji Mishima, and Toshiyuki Fukada wrote the paper. Toshiyuki Fukada approved the paper.

Conflicts of Interest: The authors declare no conflicts of interest.

Abbreviations

AE	acrodermatitis enteropathica
ATP	adenosine triphosphate
EDSSPD3	Ehlers–Danlos syndrome spondylodysplastic type 3
iWAT	inguinal white adipose tissue
MTs	metallothioneins
ZIPs	Zrt- and Irt-like proteins
ZnTs	zinc transporters

References

1. Prasad, A.S. Zinc: An overview. *Nutrition* **1995**, *11*, 93–99. [PubMed]
2. Solomons, N.W. Factors affecting the bioavailability of zinc. *J. Am. Diet. Assoc.* **1982**, *80*, 115–121. [PubMed]
3. Nielsen, F.H. History of zinc in agriculture. *Adv. Nutr.* **2012**, *3*, 783–789. [CrossRef] [PubMed]
4. Roohani, N.; Hurrell, R.; Kelishadi, R.; Schulin, R. Zinc and its importance for human health: An integrative review. *J. Res. Med. Sci.* **2013**, *18*, 144–157. [PubMed]
5. Fukada, T.; Yamasaki, S.; Nishida, K.; Murakami, M.; Hirano, T. Zinc homeostasis and signaling in health and diseases: Zinc signaling. *J. Biol. Inorg. Chem.* **2011**, *16*, 1123–1134. [CrossRef] [PubMed]
6. Prasad, A.S. Zinc: Role in immunity, oxidative stress and chronic inflammation. *Curr. Opin. Clin. Nutr. Metab. Care* **2009**, *12*, 646–652. [CrossRef] [PubMed]
7. Prasad, A.S.; Miale, A., Jr.; Farid, Z.; Sandstead, H.H.; Schulert, A.R. Zinc metabolism in patients with the syndrome of iron deficiency anemia, hepatosplenomegaly, dwarfism, and hypognadism. *J. Lab. Clin. Med.* **1963**, *61*, 537–549. [PubMed]

8. Sandstead, H.H.; Prasad, A.S.; Schulert, A.R.; Farid, Z.; Miale, A., Jr.; Bassilly, S.; Darby, W.J. Human zinc deficiency, endocrine manifestations and response to treatment. *Am. J. Clin. Nutr.* **1967**, *20*, 422–442. [CrossRef] [PubMed]

9. Lonnerdal, B. Dietary factors influencing zinc absorption. *J. Nutr.* **2000**, *130*, 1378S–1383S. [CrossRef] [PubMed]

10. Fuchs, E.; Raghavan, S. Getting under the skin of epidermal morphogenesis. *Nat. Rev. Genet.* **2002**, *3*, 199–209. [CrossRef] [PubMed]

11. Blanpain, C.; Fuchs, E. Epidermal homeostasis: A balancing act of stem cells in the skin. *Nat. Mol. Cell Biol.* **2009**, *10*, 207–217. [CrossRef] [PubMed]

12. Solanas, G.; Benitah, S.A. Regenerating the skin: A task for the heterogeneous stem cell pool and surrounding niche. *Nat. Mol. Cell Biol.* **2013**, *14*, 737–748. [CrossRef] [PubMed]

13. Agren, M.S. Studies on zinc in wound healing. *Acta Derm. Venereol.* **1990**, *154*, 1–36.

14. Schwartz, J.R.; Marsh, R.G.; Draelos, Z.D. Zinc and skin health: Overview of physiology and pharmacology. *Dermatol. Surg.* **2005**, *31*, 837–847. [CrossRef] [PubMed]

15. Lansdown, A.B.; Mirastschijski, U.; Stubbs, N.; Scanlon, E.; Agren, M.S. Zinc in wound healing: Theoretical, experimental, and clinical aspects. *Wound Repair Regen.* **2007**, *15*, 2–16. [CrossRef] [PubMed]

16. Hara, T.; Takeda, T.A.; Takagishi, T.; Fukue, K.; Kambe, T.; Fukada, T. Physiological roles of zinc transporters: Molecular and genetic importance in zinc homeostasis. *J. Physiol. Sci.* **2017**, *67*, 283–301. [CrossRef] [PubMed]

17. Fukada, T.; Kambe, T. Molecular and genetic features of zinc transporters in physiology and pathogenesis. *Metallomics* **2011**, *3*, 662–674. [CrossRef] [PubMed]

18. Taylor, K.M.; Nicholson, R.I. The LZT proteins; the LIV-1 subfamily of zinc transporters. *Biochim. Biophys. Acta* **2003**, *1611*, 16–30. [CrossRef]

19. Bin, B.H.; Fukada, T.; Hosaka, T.; Yamasaki, S.; Ohashi, W.; Hojyo, S.; Miyai, T.; Nishida, K.; Yokoyama, S.; Hirano, T. Biochemical characterization of human ZIP13 protein: A homo-dimerized zinc transporter involved in the spondylocheiro dysplastic ehlers-danlos syndrome. *J. Biol. Chem.* **2011**, *286*, 40255–40265. [CrossRef] [PubMed]

20. Taylor, K.M.; Muraina, I.A.; Brethour, D.; Schmitt-Ulms, G.; Nimmanon, T.; Ziliotto, S.; Kille, P.; Hogstrand, C. Zinc transporter ZIP10 forms a heteromer with ZIP6 which regulates embryonic development and cell migration. *Biochem. J.* **2016**, *473*, 2531–2544. [CrossRef] [PubMed]

21. Lin, W.; Chai, J.; Love, J.; Fu, D. Selective electrodiffusion of zinc ions in a Zrt-, Irt-like protein, ZIPB. *J. Biol. Chem.* **2010**, *285*, 39013–39020. [CrossRef] [PubMed]

22. Jenkitkasemwong, S.; Wang, C.Y.; Coffey, R.; Zhang, W.; Chan, A.; Biel, T.; Kim, J.S.; Hojyo, S.; Fukada, T.; Knutson, M.D. Slc39a14 is required for the development of hepatocellular iron overload in murine models of hereditary hemochromatosis. *Cell Metab.* **2015**, *22*, 138–150. [CrossRef] [PubMed]

23. Jenkitkasemwong, S.; Akinyode, A.; Paulus, E.; Weiskirchen, R.; Hojyo, S.; Fukada, T.; Giraldo, G.; Schrier, J.; Garcia, A.; Janus, C.; et al. Slc39a14 deficiency alters manganese homeostasis and excretion resulting in brain manganese accumulation and motor deficits in mice. *Proc. Natl. Acad. Sci. USA* **2018**. [CrossRef] [PubMed]

24. Liuzzi, J.P.; Aydemir, F.; Nam, H.; Knutson, M.D.; Cousins, R.J. ZIP14 (Slc39a14) mediates non-transferrin-bound iron uptake into cells. *Proc. Natl. Acad. Sci. USA* **2006**, *103*, 13612–13617. [CrossRef] [PubMed]

25. Girijashanker, K.; He, L.; Soleimani, M.; Reed, J.M.; Li, H.; Liu, Z.; Wang, B.; Dalton, T.P.; Nebert, D.W. Slc39a14 gene encodes ZIP14, a metal/bicarbonate symporter: Similarities to the ZIP8 transporter. *Mol. Pharmacol.* **2008**, *73*, 1413–1423. [CrossRef] [PubMed]

26. Dufner-Beattie, J.; Kuo, Y.M.; Gitschier, J.; Andrews, G.K. The adaptive response to dietary zinc in mice involves the differential cellular localization and zinc regulation of the zinc transporters ZIP4 and ZIP5. *J. Biol. Chem.* **2004**, *279*, 49082–49090. [CrossRef] [PubMed]

27. Dufner-Beattie, J.; Weaver, B.P.; Geiser, J.; Bilgen, M.; Larson, M.; Xu, W.; Andrews, G.K. The mouse acrodermatitis enteropathica gene Slc39a4 (ZIP4) is essential for early development and heterozygosity causes hypersensitivity to zinc deficiency. *Hum. Mol. Genet.* **2007**, *16*, 1391–1399. [CrossRef] [PubMed]

28. Weaver, B.P.; Dufner-Beattie, J.; Kambe, T.; Andrews, G.K. Novel zinc-responsive post-transcriptional mechanisms reciprocally regulate expression of the mouse Slc39a4 and Slc39a5 zinc transporters (ZIP4 and ZIP5). *Biol. Chem.* **2007**, *388*, 1301–1312. [CrossRef] [PubMed]

29. Kim, B.E.; Wang, F.; Dufner-Beattie, J.; Andrews, G.K.; Eide, D.J.; Petris, M.J. Zn^{2+}-stimulated endocytosis of the mZIP4 zinc transporter regulates its location at the plasma membrane. *J. Biol. Chem.* **2004**, *279*, 4523–4530. [CrossRef] [PubMed]

30. Kambe, T.; Andrews, G.K. Novel proteolytic processing of the ectodomain of the zinc transporter ZIP4 (Slc39a4) during zinc deficiency is inhibited by acrodermatitis enteropathica mutations. *Mol. Cell. Biol.* **2009**, *29*, 129–139. [CrossRef] [PubMed]

31. Hojyo, S.; Bin, B.H.; Fukada, T. Dysregulated zinc homeostasis in rare skin disorders. *Expert Opin. Orphan Drugs* **2017**, *5*, 865–873. [CrossRef]

32. Engelken, J.; Carnero-Montoro, E.; Pybus, M.; Andrews, G.K.; Lalueza-Fox, C.; Comas, D.; Sekler, I.; de la Rasilla, M.; Rosas, A.; Stoneking, M.; et al. Extreme population differences in the human zinc transporter ZIP4 (Slc39a4) are explained by positive selection in sub-Saharan Africa. *PLoS Genet.* **2014**, *10*, e1004128. [CrossRef] [PubMed]

33. Geiser, J.; Venken, K.J.; De Lisle, R.C.; Andrews, G.K. A mouse model of acrodermatitis enteropathica: Loss of intestine zinc transporter ZIP4 (Slc39a4) disrupts the stem cell niche and intestine integrity. *PLoS Genet.* **2012**, *8*, e1002766. [CrossRef] [PubMed]

34. Hojyo, S.; Miyai, T.; Fujishiro, H.; Kawamura, M.; Yasuda, T.; Hijikata, A.; Bin, B.H.; Irie, T.; Tanaka, J.; Atsumi, T.; et al. Zinc transporter Slc39a10/ZIP10 controls humoral immunity by modulating B-cell receptor signal strength. *Proc. Natl. Acad. Sci. USA* **2014**, *111*, 11786–11791. [CrossRef] [PubMed]

35. Miyai, T.; Hojyo, S.; Ikawa, T.; Kawamura, M.; Irie, T.; Ogura, H.; Hijikata, A.; Bin, B.H.; Yasuda, T.; Kitamura, H.; et al. Zinc transporter Slc39a10/ZIP10 facilitates antiapoptotic signaling during early B-cell development. *Proc. Natl. Acad. Sci. USA* **2014**, *111*, 11780–11785. [CrossRef] [PubMed]

36. Bin, B.H.; Bhin, J.; Takaishi, M.; Toyoshima, K.E.; Kawamata, S.; Ito, K.; Hara, T.; Watanabe, T.; Irie, T.; Takagishi, T.; et al. Requirement of zinc transporter ZIP10 for epidermal development: Implication of the ZIP10-p63 axis in epithelial homeostasis. *Proc. Natl. Acad. Sci. USA* **2017**, *114*, 12243–12248. [CrossRef] [PubMed]

37. Bin, B.H.; Bhin, J.; Seo, J.; Kim, S.Y.; Lee, E.; Park, K.; Choi, D.H.; Takagishi, T.; Hara, T.; Hwang, D.; et al. Requirement of zinc transporter slc39a7/ZIP7 for dermal development to fine-tune endoplasmic reticulum function by regulating protein disulfide isomerase. *J. Investig. Dermatol.* **2017**, *137*, 1682–1691. [CrossRef] [PubMed]

38. Fukada, T.; Civic, N.; Furuichi, T.; Shimoda, S.; Mishima, K.; Higashiyama, H.; Idaira, Y.; Asada, Y.; Kitamura, H.; Yamasaki, S.; et al. The zinc transporter slc39a13/ZIP13 is required for connective tissue development; its involvement in BMP/TGF-beta signaling pathways. *PLoS ONE* **2008**, *3*, e3642. [CrossRef]

39. Takagishi, T.; Hara, T.; Fukada, T. Recent advances in the role of SLC39A/ZIP zinc transporters in vivo. *Int. J. Mol. Sci.* **2017**, *18*, E2708. [CrossRef] [PubMed]

40. Gupta, S.; Chai, J.; Cheng, J.; D'Mello, R.; Chance, M.R.; Fu, D. Visualizing the kinetic power stroke that drives proton-coupled zinc(ii) transport. *Nature* **2014**, *512*, 101–104. [CrossRef] [PubMed]

41. Lu, M.; Fu, D. Structure of the zinc transporter YiiP. *Science* **2007**, *317*, 1746–1748. [CrossRef] [PubMed]

42. Bouron, A.; Kiselyov, K.; Oberwinkler, J. Permeation, regulation and control of expression of TRP channels by trace metal ions. *Pflüg. Arch.* **2015**, *467*, 1143–1164. [CrossRef] [PubMed]

43. Inoue, K.; O'Bryant, Z.; Xiong, Z.G. Zinc-permeable ion channels: Effects on intracellular zinc dynamics and potential physiological/pathophysiological significance. *Curr. Med. Chem.* **2015**, *22*, 1248–1257. [CrossRef] [PubMed]

44. Kagi, J.H.; Vallee, B.L. Metallothionein: A cadmium and zinc-containign protein from equine renal cortex. Ii. Physico-chemical properties. *J. Biol. Chem.* **1961**, *236*, 2435–2442. [PubMed]

45. Kagi, J.H.; Valee, B.L. Metallothionein: A cadmium- and zinc-containing protein from equine renal cortex. *J. Biol. Chem.* **1960**, *235*, 3460–3465. [PubMed]

46. Kambe, T.; Tsuji, T.; Hashimoto, A.; Itsumura, N. The physiological, biochemical, and molecular roles of zinc transporters in zinc homeostasis and metabolism. *Physiol. Rev.* **2015**, *95*, 749–784. [CrossRef] [PubMed]

47. Morgan, A.J.; Lewis, G.; Van den Hoven, W.E.; Akkerboom, P.J. The effect of zinc in the form of erythromycin-zinc complex (zineryt lotion) and zinc acetate on metallothionein expression and distribution in hamster skin. *Br. J. Dermatol.* **1993**, *129*, 563–570. [CrossRef] [PubMed]

48. Thirumoorthy, N.; Shyam Sunder, A.; Manisenthil Kumar, K.; Senthil Kumar, M.; Ganesh, G.; Chatterjee, M. A review of metallothionein isoforms and their role in pathophysiology. *World J. Surg. Oncol.* **2011**, *9*, 54. [CrossRef] [PubMed]

49. Tsujikawa, K.; Imai, T.; Kakutani, M.; Kayamori, Y.; Mimura, T.; Otaki, N.; Kimura, M.; Fukuyama, R.; Shimizu, N. Localization of metallothionein in nuclei of growing primary cultured adult rat hepatocytes. *FEBS Lett.* **1991**, *283*, 239–242. [CrossRef]

50. Cherian, M.G.; Apostolova, M.D. Nuclear localization of metallothionein during cell proliferation and differentiation. *Cell. Mol. Biol.* **2000**, *46*, 347–356. [PubMed]

51. Masters, B.A.; Kelly, E.J.; Quaife, C.J.; Brinster, R.L.; Palmiter, R.D. Targeted disruption of metallothionein i and ii genes increases sensitivity to cadmium. *Proc. Natl. Acad. Sci. USA* **1994**, *91*, 584–588. [CrossRef] [PubMed]

52. Hanada, K.; Sawamura, D.; Hashimoto, I.; Kida, K.; Naganuma, A. Epidermal proliferation of the skin in metallothionein-null mice. *J. Investig. Dermatol.* **1998**, *110*, 259–262. [CrossRef] [PubMed]

53. Iwata, M.; Takebayashi, T.; Ohta, H.; Alcalde, R.E.; Itano, Y.; Matsumura, T. Zinc accumulation and metallothionein gene expression in the proliferating epidermis during wound healing in mouse skin. *Histochem. Cell Biol.* **1999**, *112*, 283–290. [CrossRef] [PubMed]

54. Coyle, P.; Philcox, J.C.; Carey, L.C.; Rofe, A.M. Metallothionein: The multipurpose protein. *Cell. Mol. Life Sci.* **2002**, *59*, 627–647. [CrossRef] [PubMed]

55. Giedroc, D.P.; Chen, X.; Apuy, J.L. Metal response element (MRE)-binding transcription factor-1 (MTF-1): Structure, function, and regulation. *Antioxid. Redox Signal.* **2001**, *3*, 577–596. [CrossRef] [PubMed]

56. Bin, B.H.; Bhin, J.; Kim, N.H.; Lee, S.H.; Jung, H.S.; Seo, J.; Kim, D.K.; Hwang, D.; Fukada, T.; Lee, A.Y.; et al. An acrodermatitis enteropathica-associated Zn transporter, ZIP4, regulates human epidermal homeostasis. *J. Investig. Dermatol.* **2017**, *137*, 874–883. [CrossRef] [PubMed]

57. Karasawa, M.; Nishimura, N.; Nishimura, H.; Tohyama, C.; Hashiba, H.; Kuroki, T. Localization of metallothionein in hair follicles of normal skin and the basal cell layer of hyperplastic epidermis: Possible association with cell proliferation. *J. Investig. Dermatol.* **1991**, *97*, 97–100. [CrossRef] [PubMed]

58. King, J.C.; Shames, D.M.; Woodhouse, L.R. Zinc homeostasis in humans. *J. Nutr.* **2000**, *130*, 1360S–1366S. [CrossRef] [PubMed]

59. Ogawa, Y.; Kawamura, T.; Shimada, S. Zinc and skin biology. *Arch. Biochem. Biophys.* **2016**, *611*, 113–119. [CrossRef] [PubMed]

60. Inoue, Y.; Hasegawa, S.; Ban, S.; Yamada, T.; Date, Y.; Mizutani, H.; Nakata, S.; Tanaka, M.; Hirashima, N. ZIP2 protein, a zinc transporter, is associated with keratinocyte differentiation. *J. Biol. Chem.* **2014**, *289*, 21451–21462. [CrossRef] [PubMed]

61. Glover, M.T.; Atherton, D.J. Transient zinc deficiency in two full-term breast-fed siblings associated with low maternal breast milk zinc concentration. *Pediatr. Dermatol.* **1988**, *5*, 10–13. [CrossRef] [PubMed]

62. Sharma, N.L.; Sharma, R.C.; Gupta, K.R.; Sharma, R.P. Self-limiting acrodermatitis enteropathica. A follow-up study of three interrelated families. *Int. J. Dermatol.* **1988**, *27*, 485–486. [CrossRef] [PubMed]

63. Chowanadisai, W.; Lonnerdal, B.; Kelleher, S.L. Identification of a mutation in slc30a2 (ZnT-2) in women with low milk zinc concentration that results in transient neonatal zinc deficiency. *J. Biol. Chem.* **2006**, *281*, 39699–39707. [CrossRef] [PubMed]

64. Michalczyk, A.; Varigos, G.; Catto-Smith, A.; Blomeley, R.C.; Ackland, M.L. Analysis of zinc transporter, hZnT4 (slc30a4), gene expression in a mammary gland disorder leading to reduced zinc secretion into milk. *Hum. Genet.* **2003**, *113*, 202–210. [CrossRef] [PubMed]

65. Reed, S.; Qin, X.; Ran-Ressler, R.; Brenna, J.T.; Glahn, R.P.; Tako, E. Dietary zinc deficiency affects blood linoleic acid: Dihomo-gamma-linolenic acid (la:Dgla) ratio; a sensitive physiological marker of zinc status in vivo (gallus gallus). *Nutrients* **2014**, *6*, 1164–1180. [CrossRef] [PubMed]

66. Frederickson, C.J.; Koh, J.Y.; Bush, A.I. The neurobiology of zinc in health and disease. *Nat. Rev. Neurosci.* **2005**, *6*, 449–462. [CrossRef] [PubMed]

67. Kawamura, T.; Ogawa, Y.; Nakamura, Y.; Nakamizo, S.; Ohta, Y.; Nakano, H.; Kabashima, K.; Katayama, I.; Koizumi, S.; Kodama, T.; et al. Severe dermatitis with loss of epidermal langerhans cells in human and mouse zinc deficiency. *J. Clin. Investig.* **2012**, *122*, 722–732. [CrossRef] [PubMed]

68. Sharir, H.; Zinger, A.; Nevo, A.; Sekler, I.; Hershfinkel, M. Zinc released from injured cells is acting via the Zn^{2+}-sensing receptor, ZnR, to trigger signaling leading to epithelial repair. *J. Biol. Chem.* **2010**, *285*, 26097–26106. [CrossRef] [PubMed]

69. Wilson, D.; Varigos, G.; Ackland, M.L. Apoptosis may underlie the pathology of zinc-deficient skin. *Immunol. Cell Biol.* **2006**, *84*, 28–37. [CrossRef] [PubMed]

70. Lazarczyk, M.; Pons, C.; Mendoza, J.A.; Cassonnet, P.; Jacob, Y.; Favre, M. Regulation of cellular zinc balance as a potential mechanism of ever-mediated protection against pathogenesis by cutaneous oncogenic human papillomaviruses. *J. Exp. Med.* **2008**, *205*, 35–42. [CrossRef] [PubMed]

71. Dufner-Beattie, J.; Wang, F.; Kuo, Y.M.; Gitschier, J.; Eide, D.; Andrews, G.K. The acrodermatitis enteropathica gene ZIP4 encodes a tissue-specific, zinc-regulated zinc transporter in mice. *J. Biol. Chem.* **2003**, *278*, 33474–33481. [CrossRef] [PubMed]

72. Koster, M.I.; Kim, S.; Mills, A.A.; DeMayo, F.J.; Roop, D.R. P63 is the molecular switch for initiation of an epithelial stratification program. *Genes Dev.* **2004**, *18*, 126–131. [CrossRef] [PubMed]

73. McKeon, F. P63 and the epithelial stem cell: More than status quo? *Genes Dev.* **2004**, *18*, 465–469. [CrossRef] [PubMed]

74. Hashimoto, A.; Ohkura, K.; Takahashi, M.; Kizu, K.; Narita, H.; Enomoto, S.; Miyamae, Y.; Masuda, S.; Nagao, M.; Irie, K.; et al. Soybean extracts increase cell surface ZIP4 abundance and cellular zinc levels: A potential novel strategy to enhance zinc absorption by ZIP4 targeting. *Biochem. J.* **2015**, *472*, 183–193. [CrossRef] [PubMed]

75. Petris, M.J. The slc31 (ctr) copper transporter family. *Pflüg. Arch.* **2004**, *447*, 752–755.

76. Giunta, C.; Elcioglu, N.H.; Albrecht, B.; Eich, G.; Chambaz, C.; Janecke, A.R.; Yeowell, H.; Weis, M.; Eyre, D.R.; Kraenzlin, M.; et al. Spondylocheiro dysplastic form of the ehlers-danlos syndrome—An autosomal-recessive entity caused by mutations in the zinc transporter gene slc39a13. *Am. J. Hum. Genet.* **2008**, *82*, 1290–1305. [CrossRef] [PubMed]

77. Malfait, F.; Francomano, C.; Byers, P.; Belmont, J.; Berglund, B.; Black, J.; Bloom, L.; Bowen, J.M.; Brady, A.F.; Burrows, N.P.; et al. The 2017 international classification of the ehlers-danlos syndromes. *Am. J. Med. Genet. Part C Semin. Med. Genet.* **2017**, *175*, 8–26. [CrossRef] [PubMed]

78. Bin, B.H.; Hojyo, S.; Hosaka, T.; Bhin, J.; Kano, H.; Miyai, T.; Ikeda, M.; Kimura-Someya, T.; Shirouzu, M.; Cho, E.G.; et al. Molecular pathogenesis of spondylocheirodysplastic ehlers-danlos syndrome caused by mutant ZIP13 proteins. *EMBO Mol. Med.* **2014**, *6*, 1028–1042. [CrossRef] [PubMed]

79. Bin, B.H.; Hojyo, S.; Ryong Lee, T.; Fukada, T. Spondylocheirodysplastic ehlers-danlos syndrome (SCD-EDS) and the mutant zinc transporter ZIP13. *Rare Dis.* **2014**, *2*, e974982. [CrossRef] [PubMed]

80. Jeong, J.; Walker, J.M.; Wang, F.; Park, J.G.; Palmer, A.E.; Giunta, C.; Rohrbach, M.; Steinmann, B.; Eide, D.J. Promotion of vesicular zinc efflux by ZIP13 and its implications for spondylocheiro dysplastic ehlers-danlos syndrome. *Proc. Natl. Acad. Sci. USA* **2012**, *109*, E3530–E3538. [CrossRef] [PubMed]

81. Huang, L.; Kirschke, C.P.; Zhang, Y.; Yu, Y.Y. The ZIP7 gene (slc39a7) encodes a zinc transporter involved in zinc homeostasis of the golgi apparatus. *J. Biol. Chem.* **2005**, *280*, 15456–15463. [CrossRef] [PubMed]

82. Fukunaka, A.; Fukada, T.; Bhin, J.; Suzuki, L.; Tsuzuki, T.; Takamine, Y.; Bin, B.H.; Yoshihara, T.; Ichinoseki-Sekine, N.; Naito, H.; et al. Zinc transporter ZIP13 suppresses beige adipocyte biogenesis and energy expenditure by regulating C/EBP-beta expression. *PLoS Genet.* **2017**, *13*, e1006950. [CrossRef] [PubMed]

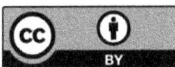

nutrients

MDPI

Article
Modifiable "Predictors" of Zinc Status in Toddlers

Lisa Daniels [1,2], Sheila M. Williams [3], Rosalind S. Gibson [1], Rachael W. Taylor [2], Samir Samman [1,4] and Anne-Louise M. Heath [1,*]

1   Department of Human Nutrition, University of Otago, Dunedin 9054, New Zealand; lisa.daniels@otago.ac.nz (L.D.); rosalind.gibson@otago.ac.nz (R.S.G.); samir.samman@sydney.edu.au (S.S.)
2   Department of Medicine, University of Otago, Dunedin 9054, New Zealand; rachael.taylor@otago.ac.nz
3   Department of Preventive and Social Medicine, University of Otago, Dunedin 9054, New Zealand; sheila.williams@otago.ac.nz
4   School of Life and Environmental Sciences, University of Sydney, Sydney, NSW 2006, Australia
*   Correspondence: anne-louise.heath@otago.ac.nz; Tel.: +64-3-479-8379

Received: 21 December 2017; Accepted: 2 March 2018; Published: 5 March 2018

Abstract: Suboptimal zinc status is common in very young children and likely associated with increased risk of infection and detrimental effects on growth. No studies have determined potentially modifiable "predictors" of zinc status in toddlers from high-income countries. This cross-sectional analysis of 115 toddlers from the Baby-Led Introduction to SolidS (BLISS) study used weighed diet records (three non-consecutive days) to assess dietary intake, and a venous blood sample (trace-element free techniques) to assess plasma zinc, at 12 months of age. "Predictors" of plasma zinc were determined by univariate analysis and multiple regression. Mean (SD) plasma zinc was 9.7 (1.5) µmol/L, 60% were below the IZiNCG reference limit of <9.9 µmol/L. Median (25th, 75th percentiles) intake of zinc was 4.4 (3.7, 5.4) mg/day. Red meat intake ($p = 0.004$), consumption of zinc-fortified infant formula (3–6 mg zinc/100 g) ($p = 0.026$), and food fussiness ($p = 0.028$) were statistically significant "predictors" of plasma zinc at 12 months. Although higher intakes of red meat, and consumption of infant formula, are potentially achievable, it is important to consider possible barriers, particularly impact on breastfeeding, cost, and the challenges of behavior modification. Of interest is the association with food fussiness—further research should investigate the direction of this association.

Keywords: zinc status; plasma zinc; toddlers; food fussiness; red meat; infant formula; zinc intake; complementary feeding

1. Introduction

During early childhood the risk of zinc deficiency is increased [1], primarily because of a higher physiological requirement for zinc due to the high growth rate during this time [2]. However, zinc intake is also an issue because the complementary foods typically offered when solids are introduced (e.g., fruit, vegetables, cereals) are generally low in absorbable zinc, and because after six months of age breast milk no longer provides sufficient zinc to meet requirements [3].

Suboptimal zinc status has frequently been reported in studies of young children from high-income countries, including New Zealand [4–13]. Inadequate zinc status during early childhood is associated with an increased risk of infection [14,15]. This is particularly important as many toddlers participate in child care programs where the exposure to illness is high [16]. Inadequate zinc status can also have detrimental effects on growth [17]. Therefore, it is also important to determine what factors may be modifiable during early childhood that might improve the zinc status of this age group.

Several international studies have indicated that various biological and methodological factors affect zinc status, including age [5,18,19], season [20,21], inflammation or infection [18,22], time of the day [22–25], and fasting status [22,24,25]. Yet, to our knowledge, no study has assessed modifiable "predictors" of zinc status in healthy infants or toddlers after standardizing these factors that are known to affect plasma zinc concentrations.

The aim of this paper was to examine associations between dietary, biochemical, and other variables, and plasma zinc concentration, and to determine potentially modifiable "predictors" of plasma zinc at 12 months of age.

2. Materials and Methods

2.1. Study Design

This is a cross-sectional analysis of data collected in the Baby-Led Introduction to SolidS (BLISS) study [26]. BLISS was a randomized controlled trial investigating the impact of a modified version of Baby-Led Weaning (BLW) on several infant outcomes including growth [27], iron [28], and zinc [29] status, and choking [30]. Written consent was obtained from all adult participants before randomization to one of two groups: BLISS (infant self-feeding using a modified version of BLW) or Control (usual care) between November 2012 and March 2014. The Lower South Regional Ethics Committee of New Zealand approved the study (LRS/11/09/037).

2.2. Outcome Assessment

2.2.1. Questionnaire Data

Demographic data, including maternal age, ethnicity, education, and parity, were collected at baseline (late pregnancy) by questionnaire. The participant's current address was used to determine household deprivation using the New Zealand Index of Deprivation (NZDep) score [31]. Infant sex, birth weight, and gestational age at birth were accessed through hospital records. Parents completed a questionnaire (self-administered) at 12 months of age which included questions from the Children's Eating Behaviour Questionnaire on food fussiness [32]. Using response options of "never", "rarely", "sometimes", "often", or "always", parents indicated whether their child enjoyed tasting new foods, consumed a wide variety of foods, were interested in tasting new foods, refused new foods, decided whether a food was disliked before tasting, and whether there was difficulty in pleasing the toddler with meals. Higher mean scores represent higher levels of food fussiness [32] and Cronbach α for our sample ranged from 0.64 to 0.88 for individual questions.

2.2.2. Anthropometric Assessment

Research staff measured toddler weight (Seca, Model 334, Hamburg, Germany) and length (Rollameter 100c length board, Harlow Healthcare, South Shields, UK) in duplicate when they were 12 months of age. Infants were weighed without clothes (wearing only a standard weight nappy which was subtracted from their weight on data entering), and length was measured with no shoes, complying with the World Health Organization (WHO) protocols [33]. Weight-for-age and length-for-age z-scores were calculated using the WHO child growth standards reference data [34].

2.2.3. Dietary Assessment

Weighed three-day diet records (WDRs) were used to assess dietary intake at 12 months of age. Parent participants were given detailed written and oral instructions for completing the WDR and then recorded all foods and beverages consumed on three randomly assigned non-consecutive days (two weekdays and one weekend day) over a three-week period. Each day of the week was represented approximately an equal number of times among participants to control for day-of-the-week effects. Dietary scales (Salter Electronic, Salter Housewares Ltd., Tonbridge, UK), accurate to ±1 g were given to each participant to complete the WDR. The completed WDRs were entered into Kai-culator (Version 1.13s, University of Otago, Dunedin, New Zealand), a New Zealand dietary analysis software program that includes dietary data from the New Zealand Food Composition Database (FOODfiles 2010, Plant and Food Research) [35]. "Meat, fish, poultry", heme iron, and non-heme iron [36] and phytate were not available in the New Zealand Food Composition Database, but were determined using values from the literature and information from the manufacturers [29].

2.2.4. Biochemical Assessment

A venous (antecubital vein) blood sample was collected from participants at 12 months of age using trace-element free lithium heparin anticoagulated tubes (7.5 mL; S-Monovette, Sarstedt, Nümbrecht, Germany) and standardized procedures, as recommended by the International Zinc Nutrition Consultative Group (IZiNCG) [37]. A local anesthetic (Ametop gel, Smith & Nephew, London, UK) was applied to the toddler's arm 1–2 h before the appointment, and infants were seated on a parent's knee for the phlebotomy. Strict procedures were used to control for known predictors of plasma zinc concentrations: time of blood collection [22–25], fasting status [22,24,25], and inflammation [18,22]. To standardize food intake prior to the blood test, parents were asked to feed their baby milk (as much as they wanted of the milk they usually have, e.g., breast milk, infant formula, or cow's milk) 90 min prior to the blood test appointment, and then to give no other food or drink until after the blood test. To reduce the impact of inflammation, if the child was unwell on the day before the scheduled blood test (i.e., presence of fever, diarrhea, or vomiting), the blood test was delayed for 14 days. A questionnaire was also administered at the blood test appointment which asked parents to confirm the timing of the milk feed, whether any illness was present and whether any zinc-containing preparations were used in the past month.

Plasma zinc was determined using flame atomic absorption spectrophotometry (Perkin Elmer AAnalyst 800), in the Department of Human Nutrition, University of Otago. The accuracy and precision of the analyses were checked using certified controls and in-house pooled samples (after every 15 samples). The analysed mean (SD, CV) value for the zinc control (UTAK Laboratories, Inc., Valencia, CA, USA) was 65.8 µmol/L (1.9 µmol/L, 2.9%), compared to the manufacturers' concentration of 65 µmol/L. Since the samples were collected from the toddlers in the morning, low plasma zinc concentrations were defined as a concentration < 9.9 µmol/L [37]. Plasma zinc concentration is used to indicate "zinc status" in this paper as has been recommended by IZiNCG [37], in the absence of a more appropriate biomarker for determining "zinc status".

C-reactive protein (CRP; a measure of acute inflammation), and α1-acid glycoprotein (AGP; a measure of chronic inflammation) were analysed using a Cobas C311 automatic electronic analyser (Roche Diagnostics, GmbH, Mannheim, Germany). These analyses were carried out in the Department of Human Nutrition laboratories (University of Otago, Dunedin, New Zealand). The mean (SD, CV) for the CRP control (Roche Diagnostics, GmbH, Mannheim, Germany) was 9.5 mg/L (0.4 mg/L, 4.6%), compared with the manufacturer's concentration of 9.1 mg/L. The multilevel controls for AGP (Roche Diagnostics, GmbH, Mannheim, Germany) were 0.5 g/L (0.01 g/L, 1.1%) and 0.8 g/L (0.01 g/L, 1.4%), compared with the manufacturer's concentrations of 0.7 g/L and 1.2 g/L, respectively.

Complete blood count, which includes hemoglobin (Sysmex XE 5000 automatic electronic analyser, Kobe, Japan) was determined by Southern Community Laboratories Ltd. (Dunedin, New Zealand), the local clinical laboratory, where external quality control measures are completed regularly.

2.3. Statistical Analysis

There were no statistically significant differences in zinc status between the two study groups (Control vs. BLISS) of the BLISS study [29], so the data were combined to enable this cross-sectional analysis. Medians and lower and upper percentiles (25th and 75th) were used to describe the dietary variables. Participant characteristics are presented as means and standard deviations.

Plasma zinc was adjusted for inflammation using the Biomarkers Reflecting Inflammation and Nutrition Determinants of Anemia (BRINDA) multiple linear regression approach described by Larson and colleagues [38]. The adjustment has two components: slopes of the associations between the inflammation markers and plasma zinc concentration, and difference between observed values and the 10th percentile (to avoid over-adjustment amongst individuals with low levels of inflammation). For the first component, two linear regression models were conducted using the natural log of plasma zinc concentration as the dependent variable and natural logs of CRP and AGP as the independent variables to determine the slope of the association (i.e., β1 and β2). For the second component, the 10th percentile for the natural logs of CRP and AGP were determined and the difference between the natural log of the observed value and this 10th percentile was calculated for each participant (e.g., lnCRPdiff). The adjusted plasma zinc was then calculated for each participant: Adjusted plasma zinc concentration = exp[unadjusted lnplasmazinc − β1(lnCRPdiff) − β2(lnAGPdiff)].

Univariate unadjusted and adjusted (for group) linear regression analyses were used to describe associations between potential "predictor" variables and plasma zinc concentration. The "predictor" variables were decided *a priori* to be of interest, either based on previous associations described in the literature, or because they were considered to potentially have an association with zinc status in toddlers. The variables from baseline that were investigated were: parity, maternal education, socioeconomic status (SES; assessed as the level of household deprivation (NZDep score) [31]), and infant sex. The variables from 12 months that were investigated were: hemoglobin concentration, weight-for-age *z*-score, length-for-age *z*-score, food fussiness score, topical zinc preparation use in the past month; and the intake of: energy, total dietary zinc, phytate, "meat, fish, poultry", red meat, cow's milk, dairy (excluding cow's milk). It was not possible to model breast milk and infant formula intake because there were so many non-consumers, so breast milk, and infant formula (all formulas in New Zealand are iron- and zinc-fortified), were used as dichotomous (i.e., yes vs. no) variables. The age when complementary foods were introduced was also investigated. Although other variables are also known to predict zinc status in childhood (e.g., age, season, time of blood collection, and fasting status), these factors were standardized during data collection and therefore not included in the analyses. Plasma zinc concentration was adjusted for inflammation as described above.

Variables that had an adjusted association of $p < 0.10$ in these univariate analyses, and that were also potentially modifiable, were considered for inclusion in the final multivariate model. This meant that hemoglobin concentration, maternal education, household deprivation, and breast milk consumption were excluded, even though they met the $p < 0.10$ criterion, because they were not considered to be modifiable. Although mothers who were breastfeeding at 12 months could potentially modify the amount their toddler was given, it was not considered to be practically possible to start breastfeeding at 12 months if the toddler had been weaned. Intervention group was not included in the final regression model as it had very little impact on the univariate analyses. Product-moment correlations were used to examine the association between the potentially modifiable "predictors" and plasma zinc concentrations. The final model used robust standard errors to overcome problems with the distribution of some of the variables.

All analyses were conducted using Stata, version 14.2 (StataCorp LP, College Station, TX, USA).

3. Results

3.1. Participant Characteristics at Baseline

Baseline maternal and infant characteristics are presented in Table 1 for participants who provided a plasma zinc sample (n = 115). Participants who provided a plasma zinc sample had similar baseline characteristics to those who did not, with none of the variables in Table 1 differing statistically significantly between those who did and did not provide a sample. Of those who provided a sample, similar proportions were primiparous and multiparous, 73% self-identified as being of New Zealand European ethnicity, and 52% had a university qualification. The level of household deprivation was high for 23% of participants (lower than the 30% expected for the New Zealand population [31]).

Table 1. Maternal and infant baseline characteristics of participants who provided plasma zinc data at 12 months of age [1].

	Total (*n* = 115)
Maternal and Household Variables at Baseline	
Maternal parity	
First child	44 (38)
Two children	47 (41)
Three or more children	24 (21)
Maternal ethnicity	
New Zealand European	84 (73)
Māori	22 (19)
Other [2]	9 (8)
Maternal education	
School only	33 (29)
Post-secondary	22 (19)
University	60 (52)
Household deprivation [3]	
1–3 (Low)	30 (26)
4–7	59 (51)
8–10 (High)	26 (23)
Infant variables at baseline	
Sex	
Female	61 (53)
Male	54 (47)
Group [4]	
Control	58 (50)
BLISS	57 (50)

[1] Data presented as *n* (%). [2] Other ethnicities were Asian and Pacific. [3] Household deprivation categorized using the NZDep scale in which decile 1 indicates the lowest level of deprivation and 10 indicates the highest [31]. [4] As part of the BLISS randomized controlled trial, participants were randomized to either the Control or BLISS group after stratification for maternal education and parity [27].

3.2. Participant Characteristics at 12 Months of Age

Dietary intake, biochemical indices, and anthropometry of toddlers who provided plasma zinc data at 12 months of age are presented in Table 2. Adjusting plasma zinc for acute (CRP) and chronic (AGP) inflammation did not alter the mean plasma zinc concentration at 12 months (Table 2).

Table 2. Characteristics of toddlers who provided plasma zinc data at 12 months of age (*n* = 115).

	Median (25th, 75th) [1]
Biochemical Variables	
Unadjusted plasma zinc, μmol/L (mean (SD))	9.7 (1.5)
Adjusted plasma zinc, μmol/L (mean (SD)) [2]	9.7 (1.5)
Hemoglobin, g/L (mean (SD)) [3]	117 (8.7)
C-reactive protein, mg/L	0.1 (0.0, 0.5)
α_1-acid glycoprotein, g/L	0.61 (0.47, 0.87)
Dietary variables [4]	
Energy, kJ/day	3543 (3090, 4168)
Zinc, mg/day	4.4 (3.7, 5.4)
Phytate, mg/day	230 (150, 318)

Table 2. Cont.

	Median (25th, 75th) [1]
Phytate:zinc molar ratio [5]	5.0 (3.4, 7.1)
"Meat, fish, poultry", g/day	18.9 (9.5, 30.5)
Red meat, g/day	4.4 (0, 11.5)
Cow's milk, g/day	21.6 (5.9, 132)
Dairy, g/day [6]	39.9 (9.5, 73.9)
Breast milk (*n* (%))	
No	47 (45)
Yes	57 (55)
Infant formula (*n* (%))	
No	59 (57)
Yes	45 (43)
Other variables	
Weight, kg (mean (SD)) [7]	9.8 (1.1)
Length, cm (mean (SD)) [7]	75.8 (2.6)
Weight-for-age z-score (mean (SD)) [7,8]	0.37 (0.96)
Length-for-age z-score (mean (SD)) [7,9]	0.26 (0.93)
Food fussiness score (mean (SD)) [7,10]	2.1 (0.6)
Age complementary foods introduced, weeks (mean (SD))	23.5 (3.6)
Topical zinc preparation use in the past month (*n* (%))	
No	56 (49)
Yes	59 (51)

[1] Data presented as median (25th, 75th), unless otherwise specified. [2] Adjusted plasma zinc = exp[unadjusted lnplasmazinc − (regression coefficient for lnCRP) * (lnCRPdiff) − (regression coefficient for lnAGP) * (lnAGPdiff)] from Larson et al. [38]. [3,4] Available data for [3] $n = 114$, [4] $n = 104$. [5] Calculated as [phytate (mg)/660]/[zinc (mg)/65.4]. [6] Excludes cow's milk. [7] Available data for $n = 114$. [8] Weight-for-age z-score calculated using the World Health Organization child growth standards reference data [34]. [9] Length-for-age z-score calculated using the World Health Organization child growth standards reference data [34]. [10] Food fussiness was determined using the six questions on food fussiness from the Children's Eating Behaviour Questionnaire [32]. Lowest score: 1.0, highest score: 5.0.

Median (25th, 75th percentiles) intakes of zinc were 4.4 (3.7, 5.4) mg/day and the phytate-to-zinc molar ratio was 5:1 (3.4:1, 7.1:1). The mean (SD) plasma zinc concentration was 9.7 (1.5) μmol/L, with 60% ($n = 69$) of toddlers below the IZiNCG morning non-fasting reference limit of <9.9 μmol/L [37]. The distribution of the plasma zinc values is presented in Figure 1.

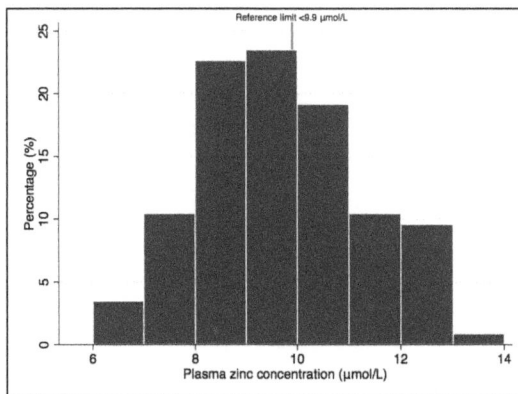

Figure 1. Plasma zinc concentrations (μmol/L) of participants ($n = 115$).

The mean (SD) BMI and BMI z-score of participants in the BLISS study groups were 16.9 (1.36) kg/m^2 and 0.20 (0.89) for the Control group, and 17.3 (1.69) kg/m^2 and 0.44 (1.13) for the BLISS group [27]. One (0.9%) participant was considered stunted (using the WHO classification of a length-for-age z-score < −2 SD [39]) and another (0.9%) was underweight (using the WHO classification of a weight-for-age z-score < −2 SD [39]) at 12 months of age.

3.3. Univariate Associations between Potential "Predictor" Variables and Plasma Zinc Concentrations

Unadjusted and adjusted univariate associations with plasma zinc concentration are presented in Table 3. Toddlers of mothers with university education had an almost 1 µmol/L lower plasma zinc concentration than toddlers whose mothers had a school education only, after adjusting for group (*p* = 0.022) (Table 3). Toddlers living in high-deprivation households had an almost 1 µmol/L higher plasma zinc concentration compared with toddlers living in low-deprivation households, after adjusting for group (*p* = 0.043) (Table 3).

Table 3. Univariate associations between potential "predictor" variables and plasma zinc concentration (µmol/L) at 12 months of age.

		Change in Plasma Zinc Concentration (µmol/L) [1] for Each Unit Change in the Potential "Predictor"				
		Unadjusted			Adjusted for Group	
	n (%)	B (95% CI)	*p*		B (95% CI)	*p*
Biochemical variables						
Hemoglobin, g/L	114 (99)	0.05 (0.01, 0.08)	**0.005**		0.05 (0.02, 0.08)	**0.004**
Dietary variables						
Energy, kJ/day	104 (90)	0.00 (−0.00, 0.00)	0.07		0.00 (−0.00, 0.00)	0.07
Zinc, mg/day	104 (90)	0.23 (0.07, 0.39)	0.005		0.23 (0.07, 0.39)	0.005
Phytate, mg/day	104 (90)	0.00 (−0.00, 0.00)	0.70		0.00 (−0.00, 0.00)	0.71
"Meat, fish, poultry", g/day	104 (90)	0.02 (0.00, 0.03)	0.015		0.02 (0.00, 0.03)	0.016
Red meat, g/day	104 (90)	0.02 (0.00, 0.03)	0.015		0.02 (0.00, 0.03)	0.016
Cow's milk, g/day	104 (90)	0.00 (−0.00, 0.00)	0.66		0.00 (−0.00, 0.00)	0.69
Dairy, g/day [2]	104 (90)	−0.00 (−0.01, 0.00)	0.50		−0.00 (−0.01, 0.00)	0.54
Breast milk						
No	47 (45)	1.00 (reference)	-		1.00 (reference)	-
Yes	57 (55)	−0.53 (−1.11, 0.06)	0.077		−0.52 (−1.11, 0.06)	0.080
Infant formula						
No	59 (57)	1.00 (reference)	-		1.00 (reference)	-
Yes	45 (43)	0.76 (0.18, 1.33)	0.010		0.77 (0.19, 1.34)	0.010
Other variables						
Maternal parity						
First child	44 (38)	1.00 (reference)	-		1.00 (reference)	-
Two children	47 (41)	−0.17 (−0.81, 0.47)	0.60		−0.16 (−0.80, 0.48)	0.62
Three or more children	24 (21)	−0.41 (−1.19, 0.36)	0.29		−0.39 (−1.18, 0.39)	0.32
Maternal education						
School only	33 (29)	1.00 (reference)	-		1.00 (reference)	-
Post-secondary	22 (19)	−0.33 (−1.15, 0.49)	0.43		−0.35 (−1.18, 0.48)	0.41
University	60 (52)	−0.77 (−1.42, −0.12)	0.020		−0.77 (−1.42, −0.11)	0.022
Household deprivation [3]						
1–3 (Low)	30 (26)	1.00 (reference)	-		1.00 (reference)	-
4–7	59 (51)	0.09 (−0.60, 0.78)	0.80		0.07 (−0.61, 0.76)	0.83
8–10 (High)	26 (23)	0.80 (0.02, 1.56)	**0.044**		0.80 (0.03, 1.57)	**0.043**
Sex						
Male	54 (47)	1.00 (reference)	-		1.00 (reference)	-
Female	61 (53)	−0.21 (−0.78, 0.36)	0.47		−0.23 (−0.81, 0.34)	0.42
Weight-for-age z-score [4]	114 (99)	0.02 (−0.28, 0.32)	0.91		0.02 (−0.28, 0.32)	0.90

Table 3. *Cont.*

		Unadjusted			Adjusted for Group	
	n (%)	B (95% CI)	*p*		B (95% CI)	*p*
		Change in Plasma Zinc Concentration (μmol/L) [1] for Each Unit Change in the Potential "Predictor"				
Length-for-age z-score [5]	114 (99)	0.14 (−0.16, 0.45)	0.35		0.16 (−0.15, 0.47)	0.32
Food fussiness score [6]	114 (99)	−0.44 (−0.89, 0.02)	**0.06**		−0.41 (−0.88, 0.06)	**0.09**
Age complementary foods introduced, weeks	115 (100)	0.03 (−0.05, 0.11)	0.39		0.03 (−0.05, 0.11)	0.47
Topical zinc preparation use in the past month						
No	59 (51)	1.00 (reference)	-		1.00 (reference)	-
Yes	56 (49)	−0.07 (−0.64, 0.50)	0.82		−0.07 (−0.64, 0.50)	0.81

Bold indicates *p* < 0.10. [1] Adjusted plasma zinc = exp[unadjusted lnplasmazinc − (regression coefficient for lnCRP) * (lnCRPdiff) − (regression coefficient for lnAGP) * (lnAGPdiff)] from Larson et al. [38]. [2] Excludes cow's milk. [3] Household deprivation categorized using the NZDep scale in which decile 1 indicates the lowest level of deprivation and 10 indicates the highest [31]. [4] Weight-for-age z-score calculated based on the World Health Organization standards [34]. [5] Length-for-age z-score calculated based on the World Health Organization standards [34]. [6] Food fussiness was determined using the six questions on food fussiness from the Children's Eating Behaviour Questionnaire [32]. Lowest score: 1.0, highest score: 5.0.

3.4. Multiple Regression Analysis of "Predictors" of Plasma Zinc Concentrations at 12 Months of Age

The correlation matrix shows the strength of the association between the continuous modifiable "predictor" variables (Table 4). Energy, zinc intake, "meat, fish, poultry", and red meat were strongly correlated with each other as well as being significantly correlated with plasma zinc, so it was only appropriate for one of them to be used in the final model. Red meat was the variable included in the final model because it was a specific component of the BLISS study intervention [26] and a component of the other variables. Therefore, the final model comprised red meat intake, consumption of infant formula (formulas contained 3–6 mg zinc per 100 g), and food fussiness score (Table 5).

Table 4. Correlations (r) between potentially modifiable "predictor" variables, and between these continuous variables and plasma zinc concentration.

		Potentially Modifiable "Predictor" Variables						
		Plasma Zinc	Energy	Zinc	Red Meat	MFP	Infant Formula	Food Fussiness
	Plasma zinc	-						
Potentially	Energy	0.18	-					
modifiable	Zinc	0.27 *	0.82 **	-				
"predictor"	Red meat	0.24 *	0.59 **	0.73 **	-			
variables	MFP	0.24 *	0.53 **	0.70 **	0.70 **	-		
	Food fussiness	−0.18	−0.15	−0.07	−0.01	0.01	0.10	-

Abbreviations: MFP, "meat, fish, poultry". * *p* < 0.05, ** *p* < 0.001.

Table 5. Multiple regression analysis of "predictors" of plasma zinc concentrations at 12 months of age (*n* = 103).

	Change in Plasma Zinc Concentration (μmol/L) [1] for Each Unit Change in the "Predictor"	
	B (SE)	*p*
Red meat intake, 10 g/day	0.12 (0.04)	**0.004**
Infant formula		
No	1.00 (reference)	-
Yes	0.64 (0.28)	**0.026**
Food fussiness score [2]	−0.49 (0.22)	**0.028**

Bold indicates a statistically significant difference at *p* < 0.05. [1] Adjusted plasma zinc = exp[unadjusted lnplasmazinc − (regression coefficient for lnCRP) * (lnCRPdiff) − (regression coefficient for lnAGP) * (lnAGPdiff)] from Larson et al. [38]. [2] Food fussiness was determined using the six questions on food fussiness from the Children's Eating Behaviour Questionnaire [32]. Lowest score: 1.0, highest score: 5.0.

Toddlers had a 0.12 μmol/L higher plasma zinc concentration per 10 g of red meat consumed per day (*p* = 0.004), and toddlers who consumed zinc-fortified infant formula had on average a 0.64 μmol/L higher plasma zinc concentration compared with those who did not consume infant formula (*p* = 0.026) (Table 5). Food fussiness was also significantly associated with plasma zinc concentration. A one-unit increase in food fussiness score (possible score range: 1.0 to 5.0, where highest scores represent increased food fussiness) was associated with a 0.49 μmol/L lower plasma zinc concentration (*p* = 0.028).

The R^2 for the final model was 0.13 (*p* < 0.001) indicating that 13% of the variance in plasma zinc concentration (μmol/L) was explained by these three "predictors".

4. Discussion

In this cross−sectional analysis, a large proportion (60%) of toddlers had plasma zinc concentrations below the recommended reference limit of <9.9 μmol/L [37]. Red meat intake, consumption of infant formula, and food fussiness were significant potentially-modifiable "predictors" of zinc status at 12 months of age.

Whether the high proportion of toddlers with plasma zinc values below the reference limit is of concern is uncertain. The current reference limit applied here was not based on data for children less than three years of age [2] and, hence, may be inappropriate for toddlers aged 12 months [40,41].

Several variables were significantly associated with plasma zinc concentration in the univariate analysis including hemoglobin, maternal education, household deprivation, dietary intakes of: energy, zinc, "meat, fish, poultry", red meat, and consumption of breast milk and infant formula. In contrast to findings from previous studies [18,24,42,43], no association was seen between plasma zinc concentration and growth indicators (length-for-age and weight-for-age z-scores), or dietary phytate intake. However, in the final regression model, the variables that were significantly associated with plasma zinc concentration at 12 months, and were potentially modifiable, were red meat intake, consumption of zinc-fortified infant formula, and food fussiness score.

The magnitude of the association between plasma zinc concentration and red meat was small (0.12 μmol/L per 10 g of intake). This small effect can be illustrated by the increase in red meat consumption required to theoretically produce an increase in plasma zinc concentration from the observed mean of 9.7 μmol/L to the recommended reference level of 9.9 μmol/L [37]. At 17 g/day, this increase in red meat intake is substantially higher than the median intake of this group (4.4 g/day), indicating that such an increase would be challenging. Although a previous intervention in New Zealand toddlers reported a 17 g per day increase in red meat consumption, the meals were provided ready-prepared and free of charge to the parents [44]. This suggests that modifying red meat intake alone is unlikely to be sufficient to increase plasma zinc concentrations meaningfully at 12 months of age. Although there have been concerns about the possible health effects of excessive intakes of red meat in adults [45], we are aware of no published studies that have investigated whether there may be detrimental effects of an increased intake of red meat in infants and toddlers. An increase in red meat intake of 17 g/day, as discussed in the current study, would result in total intakes of approximately 150 g/week—substantially lower than the recommended safe level for adults of 500 g/week (no corresponding figures exist for infants). The saturated fat content of red meat may also be a concern. However, in adults, an increased intake of lean red meat in an otherwise healthy diet does not appear to adversely affect serum lipids [46].

Toddlers consuming zinc-fortified infant formula had a 0.64 μmol/L higher plasma zinc concentration than toddlers who did not consume formula. While consuming infant formula may seem achievable for toddlers, it is important to consider whether the consumption of infant formula would then replace other milk feeding (particularly breast milk), and the cost. It is also not clear from the analyses we have been able to carry out here how much infant formula is needed to have a meaningful impact on zinc status—presumably there is a dose−response relationship of some sort, and intakes were as high as 908 mL per day in some of these toddlers.

The relationship between food fussiness and zinc concentrations is potentially exciting. A one-point lower food fussiness score was associated with a plasma zinc concentration that was 0.49 µmol/L higher in this group of toddlers. This suggests that either a decrease in food fussiness score could result in an increase in plasma zinc concentration (Figure 2A: direction 1), or an increase in plasma zinc concentration could result in a lower food fussiness score (Figure 2A: direction 2). Unfortunately, it is not possible to determine from this observational analysis whether food fussiness caused lower plasma zinc concentration, or vice versa. There is very limited research in this area, but it does appear that increased food fussiness may result in decreased zinc intake (Figure 2B: pathway 1) [47] and there is a plausible mechanism for this association—if an infant or toddler is more food fussy, then they may eat fewer foods that are high in zinc, and may also consume fewer foods that enhance zinc absorption (e.g., meat). In turn, decreased zinc intakes may result in poorer zinc status (Figure 2B: pathway 2). However, there is also evidence for the opposite pathway from low zinc status to increased food fussiness. Lower zinc status may result in impaired taste acuity in children [42,48,49] which may, in turn, result in higher food fussiness [50] (Figure 2B: pathways 3 and 4).

The only way to resolve the uncertainty about the direction of the association reported in the current study would be to conduct a randomized controlled trial of zinc supplementation, with the measurement of changes in taste acuity and food fussiness; or an intervention to reduce food fussiness (such as the behavioral intervention by Birch et al. [51], which achieved an improvement in children's food preference by increasing the frequency of their exposure to a food) with measurement of the subsequent impact on zinc intake and plasma zinc concentration.

The final regression model comprising red meat intake, infant formula consumption, and food fussiness, explained 13% of the variance in plasma zinc concentrations. This highlights that many other factors are contributing to zinc status in toddlers that were not included in this final model. More work is necessary to determine further factors that have the potential to affect plasma zinc concentrations in this age group, and whether any of these are potentially modifiable.

This study has a number of strengths, including rigorous dietary data collection using weighed diet records, a method that is recommended for estimating dietary intakes of very young children [52]. The quality of the dietary assessment data is reflected in our ability to detect a significant association between dietary zinc intake and zinc status. We used strict trace element-free methods to collect and separate blood samples for determining plasma zinc concentrations, as recommended by IZiNCG [40]. Additionally, we were able to minimize variability due to fasting status by using a rigorous pre-sample protocol that included encouraging parents to feed their child milk 90 min before the blood test, and then no other food or drink until after the blood sample was collected; and to minimize the impact of infection on plasma zinc concentrations, by delaying the blood test for 14 days if the child was unwell.

It is important to note the limitations of the current study which include that this was a cross-sectional secondary analysis using data from the BLISS study—a randomized, controlled trial that was not specifically designed to determine predictors of zinc status. Additionally, although the biochemical and dietary data were both collected at, or soon after, the toddlers turned 12 months of age, the dietary data were collected over a three-week period, and some participants' blood samples were delayed if they had been unwell, so the intakes presented here may not be a true reflection of dietary intakes immediately before the blood sample was collected. Lastly, conclusions from this study should be treated with caution as this was an observational study, so causation and the direction of associations cannot be determined.

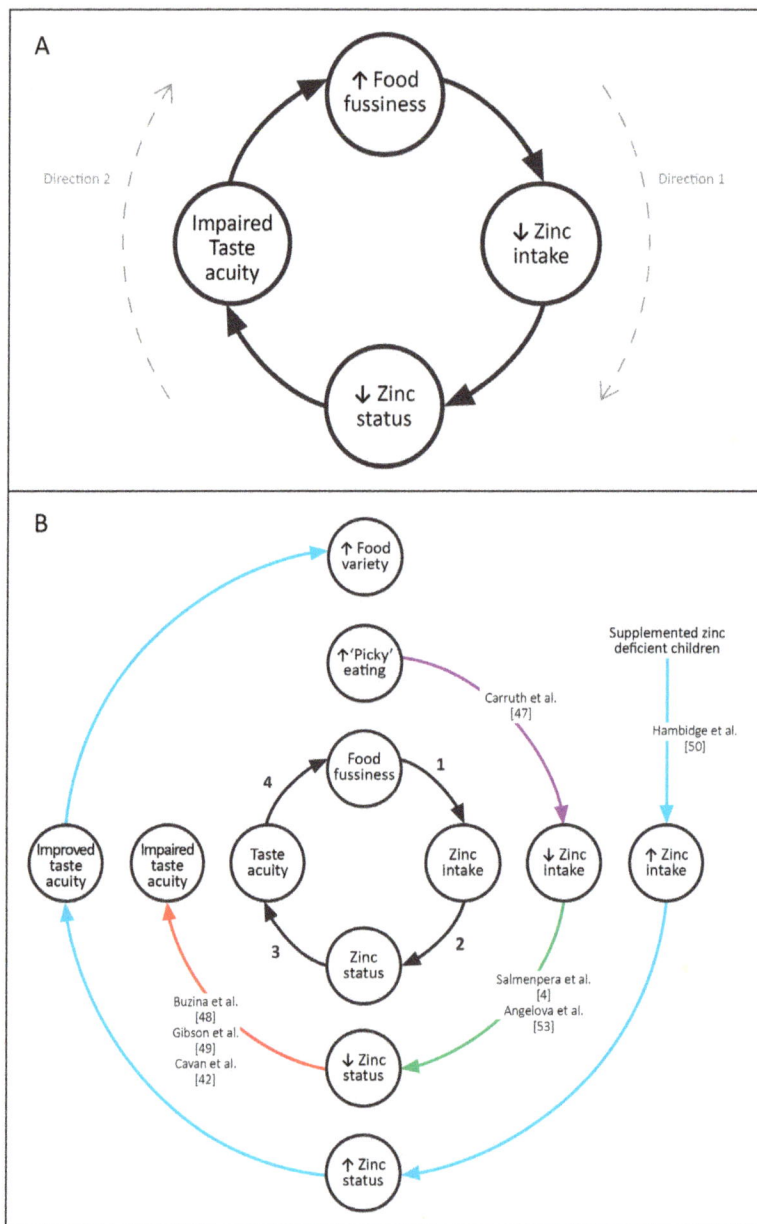

Figure 2. Four plausible pathways in the association between food fussiness and zinc status (**A**); with existing evidence for these associations [4,42,47–50,53] (**B**).

5. Conclusions

In this cross-sectional analysis, intake of red meat and the consumption of zinc-fortified infant formula were positively associated with plasma zinc concentrations, whereas food fussiness score was inversely associated with plasma zinc. Although higher intakes of red meat and the consumption of infant formula are potentially achievable in the diets of toddlers, it is important to consider the potential barriers associated with increasing intakes of both of these foods—particularly the possible impact on breastfeeding, cost, and parents' and toddlers' willingness to modify their behavior. This analysis provides compelling evidence for an association between food fussiness and zinc status, however, further studies are required to determine the direction of this association.

Acknowledgments: We would like to acknowledge all the families who participated in the BLISS study, as well as the research staff involved from the Departments of Human Nutrition and Medicine at the University of Otago. Funders: Meat & Livestock Australia, Lottery Health Research, Karitane Products Society, Perpetual Trustees, the University of Otago, and the New Zealand Federation of Women's Institutes. The funders provided funds only and played no role in carrying out the study or the analysis or interpretation of results. Heinz—Wattie's provided baby rice cereal for participants in the intervention group. Part of R.W.T.'s salary is from a Karitane Products Society (KPS) Fellowship that is paid via the University of Otago. L.D. was supported by a University of Otago Doctoral Scholarship, and a University of Otago Postgraduate Publishing Bursary.

Author Contributions: L.D. contributed to the design of the biochemical methods, collected data and prepared the first full and subsequent drafts of this manuscript. A.-L.M.H. and R.W.T. are the co-principal investigators of the BLISS study, designed the research project, and made a considerable intellectual contribution to the writing of this manuscript. S.M.W. and R.S.G. advised on study design. S.M.W. performed the statistical analyses. S.M.W., R.S.G. and S.S. provided expert input and ongoing advice and support. All authors have made an important intellectual contribution to the manuscript and have read and approved the final manuscript.

Conflicts of Interest: The authors declare no conflict of interest. The funding sponsors had no role in the design of the study; in the collection, analyses, or interpretation of data; in the writing of the manuscript; or in the decision to publish the results.

References

1. Gibson, R.; Heath, A.-L.M. Population groups at risk of zinc deficiency in Australia and New Zealand. *Nutr. Diet.* **2011**, *68*, 97–108. [CrossRef]
2. Institute of Medicine; Food and Nutrition Board. *Dietary Reference Intakes: Vitamin A, Vitamin K, Arsenic, Boron, Chromium, Copper, Iodine, Iron, Manganese, Molybdenum, Nickel, Silicon, Vanadium, and Zinc*; National Academy Press: Washington, DC, USA, 2001.
3. World Health Organization. *Guiding Principles of Complementary Feeding of the Breastfed Child*; World Health Organization: Geneva, Switzerland, 2004; pp. 1–38.
4. Salmenperä, L.; Perheentupa, J.; Näntö, V.; Siimes, M.A. Low Zinc Intake during Exclusive Breast-Feeding Does Not Impair Growth. *J. Pediatr. Gastroenterol. Nutr.* **1994**, *18*, 361–370. [CrossRef] [PubMed]
5. Michaelsen, K.F.; Samuelson, G.; Graham, T.W.; Lönnerdal, B. Zinc intake, zinc status and growth in a longitudinal study of healthy Danish infants. *Acta Paediatr. Scand.* **1994**, *83*, 1115–1121. [CrossRef]
6. Persson, L.Å.; Lundström, M.; Lönnerdal, B.; Hernell, O. Are weaning foods causing impaired iron and zinc status in 1-year-old Swedish infants? A cohort study. *Acta Paediatr. Scand.* **1998**, *87*, 618–622. [CrossRef]
7. Bouglé, D.; Laroche, D.; Bureau, F. Zinc and iron status and growth in healthy infants. *Eur. J. Clin. Nutr.* **2000**, *54*, 764–767. [CrossRef] [PubMed]
8. Kattelmann, K.K.; Ho, M.; Specker, B.L. Effect of Timing of Introduction of Complementary Foods on Iron and Zinc Status of Formula Fed Infants at 12, 24 and 36 Months of Age. *J. Am. Diet. Assoc.* **2001**, *101*, 443–447. [CrossRef]
9. Taylor, A.; Redworth, E.W.; Morgan, J.B. Influence of diet on iron, copper, and zinc status in children under 24 months of age. *Biol. Trace Elem. Res.* **2004**, *97*, 197–214. [CrossRef]
10. Torrejón, C.S.; Castillo-Durán, C.; Hertrampf, E.D.; Ruz, M. Zinc and iron nutrition in Chilean children fed fortified milk provided by the Complementary National Food Program. *Nutr. Rev.* **2004**, *20*, 177–180. [CrossRef] [PubMed]
11. Krebs, N.F.; Westcott, J.E.; Butler, T.; Robinson, C.; Bell, M.; Hambidge, K.M. Meat as a first complementary food for breastfed infants: Feasibility and impact on zinc intake and status. *J. Pediatr. Gastroenterol. Nutr.* **2006**, *42*, 207–214. [PubMed]
12. Morgan, E.J.; Heath, A.-L.M.; Szymlek-Gay, E.; Gibson, R.S.; Gray, A.R.; Bailey, K.B.; Ferguson, E.L. Red meat and a fortified manufactured toddler milk drink increase dietary zinc intakes without affecting zinc status of New Zealand toddlers. *J. Nutr.* **2010**, *140*, 2221–2226. [CrossRef] [PubMed]

13. Han, Y.-H.; Yon, M.; Han, H.-S.; Johnston, K.E.; Tamura, T.; Hyun, T. Zinc status and growth of Korean infants fed human milk, casein-based, or soy-based formula: Three-year longitudinal study. *Nutr. Res. Pract.* **2011**, *5*, 46–51. [CrossRef] [PubMed]
14. Shankar, A.H.; Prasad, A.S. Zinc and immune function: the biological basis of altered resistance to infection. *Am. J. Clin. Nutr.* **1998**, *68*, 447S–463S. [CrossRef] [PubMed]
15. Fraker, P.J.; King, L.E.; Laakko, T.; Vollmer, T.L. The dynamic link between the integrity of the immune system and zinc status. *J. Nutr.* **2000**, *130*, 1399S–1406S. [CrossRef] [PubMed]
16. Cross, A.J.; Heath, A.; Ferguson, E.L. Rates of common communicable illnesses in non-anaemic 12–24 month old South Island, New Zealand children. *N. Z. Med. J.* **2009**, *122*, 24–35. [PubMed]
17. Nissensohn, M.; Sánchez-Villegas, A. Effect of zinc intake on growth in infants: A meta-analysis. *Crit. Rev. Food Sci. Nutr.* **2016**, *56*, 350–363. [CrossRef] [PubMed]
18. Brown, K.H.; Lanata, C.F.; Yuen, M.L.; Peerson, J.M.; Butron, B.; Lönnerdal, B. Potential magnitude of the misclassification of a population's trace element status due to infection: example from a survey of young Peruvian children. *Am. J. Clin. Nutr.* **1993**, *58*, 549–554. [CrossRef] [PubMed]
19. Hemalatha, P.; Bhaskaram, P.; Kumar, P.A.; Khan, M.M.; Islam, M.A. Zinc status of breastfed and formula-fed infants of different gestational ages. *J. Trop. Pediat.* **1997**, *43*, 52–54. [CrossRef]
20. Gibson, R.S.; Ferguson, E.F.; Vanderkooy, P.; MacDonald, A.C. Seasonal variations in hair zinc concentrations in Canadian and African children. *Sci. Total Environ.* **1989**, *84*, 291–298. [CrossRef]
21. Wilhelm, M.; Hafner, D.; Lombeck, I.; Ohnesorge, F.K. Monitoring of cadmium, copper, lead and zinc status in young children using toenails: Comparison with scalp hair. *Sci. Total Environ.* **1991**, *103*, 199–207. [CrossRef]
22. Arsenault, J.E.; Wuehler, S.E.; de Romaña, D.L.; Penny, M.E.; Sempertegui, F.; Brown, K.H. The time of day and the interval since previous meal are associated with plasma zinc concentrations and affect estimated risk of zinc deficiency in young children in Peru and Ecuador. *Eur. J. Clin. Nutr.* **2011**, *65*, 184–190. [CrossRef] [PubMed]
23. Gibson, R.S.; Bailey, K.B.; Parnell, W.R.; Wilson, N.; Ferguson, E.L. Higher risk of zinc deficiency in New Zealand Pacific school children compared with their Māori and European counterparts: A New Zealand national survey. *Br. J. Nutr.* **2010**, *105*, 436–446. [CrossRef] [PubMed]
24. Engle-Stone, R.; Ndjebayi, A.O.; Nankap, M.; Killilea, D.W.; Brown, K.H. Stunting Prevalence, Plasma Zinc Concentrations, and Dietary Zinc Intakes in a Nationally Representative Sample Suggest a High Risk of Zinc Deficiency among Women and Young Children in Cameroon. *J. Nutr.* **2014**, *144*, 382–391. [CrossRef] [PubMed]
25. Galetti, V.; Mitchikpè, C.E.S.; Kujinga, P.; Tossou, F.; Hounhouigan, D.J.; Zimmermann, M.B.; Moretti, D. Rural Beninese Children Are at Risk of Zinc Deficiency According to Stunting Prevalence and Plasma Zinc Concentration but Not Dietary Zinc Intakes. *J. Nutr.* **2016**, *146*, 114–123. [CrossRef] [PubMed]
26. Daniels, L.; Heath, A.-L.M.; Williams, S.M.; Cameron, S.L.; Fleming, E.A.; Taylor, B.J.; Wheeler, B.J.; Gibson, R.S.; Taylor, R.W. Baby-Led Introduction to SolidS (BLISS) study: A randomised controlled trial of a baby-led approach to complementary feeding. *BMC Pediatr.* **2015**, *15*, 1–15. [CrossRef] [PubMed]
27. Taylor, R.W.; Williams, S.M.; Fangupo, L.J.; Wheeler, B.J.; Taylor, B.J.; Daniels, L.; Fleming, E.A.; McArthur, J.; Morison, B.; Erickson, L.W.; et al. Effect of a Baby-Led Approach to Complementary Feeding on Infant Growth and Overweight. *JAMA Pediatr.* **2017**, *171*, 838–846. [CrossRef] [PubMed]
28. Daniels, L.; Taylor, R.W.; Williams, S.M.; Gibson, R.S.; Fleming, E.A.; Wheeler, B.J.; Taylor, B.J.; Haszard, J.J.; Heath, A.-L.M. Impact of a modified version of Baby-Led Weaning on iron intake and status: A randomised controlled trial. *BMJ Open* **2018**, in press.
29. Daniels, L.; Taylor, R.W.; Williams, S.M.; Gibson, R.S.; Samman, S.; Wheeler, B.J.; Taylor, B.J.; Fleming, E.A.; Heath, A.-L.M. Modified version of Baby-Led Weaning does not result in lower zinc intake or status in infants: A randomized controlled trial. *J. Acad. Nutr. Diet.* **2018**, in press.
30. Fangupo, L.J.; Heath, A.-L.M.; Williams, S.M.; Erickson Williams, L.W.; Morison, B.J.; Fleming, E.A.; Taylor, B.J.; Wheeler, B.J.; Taylor, R.W. A Baby-Led Approach to Eating Solids and Risk of Choking. *Pediatrics* **2016**, *138*, 1–10. [CrossRef] [PubMed]
31. Atkinson, J.; Salmond, C.; Crampton, P. *NZDep2013 Index of Deprivation User's Manual*; Department of Public Health, University of Otago: Wellington, New Zealand; Division of Health Sciences, University of Otago: Dunedin, New Zealand, 2014.

32. Wardle, J.; Guthrie, C.A.; Sanderson, S.; Rapoport, L. Development of the children's eating behaviour questionnaire. *J. Child Psychol. Psychiatry* **2001**, *42*, 963–970. [CrossRef] [PubMed]

33. De Onis, M.; Onyango, A.W.; Van den Broeck, J.; Chumlea, W.C.; Martorell, R. Measurement and standardization protocols for anthropometry used in the construction of a new international growth reference. *Food Nutr. Bull.* **2004**, *25*, S27–S36. [CrossRef] [PubMed]

34. De Onis, M.; Martorell, R.; Garza, C.; Lartey, A.; Reference, W.M.G. WHO Child Growth Standards based on length/height, weight and age. *Acta Paediatr. Scand.* **2006**, *95*, 76–85.

35. Ministry of Health New Zealand Food Composition Database (FOODfiles). Available online: www.foodcomposition.co.nz/foodfiles (accessed on 4 July 2014).

36. Barris, A. Meat and Haem Iron Intakes of New Zealand Toddlers Aged 12–24 Months. Master of Dietetics, University of Otago: Dunedin, New Zealand, 2012. Available online: http://hdl.handle.net/10523/3839 (accessed on 15 September 2017).

37. International Zinc Nutrition Consultative Group (IZiNCG). *IZiNCG Technical Brief 2007: Assessing Population Zinc Status with Serum Zinc Concentration*; International Zinc Nutrition Consultative Group (IZiNCG): Davis, CA, USA, 2007.

38. Larson, L.M.; Addo, O.Y.; Sandalinas, F.; Faigao, K.; Kupka, R.; Flores-Ayala, R.; Suchdev, P.S. Accounting for the influence of inflammation on retinol-binding protein in a population survey of Liberian preschool-age children. *Matern. Child Nutr.* **2017**, *13*, 1–10. [CrossRef] [PubMed]

39. Gorstein, J.; Sullivan, K.; Yip, R.; de Onis, M.; Trowbridge, F.; Fajans, P.; Clugston, G. Issues in the assessment of nutritional status using anthropometry. *Bull. World Health Organ.* **1994**, *72*, 273–283. [PubMed]

40. Brown, K.H.; Rivera, J.A.; Bhutta, Z.; Gibson, R.S.; King, J.C.; Lönnerdal, B.; Ruel, M.T.; Sandström, B.; Wasantwisut, E.; Hotz, C. International Zinc Nutrition Consultative Group (IZiNCG) Technical Document #1 Assessment of the Risk of Zinc Deficiency in Populations and Options for its Control. *Food Nutr. Bull.* **2004**, *25* (Suppl. 2), S91–S203.

41. Hotz, C.; Peerson, J.M.; Brown, K.H. Suggested lower cutoffs of serum zinc concentrations for assessing zinc status: reanalysis of the second National Health and Nutrition Examination Survey data (1976–1980). *Am. J. Clin. Nutr.* **2003**, *78*, 756–764. [CrossRef] [PubMed]

42. Cavan, K.R.; Gibson, R.S.; Grazioso, C.F.; Isalgue, A.M.; Ruz, M.; Solomons, N.W. Growth and Body Composition of Periurban Guatemalan Children in Relation to Zinc Status—A Cross-Sectional Study. *Am. J. Clin. Nutr.* **1993**, *57*, 334–343. [CrossRef] [PubMed]

43. Ferguson, E.L.; Parackal, S.; Gibson, R.S. Zinc status of 6–24 month old New Zealand children and their mothers. In Proceedings of the IZiNCG Symposium—Moving Zinc into the Micronutrient Program Agenda, Lima, Peru, 19 November 2004.

44. Szymlek-Gay, E.A.; Ferguson, E.L.; Heath, A.-L.M.; Gray, A.R.; Gibson, R.S. Food-based strategies improve iron status in toddlers: A randomized controlled trial. *Am. J. Clin. Nutr.* **2009**, *90*, 1541–1551. [CrossRef] [PubMed]

45. World Cancer Research Fund; American Institute for Cancer Research. *Food, Nutrition, Physical Activity, and the Prevention of Cancer: A Global Perspective*; American Institute for Cancer Research (AICR): Washington, DC, USA, 2007.

46. Roussell, M.A.; Hill, A.M.; Gaugler, T.L.; West, S.G.; Vanden Heuvel, J.P.; Alaupovic, P.; Gillies, P.J.; Kris-Etherton, P.M. Beef in an Optimal Lean Diet study: effects on lipids, lipoproteins, and apolipoproteins. *Am. J. Clin. Nutr.* **2012**, *95*, 9–16. [CrossRef] [PubMed]

47. Carruth, B.R.; Ziegler, P.J.; Gordon, A.; Barr, S.I. Prevalence of picky eaters among infants and toddlers and their caregivers' decisions about offering a new food. *J. Am. Diet. Assoc.* **2004**, *104*, S57–S64. [CrossRef] [PubMed]

48. Buzina, R.; Jusić, M.; Sapunar, J.; Milanović, N. Zinc nutrition and taste acuity in school children with impaired growth. *Am. J. Clin. Nutr.* **1980**, *33*, 2262–2267. [CrossRef] [PubMed]

49. Gibson, R.S.; Vanderkooy, P.; MacDonald, A.C.; Goldman, A.; Ryan, B.A.; Berry, M. A Growth-Limiting, Mild Zinc-Deficiency Syndrome in Some Southern Ontario Boys with Low Height Percentiles. *Am. J. Clin. Nutr.* **1989**, *49*, 1266–1273. [CrossRef] [PubMed]

50. Hambidge, K.M.; Hambidge, C.; Jacobs, M.; Baum, J.D. Low-Levels of Zinc in Hair, Anorexia, Poor Growth, and Hypogeusia in Children. *Pediatr. Res.* **1972**, *6*, 868–874. [CrossRef] [PubMed]

51. Birch, L.L.; Marlin, D.W. I don't like it; I never tried it: Effects of exposure on two-year-old children's food preferences. *Appetite* **1982**, *3*, 353–360. [CrossRef]

52. Burrows, T.L.; Martin, R.J.; Collins, C.E. A Systematic Review of the Validity of Dietary Assessment Methods in Children when Compared with the Method of Doubly Labeled Water. *J. Am. Diet. Assoc.* **2010**, *110*, 1501–1510. [CrossRef] [PubMed]

53. Angelova, M.G.; Petkova-Marinova, T.V.; Pogorielov, M.V.; Loboda, A.N.; Nedkova-Kolarova, V.N.; Bozhinova, A.N. Trace Element Status (Iron, Zinc, Copper, Chromium, Cobalt, and Nickel) in Iron-Deficiency Anaemia of Children under 3 Years. *Anemia* **2014**, *2014*, 718089, 8p.

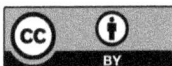

![nutrients logo] *nutrients*

MDPI

Review

Zinc, Magnesium, Selenium and Depression: A Review of the Evidence, Potential Mechanisms and Implications

Jessica Wang [1,†]**, Phoebe Um** [1,†]**, Barbra A. Dickerman** [2] **and Jianghong Liu** [1,*]

[1] University of Pennsylvania School of Nursing, Philadelphia, PA 19104, USA; jeswang@sas.upenn.edu (J.W.); phoebeum@sas.upenn.edu (P.U.)
[2] Harvard T. H. Chan School of Public Health, Boston, MA 02115, USA; bad788@mail.harvard.edu
*   Correspondence: jhliu@nursing.upenn.edu; Tel.: +1-(215)-898-8293
†   Co-first authors.

Received: 5 April 2018; Accepted: 3 May 2018; Published: 9 May 2018

Abstract: Micronutrient deficiency and depression are major global health problems. Here, we first review recent empirical evidence of the association between several micronutrients—zinc, magnesium, selenium—and depression. We then present potential mechanisms of action and discuss the clinical implications for each micronutrient. Collectively, empirical evidence most strongly supports a positive association between zinc deficiency and the risk of depression and an inverse association between zinc supplementation and depressive symptoms. Less evidence is available regarding the relationship between magnesium and selenium deficiency and depression, and studies have been inconclusive. Potential mechanisms of action involve the HPA axis, glutamate homeostasis and inflammatory pathways. Findings support the importance of adequate consumption of micronutrients in the promotion of mental health, and the most common dietary sources for zinc and other micronutrients are provided. Future research is needed to prospectively investigate the association between micronutrient levels and depression as well as the safety and efficacy of micronutrient supplementation as an adjunct treatment for depression.

Keywords: nutrition; micronutrient; diet; depression; zinc; magnesium; selenium; microbiota

1. Introduction

Micronutrient deficiencies and depression are major global health problems, with more than two billion people in the world estimated to be deficient in key vitamins and minerals [1] and more than 300 million people suffering from depression [2]. Micronutrients have been consistently linked with health outcomes such as cognitive functioning [3,4], cancer [5,6], obesity [7,8], and immune functioning [9,10]. However, the role of micronutrients in the etiology and progression of depression remains unclear. Given that micronutrient deficiency is both prevalent and modifiable, even a modest association with risk of depression would be of public health interest.

Micronutrient deficiencies may play a role in the development of depression, and several studies have explored micronutrient supplementation as an adjunct to antidepressant therapy. Zinc and magnesium have been most commonly studied with respect to depression, and it has been suggested that these micronutrients might influence depression through similar biological mechanisms. Recent studies have suggested that selenium may also play a role in the development of depression, although evidence is sparse and inconsistent.

The aim of the present review is to (1) examine empirical evidence of the association between micronutrients (zinc, magnesium, selenium) and depression; (2) discuss possible mechanisms of action; and (3) explore the clinical implications of such findings. As micronutrient deficiency and mental health are of great global public health importance, understanding the possible roles of micronutrients in depression will help elucidate the mechanisms underlying this condition and inform primary and secondary prevention strategies.

2. Zinc

Zinc is an essential trace element important for many biochemical and physiological processes related to brain growth and function [11,12], as well as cellular metabolism [13,14]. Zinc is acquired through dietary intake of foods such as red meat, oysters and crab, and zinc deficiency can occur with reduced intake, insufficient absorption, and/or increased zinc utilization or expenditure. Normal serum zinc levels range from 0.66 to 1.10 µg/mL in adults [15]. The balance of intracellular and extracellular zinc levels is crucial for maintaining zinc homeostasis in many brain regions, including those involved in the physiopathology of depression, such as the hippocampus, amygdala, and the cerebral cortex [13,14,16].

An association between zinc and depression was first suggested in the late 1980s [17]. Since then, the association between zinc and depression has been extensively studied in both animals and humans. Rodent studies have reported associations between zinc deficiency and depressive symptoms [18–21]. Researchers have also reported lower serum zinc levels in animals more resistant to antidepressant treatment [18,20]. Observational studies have supported these findings [14,22–24]. A meta-analysis of 17 observational studies found that blood zinc concentrations were approximately 0.12 µg/mL lower in depressed subjects than in control subjects [25]. Cross-sectional studies among female adolescents [22,23], postmenopausal women [26] and patients on hemodialysis [27] have reported a positive association between zinc deficiency and depression severity. Interestingly, in their 2012 cross-sectional study, Maserejian et al. [14] found an association between zinc deficiency and depressive symptoms among women, but not men. A prospective cohort study similarly found no significant association between dietary zinc intake and the risk of depression among middle-aged men [28].

Intervention studies in both humans and rodents involving dietary or supplemental zinc have reported antidepressant-like and mood-enhancing activities of zinc [29–31]. In animal models, adult rats fed a zinc-deficient diet demonstrated more depressive symptoms than adult rats fed a zinc-sufficient diet, as assessed by the forced swim test, the tail suspension test as well as demonstrated anorexia and anhedonia [20,21]. Similarly, depressive symptoms induced in mice through chronic restraint stress (CRS) were alleviated by treatment by zinc (30 mg/kg) or imipramine, a traditional antidepressant [32]. Randomized controlled trials among individuals with depression have demonstrated decreases in depressive symptoms when supplementing antidepressant drug treatments with zinc compared to antidepressants alone [29,31]. Among healthy young women, those who received zinc and multivitamin supplements showed greater reductions in depression-dejection scores of the Profile of Moods State (POMS) assessment than those who had only received multivitamin supplementation [30].

2.1. Mechanisms

The potential mechanisms underlying the association between low serum zinc and depression remain unclear, but may involve the regulation of neurotransmitter, endocrine and neurogenesis pathways. Such mechanisms are outlined in Table 1.

In the hippocampus and cortex, zinc ions regulate synaptic transmission or act as neurotransmitters [33], modulating many ligand- and voltage-gated ion channels [34–40]. Disruption of zinc homeostasis in these regions has been implicated in many disturbances in cognition, behavioral and emotional regulation [41] through mechanisms of decreased neurogenesis [42,43] and neuronal plasticity [43].

Zinc deficiency has also been implicated in the endocrine pathway of depression. Takeda et al. [44] reported that a zinc-deficient diet induced high levels of serum cortisol concentration in rats. Persistently high levels of cortisol have been implicated in the development of depression via hyperactivity of the hypothalamic–pituitary–adrenal (HPA) axis [45,46]. Increased plasma cortisol levels could, therefore, potentially mediate the relationship between zinc deficiency and depression.

Further, recent research has highlighted the role of zinc transporters (ZincTs) and zinc-sensing GPR39 receptors in the development and treatment of depression [47]. Zinc transporter-3 knockout mice lack vesicular zinc and demonstrated fewer proliferating progenitor cells and immature neurons [48]. A reduced hippocampal volume has been extensively reported in association with depression [49,50], thus implicating the disruption of Zinct-3-dependent neurogenesis in the etiology of depression. In addition, GPR39 receptors have been increasingly associated with the serotonergic system, as recent studies have established links between GPR39 proteins and serotonin synthesis [51] and receptor signaling [52]. Moreover, GPR39 receptors have also been reported to play a role in the action of antidepressants. GPR39 knockout mice have been shown to be resistant to the normalizing effects of imipramine and escitalopram in the forced swim test (FST) [53]. Moreover, studies have shown that the binding of zinc to GPR39 receptors activates downstream cyclic AMP-response element (CRE)-dependent gene transcription, resulting in higher levels of brain-derived neurotrophic factor (BDNF) in the hippocampus and cortex [54]. The action of zinc mimics the actions of traditional antidepressants, and previous studies have shown normalization of low BDNF levels in depressed patients treated with antidepressants [55,56].

Another possible reason for the antidepressant effects of zinc may be the anti-inflammatory and antioxidant properties of zinc supplementation. Previous studies have reported that zinc supplementation decreases C-reactive protein (CRP) levels in humans [57,58]. Increased CRP levels have been previously associated with depression [59,60], and a recent study found that the effectiveness of the antidepressant, agomelatine, was associated with a reduction in CRP levels [61]. Similarly, zinc has demonstrated protective effects against lipid peroxidation [62,63]. Recent evidence has supported a relationship between lipid peroxidation and major depression [64], suggesting that the observed antidepressant properties of zinc result, in part, from its antioxidant effects.

Lastly, the potential antidepressant properties of zinc may be related to its function as an antagonist of the glutamatergic *N*-methyl-D-aspartate (NMDA) receptor and involvement in the L-arginine–nitric oxide (NO) pathway as a nitric oxide synthase (NOS) inhibitor. NMDA has been therapeutically targeted in clinical and preclinical studies of depression treatment, as growing evidence supports the presence of disrupted glutamate homeostasis and neurotransmission in depressed subjects [65]. In a study that measured depressive symptomology in mice, both blockage of NMDA receptors and addition of NOS substrate independently negated the beneficial effects of zinc–chloride on the reduction of depressive symptoms, suggesting that the antidepressant properties of zinc–chloride may have been partially mediated by zinc's inhibition of NOS and NMDA receptors [66].

Table 1. Potential Mechanisms, Food Sources, and Normal Serum Levels of Zinc (Zn), Magnesium (Mg), and Selenium (Se).

	Potential Mechanisms		Food Sources	Normal Serum Levels in Adults
	Development of Depression	Antidepressant Action		
Zn	Increased cortisol; decreased neurogenesis and neural plasticity; disruption of glutamate homeostasis	N-methyl-D-aspartate (NMDA) antagonist; elevated expression of hippocampal and cortical brain-derived neurotrophic factor (BDNF)	Oysters, beans, nuts, red meat, certain types of seafood (crab and lobster), whole grains, fortified breakfast cereals, dairy products	0.66–1.10 µg/mL
Mg	Dysregulation of hypothalamic–pituitary–adrenal (HPA axis); increased Ca^{2+} in brain; increased inflammatory response	NMDA antagonist; serotonin, dopamine, noradrenaline modulation; increased BDNF expression; modulation of sleep–wake cycle	Green leafy vegetables (spinach), some legumes (beans and peas), nuts and seeds, whole grains	0.62–1.02 mmol/L
Se	Dysregulation of thyroid function; dysregulation of oxidative and inflammatory pathways	Serotonin, dopamine, noradrenaline modulation; attenuation of inflammation	Seafood, bread, grains, meat, poultry, fish, eggs	70–90 µg/L

2.2. Discussion and Implications

Several methodological considerations underlie the evaluation of the research studies reviewed here. First, the measurement error of zinc status should be considered. While the measurement of serum zinc levels has been shown to be a useful biomarker of population zinc status, its reliability as an indicator of individual zinc status has not been demonstrated [67]. The relationship between serum zinc levels and depression could be partially explained by reverse causation, whereby depression influences the intake [68], bioavailability or biological regulation of zinc [20,32,69]. Oxidative stress and its accompanying immune-inflammatory response have been linked to the pathophysiology of depression [70]. In response to oxidative stress, levels of pro-inflammatory cytokines (e.g., interleukin 1 (IL-1) and IL-6) increase and, in turn, decrease of the level of albumin and increase the synthesis of metallothioneins [71]. Albumin is the main zinc transporter [72], and a decrease in albumin coupled with an increase in metallothioneins may compound to decrease serum levels of zinc. Future studies should include oxidative stress markers to further assess the directionality of the relationship between zinc status and depression status.

Finally, potential confounding by socioeconomic status and diet should be considered, as these factors could influence both zinc status and the risk of depression. Hair cortisol and parental education status have been found to be associated with hair zinc levels in a population of Canadian preschoolers [73], thus pointing towards a possible mechanism through which socioeconomic status could influence both zinc levels and depression. Dietary factors, such as the consumption of phytates, a compound present in many grains, have been shown to reduce zinc absorption in the intestine [74]. Furthermore, as zinc is primarily consumed through red meats and seafood, diets that limit the consumption of these foods (e.g., vegetarianism, veganism) may alter serum zinc levels.

Further prospective studies are needed to investigate potential biologic mechanisms that may underlie the association between zinc and depression. Zinc deficiency may increase the vulnerability to psychological stress by depressing levels of neurogenesis and plasticity, and maintaining electrophysiological balance in various brain regions. These psychological and biological changes may act in concert to influence the development of depression, which itself could further reduce serum zinc levels. If evidence for a causal effect of zinc on depression risk accumulates, future studies exploring the safety and effectiveness of zinc as a potential supplement to antidepressants could also be warranted. Future intervention treatments should note that the presence of excess zinc can be potentially problematic. Secondary copper deficiency has been demonstrated as a potential consequence of a high dietary intake of zinc [75]. As a result, it is recommended that dietary zinc intake is limited to the recommended amount or that zinc supplementation is coupled with adequate copper supplementation. In the Age-Related Eye Disease Study, supplementation of zinc was given with a small amount of copper (80 mg zinc oxide, 2 mg cupric oxide) [76].

3. Magnesium

Magnesium is a micronutrient that is essential for the proper activity of many biochemical and physiological processes, including DNA replication, transcription and translation [77,78]. It is a bivalent intracellular cation that acts as a coenzyme or an activator for over 300 enzymatic systems, many of which are important for proper brain function [79]. Magnesium is usually consumed through nuts, seeds, green leafy vegetables and whole grains. Normal serum magnesium levels range from 0.62 to 1.02 mmol/L [80]. A 2005 study that leveraged dietary surveys suggested that 68% of Americans consume less than the recommended daily allowance of magnesium [81]. Magnesium levels are important for central nervous system (CNS) function and may play a role in Alzheimer's disease, diabetes, stroke, hypertension, migraines and attention deficit hyperactivity deficit [82]. Previous studies have associated magnesium with various brain regions in the limbic system [83], thus implicating a possible role for magnesium in the etiology and progression of depression.

A positive association between magnesium deficiency and depression has been documented in both animal and human studies. Mice subjected to magnesium deficient diets have shown behavioral deficits associated with depression [84–86]. Likewise, cross-sectional studies [26,87–89] have reported an inverse relationship between depressive symptoms and magnesium levels and magnesium intake, which persisted after adjustment for age, body mass index, and education. However, prospective cohort studies have failed to find an association between magnesium status and later risk of depression. A study performed in the SUN Mediterranean cohort of 15,863 men and women without any history of depression found no significant association between magnesium intake, as assessed by diet, and risk of depression 10 years later [90]. Another study of approximately 13,000 Spanish university graduates free of depression at baseline reported an inverse association between magnesium intake and depression incidence 6 years later [91].

Some intervention studies have suggested a beneficial role of magnesium supplementation in the treatment of depression [92,93], while others have not [94,95]. A recent randomized clinical trial in a population of adults diagnosed with mild-to-moderate depression found that the consumption of 248 mg of magnesium per day for 6 weeks resulted in a clinically-significant 6 point decrease ($p < 0.001$) in depressive symptoms, as measured by the Patient Health Questionnaire-9 (PHQ-9) compared to those receiving a placebo treatment [93]. Similarly, a randomized controlled trial of 60 individuals with depression and hypomagnesemia demonstrated that daily consumption of 500 mg magnesium oxide led to significant improvements in Beck Depression Inventory scores, compared to individuals with depression and hypomagnesemia who received a placebo [92]. However, intervention studies among postpartum women [95] and an elderly population with hypomagnesemia [94] found no effect of magnesium supplements, of 328 mg/day and 50 mg/day, respectively, on the depression statuses of these individuals.

3.1. Mechanisms

The biological mechanisms that potentially underlie the association between low serum magnesium levels and depression remain unclear but may involve the central nervous system, stress axis, and oxidative pathways. These mechanisms are outlined in Table 1.

Magnesium deficiency has been shown to lead to changes in the functioning of the central nervous system (CNS), especially in the glutamatergic transmission in the limbic system and cerebral cortex [54]—brain regions that play important roles in the etiopathogenesis of depression [96–98]. Magnesium is particularly well known for its importance as an antagonist of the NMDA glutamate receptor, which has long been understood as a key player in synaptic potentiation, learning and memory [99,100]. However, despite magnesium's well-known involvement in the voltage gating function of the receptor, evidence pointing towards direct magnesium-induced changes in NMDA channels in the expression of depression-like behavior is scarce. A recent mouse study found that dietary magnesium restriction reduced levels of the GluN1 NMDA receptor subunit in the amygdala and hypothalamus [101], a phenomenon that mirrors the GluN1 reduction response to chronic stress [102]. Further, because NMDA channels mainly conduct calcium and sodium currents, a depletion of magnesium could allow for excess calcium current. Evidence supports the possibility that magnesium deficiency disrupts neuronal function by means of increasing neuronal calcium flow, thereby resulting in increased nitric oxide, a toxic reactive oxygen species that leads to neuronal swelling and death [103–105]. While the mechanism has yet to be elucidated, studies have demonstrated that the ameliorative effects of magnesium on depressive symptoms in mice can be reversed by NMDA-receptor agonists [106], thus pointing to a possible interaction between magnesium and the NMDA receptor as a therapeutic target for the treatment of depression.

Another possible mechanism for magnesium's protective effect against depression could involve magnesium's modification of the stress response. Magnesium's ability to reduce the release of adrenocorticotrophic hormone (ACTH) and modulate adrenocorticotropic sensitivity to ACTH is preventative against the hyperactivation of the HPA axis. Dysregulation of the HPA axis in adults has been robustly linked to stress and depression; elevated cortisol and dysregulated HPA activity are highly over-represented in depressed populations [107,108]. Glucocorticoids have been continuously demonstrated to exhibit neurotoxic effects in the hippocampus, thus suggesting a role for excess glucocorticoids in the hippocampal cell death observed in depression [109,110]. If HPA axis dysfunction plays a mechanistic role in depression, magnesium deficiency could be a risk factor making individuals vulnerable to chronic elevated cortisol and its neurodegenerative effects.

Magnesium's role in the gut microbiota (GM) has been of recent interest, as alterations in GM have been linked to depression [111,112]. Magnesium-induced changes in microbiota have also been associated with changes in the oxidative and inflammatory response, characterized by increased cytokines and biomarkers of cellular stress [113]. A recent study examining depression in mice demonstrated that 6 weeks of a magnesium-deficient diet induced depressive symptoms in the FST, which was associated with changes in GM and hippocampal interleukin-6 [86]. Previous studies have also demonstrated an inverse association between dietary magnesium intake and levels of inflammatory markers, such as serum C-reactive protein, interleukin-6 and tumor necrosis factor-α receptor 2 [114,115]. As evidence for the potential roles of inflammation and oxidative stress in the pathogenesis [116,117] and the progression of depression [118] continues to accumulate, it may be important to consider magnesium's immune modulatory role.

Magnesium could potentially exert antidepressant effects through its role in serotonergic, noradrenergic and dopaminergic neurotransmission [119,120], increased expression of BDNF [121] and modulation of the sleep–wake cycle through augmentation of the biosynthesis of melatonin [122].

3.2. Discussion and Implications

Overall, the majority of evidence supports an inverse association between magnesium and the development of depression, as well as the antidepressant properties of magnesium. Methodologically, it is important to note that erythrocyte magnesium levels have been demonstrated to be more reliable in determining magnesium deficiency than serum levels [123]. Because only about 1% of total body magnesium is typically found extracellularly in the serum, serum magnesium levels are not necessarily representative of total body magnesium or the concentration of magnesium found intracellularly that is available for cellular use [124]. Magnesium homeostasis is maintained by the intestine, the bones and the kidneys; magnesium should still be consumed regularly in sufficient amount to prevent deficiency [125]. As a result of active biological regulation of magnesium levels, magnesium deficiency is likely an indicator of poor nutrition or ailments that affect magnesium absorption or excretion, such as diabetes mellitus [125]. The reviewed studies using serum magnesium can thus be viewed as reliable indicators of persistent hypomagnesemia in individuals, rather than a daily fluctuation in magnesium intake.

Potential confounding by obesity, comorbidities, medication or diet should be considered, as these factors may be common causes of a low magnesium status and depression. Potential confounding by vitamin D and calcium levels is also possible. Magnesium is known to play a role in calcium balance as well as vitamin D metabolism [126], and dysregulation of these two compounds has also been implicated in depression [127,128]. Lastly, reverse causation may again be considered, whereby magnesium deficiency may be secondary to depression-related behavioral changes, such as reduced food intake [20].

Going forward, additional studies are needed to investigate the potential mechanisms that may underlie the association between magnesium and depression, as well as individual-level factors that might explain the variable associations found for magnesium supplementation. The evaluated studies varied with regard to magnesium dosage, ranging from 50 to 500 mg/day, and there is no clear trend between magnesium dosage and antidepressant effects. Similarly, the studies also varied with regard to patient population and duration of treatment as well as the unreliability of magnesium intake reports, which could, in turn, affect the discrepant findings. Furthermore, there is no observed relationship between the effect of magnesium supplementation and pre-treatment with magnesium or depressive status. Additional intervention studies might clarify whether magnesium supplementation can confer any benefits in the treatment of depression.

4. Selenium

Selenium is an essential trace element that is vital for the proper functioning of several selenoproteins involved in antioxidant defenses within the brain and nervous system [129–131]. Currently, the recommended daily allowance of selenium is 55 µg/day [132]. Optimal serum selenium levels are defined as being between 70 µg/L and 90 µg/L [133]. As the source of selenium intake is through the consumption of grains, selenium intake is highly dependent on the selenium content in food, which is, in turn, dependent on the selenium content of the soils in which it is grown. As a result, selenium deficiency often results from suboptimal presence in regional soil, thus making selenium deficiency often an endemic problem. It is estimated that one in seven people have low dietary selenium intake [134], and selenium deficiency has been implicated in a variety of conditions, such as renal disease [135] and obesity [136].

Given its neuromodulatory role in brain function [137–139], recent studies have investigated a relationship between selenium levels and depression. A rodent study found an association between selenium deficiency and decreased BDNF concentrations [140]. As a neurotrophic factor that has been extensively associated with the pathophysiology of major depressive disorder [141,142], it is plausible that BDNF concentrations could mediate the relationship between selenium deficiency and depression. In an intervention study performed on mice, Brüning et al. [143] showed that the administration of m-trifluoromethyl-diphenyl diselenide (m-CF$_3$–PhSe)$_2$, a multi-target selenium-based compound, reduced depressive symptoms as measured by immobility time in a forced swimming test (FST), in female mice, suggesting a potential antidepressant effect of selenium.

Observational studies have also investigated the relationship between selenium and depressive symptomology or risk of depression but have provided inconsistent results. A cross sectional study performed in a middle-aged population in West Texas demonstrated an inverse relationship between selenium level and depressive symptoms as measured by the Geriatric Depression Scale (GDS) [144]. Similarly, data from a nested case-control study on 1494 women aged 20–89 years reported that lower dietary selenium intake (<8.9 µg/day) was associated with a higher risk of developing major depressive disorder [139]. However, the results of two cross-sectional studies performed among a geriatric population in rural China [137] as well as a population of hemodialysis patients [145] found no significant association between selenium levels and depression scores after controlling for chronic kidney disease and cognitive function. Conversely, several studies have found a positive association between selenium serum levels and depressive symptomology. In a cross-sectional study using toenail biomarkers from 3735 participants aged 20–32 years, Colangelo et al. [146] found that higher levels of selenium exposure as assessed through toenail clippings were associated with the presence of elevated depressive symptoms. The idea that an "optimal range" with respect to depressive outcomes may exist for selenium levels was supported by Conner et al.'s [147] cross sectional study that found increased depressive symptomology below and above the serum selenium levels of 82 and 85 µg/L, with depressive symptomatology at its lowest at 85 µg/L.

Intervention studies of selenium supplementation in humans have reported similarly inconsistent findings. A randomized control trial among 166 Iranian women found that selenium supplementation during pregnancy was associated with increased selenium serum levels as well as lower scores on the Edinburgh Postnatal Depression Scale (EPDS) compared to those receiving placebo after 8 weeks of treatment [138]. However, Rayman et al. [148] reported the results of a randomized control trial to evaluate the effect of selenium supplementation on mood using the Profile of Moods States-Bipolar Form (POMS-BI) questionnaire and found that supplementation of selenium significantly increased plasma selenium levels without influencing mood scores after six months of supplementation.

4.1. Mechanism of Action

The association between selenium and depression has been less explored than the associations between zinc and magnesium with depression. However, research has suggested several possible hypotheses regarding selenium's mood-enhancing effects, including its role in maintaining metabolic, oxidative and central nervous system functioning. These are outlined in Table 1.

Selenium's modulatory effects on metabolism may influence an individual's susceptibility to developing depression. Selenium, which is incorporated into iodothyronine deiodinases (DIOs), is essential for the proper synthesis and metabolism of thyroid hormones. It has been long recognized by clinical investigators that thyroid function is associated with neuropsychiatric manifestation, such as mood disorders, cognitive dysfunction and other psychiatric symptoms [149]. Selenium deficiency and resulting deregulation of thyroid function may play a role in the development of depression [150].

The results from our review also indicate that an increasing amount of evidence points towards an "optimum range" of serum selenium levels in relation to depressive symptomology [146,147]. Studies have found that both high and low selenium levels have been linked with dysregulation of oxidative and inflammatory pathways, offering another potential mechanism that could explain the observed association between selenium levels and depression. Selenoproteins, such as glutathione peroxidases, thioredoxin reductases and selenoprotein P, are known to provide protection against lipoperoxidation and oxidative cell damage. A low selenium concentration has been associated with an increased level of pro-inflammatory cytokines, such as interleukin-6 (IL-6), C-reactive protein, and growth differentiation factor-5 (GDF-5) [151–153]. Additionally, a 2017 study demonstrated an association between low levels of cholesterol and increased risks of depression and suicidality [154], suggesting a possible role for selenium's anti-lipoperoxidative actions in its protective effect against depression. However, at an optimum level of selenium supplementation, there is an enzymatic and protein saturation effect that sends excess selenium into a metabolic process to restrict the further creation of selenoproteins. The metabolites of this excess selenium metabolism have been demonstrated to be pro-oxidative and result in increased levels of damaging reactive oxygen species (ROS) [155] Recent studies have shown that depression is associated with increased levels of oxidative stress biomarkers, strengthening the hypothesis that oxidative stress and inflammation may be significant factors in the pathogenesis of depression [149]. In light of selenium's dual antioxidant and pro-oxidative properties, it is conceivable that hyperactivity of oxidative and inflammatory pathways can contribute to the pathophysiology of depression.

Lastly, selenium could potentially exert antidepressant effects through its modulatory role in various neurotransmitter systems. Selenium has been found to have significant modulatory effects on the dopaminergic, serotonergic, and noradrenergic systems [156], which are all involved in the physiopathology of depression and other psychiatric illnesses [157]. Neurochemical data indicate that $(m\text{-}CF_3\text{-}PhSe)_2$ modulates the serotonergic system through mechanisms that involve selective inhibition of monoamine oxidase A (MAO-A), an enzyme implicated in 5-HT degradation, resulting in an overall increase of 5-HT availability in the synaptic cleft, contributing to its pharmacological effects [158]. Similarly, dopaminergic neurons vulnerable to oxidative stress have been shown to be modulated by selenoprotein, thus allowing selenium to play a preventative role in neurodegeneration [159]. While more studies are needed to clarify the relationship between selenium and depression, these findings suggest several plausible mechanisms through which selenium could be protective against depression.

4.2. Discussion and Implications

Studies examining the association between depression and selenium have been largely inconclusive. Overall, selenium deficiency seems to correlate with depression symptoms. However, this result was not observed in hemodialysis patients or in a rural elderly population in China. It is important to note that dialysis patients are at increased risk of selenium depletion due to low diffusion of selenium over the dialyzer membrane [160]. Moreover, comorbidities and other confounders, such as age and geographic location, may contribute to the discrepant findings. Alcohol is another potentially important confounder of this relationship as chronic alcoholism leads to lower plasma selenium through a reduction of selenium deposits as well as depression of selenoprotein expression and activity [161]. Longitudinal and cross sectional studies have further found associations between alcohol abuse and depression [162,163], In addition, zinc [25] and iron [164] may serve as confounders as both have been associated with depression status. Zinc has been shown to modulate the bioavailability of selenium, although the mechanism for this relationship is unclear [165].

Selenium exposure classification also varied within the reviewed studies. The majority of the reviewed studies utilized serum selenium or dietary intake of selenium as measurements of selenium levels. Selenium is regulated through excretion, and a direct relationship is evident between selenium intake and excretion [166]. As a result, selenium must be consumed regularly to maintain adequate selenium levels. However, the brain retains selenium better than any other tissue [167] and thus, measurement of selenium serum deficiency may not be indicative of brain selenium levels. Similarly, utilizing dietary recall incurs the risk of unreliability and recall bias that could potentially confound the results.

Further prospective investigations are needed to clarify the relationship between selenium and depression and to investigate reasons for the discrepant findings noted in this review. The inconsistent findings could be a result of different participant characteristics, such as geographic location, which plays a role in the amount of selenium available in local produce and subsequent selenium intake. Similarly, differing methods of the measurement of depression outcome as well as the duration of selenium treatment could potentially explain discrepant findings. For future intervention trials, it is important to note that high levels of selenium are toxic, as high dose selenium supplementation at or above 1600 µg/day has been shown to induce symptoms of selenium toxicity [168].

5. Conclusions

In this integrated review, we examined several lines of evidence, including animal, observational, and intervention studies, which provided evidence for a potential role of micronutrients in the development and progression of depression. The literature most strongly supports a role for zinc deficiency in increasing the risk of depression as well as the mood-enhancing effects of zinc supplementation in populations both with and without depression. While studies examining the magnesium–depression relationship have reported mixed findings, evidence generally supports a relationship between magnesium deficiency and the risk of depression as well as its antidepressant properties. The fewest number of studies have examined the link between selenium and depression, as most of the literature studying micronutrients has focused on zinc and magnesium. Studies examining the selenium–depression relationship have reported inconsistent findings, and future studies are needed to understand the effects of selenium deficiency on the etiology and treatment of depression. Although selenium deficiency is quite rare and regionally-specific, it has been recognized as an imminent public health problem due to the effects of climate change [169]. More prospective cohort and intervention studies are needed to assess the relationship between serum micronutrient levels and later risk of depression as well as the potential mechanisms underlying the observed associations. If evidence for a causal effect of these micronutrients on depression outcomes accumulates, the safety and efficacy of micronutrient supplementation as an adjust treatment for depression could also be explored. A balanced diet including adequate intake of foods containing zinc and other micronutrients could be an effective supplement to antidepressants for alleviating depressive symptoms.

Author Contributions: J.W., P.U. and B.A.D. performed the literature searches and the article retrieval, analyzed the data, and wrote and revised the article. J.L. developed the idea for the study. J.L. and B.A.D. mentored the review process, including conceptualizing the research question, the literature search, the interpretation of results and giving critical review.

Acknowledgments: The authors would like to thank Jenny Dharmawirya for performing initial literature searches and synthesis. This study was funded by the National Institutes of Environmental Health Sciences and the National Institutes of Health (R01-ES-018858, K02-ES-019878, K01-ES015877, and R25-ES021649).

Conflicts of Interest: The authors declare no conflicts of interest.

References

1. Sijbesma, F.; Sheeran, J. Micronutrients, Macro Impact: The Story of Vitamins and a Hungry World. Waldkirch: Sight and Life. 2011. Available online: http://www.sightandlife.org/fileadmin/data/Books/Micronutrients_Macro_Impact.pdf (accessed on 1 June 2017).
2. Depression. Available online: http://www.who.int/mediacentre/factsheets/fs369/en/ (accessed on 1 June 2017).
3. Black, M.M. Micronutrient deficiencies and cognitive functioning. *J. Nutr.* **2003**, *133*, 3927S–3931S. [CrossRef] [PubMed]
4. Jáuregui-Lobera, I. Iron deficiency and cognitive functions. *Neuropsychiatr. Dis. Treat.* **2014**, *10*, 2087–2095. [CrossRef] [PubMed]
5. Ames, B.N. DNA damage from micronutrient deficiencies is likely to be a major cause of cancer. *Mutat. Res. Fundam. Mol. Mech. Mutagen.* **2001**, *475*, 7–20. [CrossRef]
6. Kristal, A.R.; Darke, A.K.; Morris, J.S.; Tangen, C.M.; Goodman, P.J.; Thompson, I.M.; Meyskens, F.L.; Goodman, G.E.; Minasian, L.M.; Parnes, H.L. Baseline selenium status and effects of selenium and vitamin e supplementation on prostate cancer risk. *J. Natl. Cancer Inst.* **2014**, *106*. [CrossRef] [PubMed]
7. García, O.P.; Long, K.Z.; Rosado, J.L. Impact of micronutrient deficiencies on obesity. *Nutr. Rev.* **2009**, *67*, 559–572. [CrossRef] [PubMed]
8. Asfaw, A. Micronutrient deficiency and the prevalence of mothers' overweight/obesity in Egypt. *Econ. Hum. Biol.* **2007**, *5*, 471–483. [CrossRef] [PubMed]
9. Shankar, A.H.; Prasad, A.S. Zinc and immune function: The biological basis of altered resistance to infection. *Am. J. Clin. Nutr.* **1998**, *68*, 447S–463S. [CrossRef] [PubMed]
10. Wintergerst, E.S.; Maggini, S.; Hornig, D.H. Contribution of selected vitamins and trace elements to immune function. *Ann. Nutr. Metab.* **2007**, *51*, 301–323. [CrossRef] [PubMed]
11. Jurowski, K.; Szewczyk, B.; Nowak, G.; Piekoszewski, W. Biological consequences of zinc deficiency in the pathomechanisms of selected diseases. *J. Biol. Inorg. Chem.* **2014**, *19*, 1069–1079. [CrossRef] [PubMed]
12. Szewczyk, B.; Kubera, M.; Nowak, G. The role of zinc in neurodegenerative inflammatory pathways in depression. *Prog. Neuro-Psychopharmacol. Biol. Psychiatry* **2011**, *35*, 693–701. [CrossRef] [PubMed]
13. Bitanihirwe, B.K.; Cunningham, M.G. Zinc: The brain's dark horse. *Synapse* **2009**, *63*, 1029–1049. [CrossRef] [PubMed]
14. Maserejian, N.N.; Hall, S.A.; McKinlay, J.B. Low dietary or supplemental zinc is associated with depression symptoms among women, but not men, in a population-based epidemiological survey. *J. Affect. Disord.* **2012**, *136*, 781–788. [CrossRef] [PubMed]
15. Tucker, S.B.; Schroeter, A.L.; Brown, P.W.; McCall, J.T. Acquired zinc deficiency: Cutaneous manifestations typical of acrodermatitis enteropathica. *JAMA* **1976**, *235*, 2399–2402. [CrossRef] [PubMed]
16. Nowak, G.; Szewczyk, B.; Pilc, A. Zinc and depression. An update. *Pharmacol. Rep.* **2005**, *57*, 713–718. [PubMed]
17. Little, K.Y.; Castellanos, X.; Humphries, L.L.; Austin, J. Altered zinc metabolism in mood disorder patients. *Biol. Psychiatry* **1989**, *26*, 646–648. [CrossRef]
18. Młyniec, K.; Nowak, G. Zinc deficiency induces behavioral alterations in the tail suspension test in mice. Effect of antidepressants. *Pharmacol. Rep.* **2012**, *64*, 249–255. [CrossRef]
19. Tamano, H.; Kan, F.; Kawamura, M.; Oku, N.; Takeda, A. Behavior in the forced swim test and neurochemical changes in the hippocampus in young rats after 2-week zinc deprivation. *Neurochem. Int.* **2009**, *55*, 536–541. [CrossRef] [PubMed]
20. Tassabehji, N.M.; Corniola, R.S.; Alshingiti, A.; Levenson, C.W. Zinc deficiency induces depression-like symptoms in adult rats. *Physiol. Behav.* **2008**, *95*, 365–369. [CrossRef] [PubMed]
21. Whittle, N.; Lubec, G.; Singewald, N. Zinc deficiency induces enhanced depression-like behaviour and altered limbic activation reversed by antidepressant treatment in mice. *Amino Acids* **2009**, *36*, 147–158. [CrossRef] [PubMed]
22. Amani, R.; Saeidi, S.; Nazari, Z.; Nematpour, S. Correlation between dietary zinc intakes and its serum levels with depression scales in young female students. *Biol. Trace Elem. Res.* **2010**, *137*, 150–158. [CrossRef] [PubMed]
23. Kim, T.-H.; Choi, J.-y.; Lee, H.-H.; Park, Y. Associations between dietary pattern and depression in Korean adolescent girls. *J. Pediatr. Adolesc. Gynecol.* **2015**, *28*, 533–537. [CrossRef] [PubMed]

24. Liu, J.; Hanlon, A.; Ma, C.; Zhao, S.R.; Cao, S.; Compher, C. Low blood zinc, iron, and other sociodemographic factors associated with behavior problems in preschoolers. *Nutrients* **2014**, *6*, 530–545. [CrossRef] [PubMed]
25. Swardfager, W.; Herrmann, N.; Mazereeuw, G.; Goldberger, K.; Harimoto, T.; Lanctôt, K.L. Zinc in depression: A meta-analysis. *Biol. Psychiatry* **2013**, *74*, 872–878. [CrossRef] [PubMed]
26. Stanisławska, M.; Szkup-Jabłońska, M.; Jurczak, A.; Wieder-Huszla, S.; Samochowiec, A.; Jasiewicz, A.; Noceń, I.; Augustyniuk, K.; Brodowska, A.; Karakiewicz, B. The severity of depressive symptoms vs. serum Mg and Zn levels in postmenopausal women. *Biol. Trace Elem. Res.* **2014**, *157*, 30–35. [CrossRef] [PubMed]
27. Roozbeh, J.; Sharifian, M.; Ghanizadeh, A.; Sahraian, A.; Sagheb, M.M.; Shabani, S.; Jahromi, A.H.; Kashfi, M.; Afshariani, R. Association of zinc deficiency and depression in the patients with end-stage renal disease on hemodialysis. *J. Renal Nutr.* **2011**, *21*, 184–187. [CrossRef] [PubMed]
28. Lehto, S.M.; Ruusunen, A.; Tolmunen, T.; Voutilainen, S.; Tuomainen, T.-P.; Kauhanen, J. Dietary zinc intake and the risk of depression in middle-aged men: A 20-year prospective follow-up study. *J. Affect. Disord.* **2013**, *150*, 682–685. [CrossRef] [PubMed]
29. Lai, J.; Moxey, A.; Nowak, G.; Vashum, K.; Bailey, K.; McEvoy, M. The efficacy of zinc supplementation in depression: Systematic review of randomised controlled trials. *J. Affect. Disord.* **2012**, *136*, e31–e39. [CrossRef] [PubMed]
30. Sawada, T.; Yokoi, K. Effect of zinc supplementation on mood states in young women: A pilot study. *Eur. J. Clin. Nutr.* **2010**, *64*, 331–333. [CrossRef] [PubMed]
31. Siwek, M.; Dudek, D.; Paul, I.A.; Sowa-Kućma, M.; Zięba, A.; Popik, P.; Pilc, A.; Nowak, G. Zinc supplementation augments efficacy of imipramine in treatment resistant patients: A double blind, placebo-controlled study. *J. Affect. Disord.* **2009**, *118*, 187–195. [CrossRef] [PubMed]
32. Ding, Q.; Li, H.; Tian, X.; Shen, Z.; Wang, X.; Mo, F.; Huang, J.; Shen, H. Zinc and imipramine reverse the depression-like behavior in mice induced by chronic restraint stress. *J. Affect. Disord.* **2016**, *197*, 100–106. [CrossRef] [PubMed]
33. Huang, E.P. Metal ions and synaptic transmission: Think zinc. *Proc. Natl. Acad. Sci. USA* **1997**, *94*, 13386–13387. [CrossRef] [PubMed]
34. Chen, N.; Moshaver, A.; Raymond, L.A. Differential Sensitivity of RecombinantN-Methyl-D-Aspartate Receptor Subtypes to Zinc Inhibition. *Mol. Pharmacol.* **1997**, *51*, 1015–1023. [CrossRef] [PubMed]
35. Frederickson, C.J. Neurobiology of zinc and zinc-containing neurons. In *International Review of Neurobiology*; Elsevier: New York, NY, USA, 1989; Volume 31, pp. 145–238.
36. Kalappa, B.I.; Anderson, C.T.; Goldberg, J.M.; Lippard, S.J.; Tzounopoulos, T. AMPA receptor inhibition by synaptically released zinc. *Proc. Natl. Acad. Sci. USA* **2015**, *112*, 15749–15754. [CrossRef] [PubMed]
37. Marchetti, C. Interaction of metal ions with neurotransmitter receptors and potential role in neurodiseases. *Biometals* **2014**, *27*, 1097–1113. [CrossRef] [PubMed]
38. Satała, G.; Duszyńska, B.; Stachowicz, K.; Rafalo, A.; Pochwat, B.; Luckhart, C.; Albert, P.R.; Daigle, M.; Tanaka, K.F.; Hen, R. Concentration-dependent dual mode of Zn action at serotonin 5-HT1A receptors: In vitro and in vivo studies. *Mol. Neurobiol.* **2016**, *53*, 6869–6881. [CrossRef] [PubMed]
39. Szewczyk, B.; Pałucha-Poniewiera, A.; Poleszak, E.; Pilc, A.; Nowak, G. Investigational NMDA receptor modulators for depression. *Expert Opin. Investig. Drugs* **2012**, *21*, 91–102. [CrossRef] [PubMed]
40. Veran, J.; Kumar, J.; Pinheiro, P.S.; Athané, A.; Mayer, M.L.; Perrais, D.; Mulle, C. Zinc potentiates GluK3 glutamate receptor function by stabilizing the ligand binding domain dimer interface. *Neuron* **2012**, *76*, 565–578. [CrossRef] [PubMed]
41. Takeda, A. Movement of zinc and its functional significance in the brain. *Brain Res. Rev.* **2000**, *34*, 137–148. [CrossRef]
42. Gao, H.-L.; Zheng, W.; Xin, N.; Chi, Z.-H.; Wang, Z.-Y.; Chen, J.; Wang, Z.-Y. Zinc deficiency reduces neurogenesis accompanied by neuronal apoptosis through caspase-dependent and -independent signaling pathways. *Neurotox. Res.* **2009**, *16*, 416–425. [CrossRef] [PubMed]
43. Pfaender, S.; Föhr, K.; Lutz, A.-K.; Putz, S.; Achberger, K.; Linta, L.; Liebau, S.; Boeckers, T.M.; Grabrucker, A.M. Cellular zinc homeostasis contributes to neuronal differentiation in human induced pluripotent stem cells. *Neural Plast.* **2016**, *2016*. [CrossRef] [PubMed]
44. Takeda, A.; Tamano, H.; Ogawa, T.; Takada, S.; Ando, M.; Oku, N.; Watanabe, M. Significance of serum glucocorticoid and chelatable zinc in depression and cognition in zinc deficiency. *Behav. Brain Res.* **2012**, *226*, 259–264. [CrossRef] [PubMed]

45. Jokinen, J.; Nordström, P. HPA axis hyperactivity and attempted suicide in young adult mood disorder inpatients. *J. Affect. Disord.* **2009**, *116*, 117–120. [CrossRef] [PubMed]

46. Pariante, C.M.; Lightman, S.L. The HPA axis in major depression: Classical theories and new developments. *Trends Neurosci.* **2008**, *31*, 464–468. [CrossRef] [PubMed]

47. Doboszewska, U.; Wlaź, P.; Nowak, G.; Radziwoń-Zaleska, M.; Cui, R.; Młyniec, K. Zinc in the monoaminergic theory of depression: Its relationship to neural plasticity. *Neural Plast.* **2017**, *2017*. [CrossRef] [PubMed]

48. Suh, S.W.; Won, S.J.; Hamby, A.M.; Yoo, B.H.; Fan, Y.; Sheline, C.T.; Tamano, H.; Takeda, A.; Liu, J. Decreased brain zinc availability reduces hippocampal neurogenesis in mice and rats. *J. Cereb. Blood Flow Metab.* **2009**, *29*, 1579–1588. [CrossRef] [PubMed]

49. Malykhin, N.; Coupland, N. Hippocampal neuroplasticity in major depressive disorder. *Neuroscience* **2015**, *309*, 200–213. [CrossRef] [PubMed]

50. Czéh, B.; Michaelis, T.; Watanabe, T.; Frahm, J.; de Biurrun, G.; van Kampen, M.; Bartolomucci, A.; Fuchs, E. Stress-induced changes in cerebral metabolites, hippocampal volume, and cell proliferation are prevented by antidepressant treatment with tianeptine. *Proc. Natl. Acad. Sci. USA* **2001**, *98*, 12796–12801. [CrossRef] [PubMed]

51. Młyniec, K.; Gaweł, M.; Librowski, T.; Reczyński, W.; Bystrowska, B.; Holst, B. Investigation of the GPR39 zinc receptor following inhibition of monoaminergic neurotransmission and potentialization of glutamatergic neurotransmission. *Brain Res. Bull.* **2015**, *115*, 23–29. [CrossRef] [PubMed]

52. Tena-Campos, M.; Ramon, E.; Borroto-Escuela, D.O.; Fuxe, K.; Garriga, P. The zinc binding receptor GPR39 interacts with 5-HT1A and GalR1 to form dynamic heteroreceptor complexes with signaling diversity. *Biochim. Biophys. Acta Mol. Basis Dis.* **2015**, *1852*, 2585–2592. [CrossRef] [PubMed]

53. Młyniec, K.; Gaweł, M.; Nowak, G. Study of antidepressant drugs in GPR39 (zinc receptor−/−) knockout mice, showing no effect of conventional antidepressants, but effectiveness of NMDA antagonists. *Behav. Brain Res.* **2015**, *287*, 135–138. [CrossRef] [PubMed]

54. Mlyniec, K. Zinc in the glutamatergic theory of depression. *Curr. Neuropharmacol.* **2015**, *13*, 505–513. [CrossRef] [PubMed]

55. Castrén, E.; Võikar, V.; Rantamäki, T. Role of neurotrophic factors in depression. *Curr. Opin. Pharmacol.* **2007**, *7*, 18–21. [CrossRef] [PubMed]

56. Schmidt, H.D.; Duman, R.S. The role of neurotrophic factors in adult hippocampal neurogenesis, antidepressant treatments and animal models of depressive-like behavior. *Behav. Pharmacol.* **2007**, *18*, 391–418. [CrossRef] [PubMed]

57. Rashidi, A.A.; Salehi, M.; Piroozmand, A.; Sagheb, M.M. Effects of zinc supplementation on serum zinc and C-reactive protein concentrations in hemodialysis patients. *J. Ren. Nutr.* **2009**, *19*, 475–478. [CrossRef] [PubMed]

58. Bao, B.; Prasad, A.S.; Beck, F.W.; Fitzgerald, J.T.; Snell, D.; Bao, G.W.; Singh, T.; Cardozo, L.J. Zinc decreases C-reactive protein, lipid peroxidation, and inflammatory cytokines in elderly subjects: A potential implication of zinc as an atheroprotective agent. *Am. J. Clin. Nutr.* **2010**, *91*, 1634–1641. [CrossRef] [PubMed]

59. Howren, M.B.; Lamkin, D.M.; Suls, J. Associations of depression with C-reactive protein, IL-1, and IL-6: A meta-analysis. *Psychosom. Med.* **2009**, *71*, 171–186. [CrossRef] [PubMed]

60. Köhler-Forsberg, O.; Buttenschøn, H.N.; Tansey, K.E.; Maier, W.; Hauser, J.; Dernovsek, M.Z.; Henigsberg, N.; Souery, D.; Farmer, A.; Rietschel, M. Association between C-reactive protein (CRP) with depression symptom severity and specific depressive symptoms in major depression. *Brain Behav. Immun.* **2017**, *62*, 344–350. [CrossRef] [PubMed]

61. De Berardis, D.; Fornaro, M.; Orsolini, L.; Iasevoli, F.; Tomasetti, C.; de Bartolomeis, A.; Serroni, N.; De Lauretis, I.; Girinelli, G.; Mazza, M. Effect of agomelatine treatment on C-reactive protein levels in patients with major depressive disorder: An exploratory study in "real-world," everyday clinical practice. *CNS Spectr.* **2017**, *22*, 342–347. [CrossRef] [PubMed]

62. Mansour, S.A.; Mossa, A.-T.H. Lipid peroxidation and oxidative stress in rat erythrocytes induced by chlorpyrifos and the protective effect of zinc. *Pestic. Biochem. Physiol.* **2009**, *93*, 34–39. [CrossRef]

63. Irmisch, G.; Schlaefke, D.; Richter, J. Zinc and fatty acids in depression. *Neurochem. Res.* **2010**, *35*, 1376–1383. [CrossRef] [PubMed]

64. Sowa-Kućma, M.; Styczeń, K.; Siwek, M.; Misztak, P.; Nowak, R.J.; Dudek, D.; Rybakowski, J.K.; Nowak, G.; Maes, M. Lipid peroxidation and immune biomarkers are associated with major depression and its phenotypes, including treatment-resistant depression and melancholia. *Neurotox. Res.* **2018**, *33*, 448–460. [CrossRef] [PubMed]

65. Pittenger, C.; Sanacora, G.; Krystal, J.H. The NMDA receptor as a therapeutic target in major depressive disorder. *CNS Neurol. Disord. Drug Targets* **2007**, *6*, 101–115. [CrossRef] [PubMed]

66. Rosa, A.O.; Lin, J.; Calixto, J.B.; Santos, A.R.S.; Rodrigues, A.L.S. Involvement of NMDA receptors and L-arginine-nitric oxide pathway in the antidepressant-like effects of zinc in mice. *Behav. Brain Res.* **2003**, *144*, 87–93. [CrossRef]

67. Hess, S.Y.; Peerson, J.M.; King, J.C.; Brown, K.H. Use of serum zinc concentration as an indicator of population zinc status. *Food Nutr. Bull.* **2007**, *28*, S403–S429. [CrossRef] [PubMed]

68. Simmons, W.K.; Burrows, K.; Avery, J.A.; Kerr, K.L.; Bodurka, J.; Savage, C.R.; Drevets, W.C. Depression-related increases and decreases in appetite: Dissociable patterns of aberrant activity in reward and interoceptive neurocircuitry. *Am. J. Psychiatry* **2016**, *173*, 418–428. [CrossRef] [PubMed]

69. Dou, X.; Tian, X.; Zheng, Y.; Huang, J.; Shen, Z.; Li, H.; Wang, X.; Mo, F.; Wang, W.; Wang, S. Psychological stress induced hippocampus zinc dyshomeostasis and depression-like behavior in rats. *Behav. Brain Res.* **2014**, *273*, 133–138. [CrossRef] [PubMed]

70. Siwek, M.; Sowa-Kućma, M.; Dudek, D.; Styczeń, K.; Szewczyk, B.; Kotarska, K.; Misztak, P.; Pilc, A.; Wolak, M.; Nowak, G. Oxidative stress markers in affective disorders. *Pharmacol. Rep.* **2013**, *65*, 1558–1571. [CrossRef]

71. Anderson, G.; Kubera, M.; Duda, W.; Lasoń, W.; Berk, M.; Maes, M. Increased IL-6 trans-signaling in depression: Focus on the tryptophan catabolite pathway, melatonin and neuroprogression. *Pharmacol. Rep.* **2013**, *65*, 1647–1654. [CrossRef]

72. Siwek, M.; Szewczyk, B.; Dudek, D.; Styczeń, K.; Sowa-Kućma, M.; Młyniec, K.; Siwek, A.; Witkowski, L.; Pochwat, B.; Nowak, G. Zinc as a marker of affective disorders. *Pharmacol. Rep.* **2013**, *65*, 1512–1518. [CrossRef]

73. Vaghri, Z.; Guhn, M.; Weinberg, J.; Grunau, R.E.; Yu, W.; Hertzman, C. Hair cortisol reflects socio-economic factors and hair zinc in preschoolers. *Psychoneuroendocrinology* **2013**, *38*, 331–340. [CrossRef] [PubMed]

74. Lönnerdal, B. Dietary factors influencing zinc absorption. *J. Nutr.* **2000**, *130*, 1378S–1383S. [CrossRef] [PubMed]

75. Scheiber, I.; Dringen, R.; Mercer, J.F. Copper: Effects of deficiency and overload. In *Interrelations between Essential Metal Ions and Human Diseases*; Springer: Berlin, Germany, 2013; pp. 359–387.

76. Age-Related Eye Disease Study Research Group. A randomized, placebo-controlled, clinical trial of high-dose supplementation with vitamins C and E, beta carotene, and zinc for age-related macular degeneration and vision loss: AREDS report No. 8. *Arch. Ophthalmol.* **2001**, *119*, 1417–1436.

77. Kaplan, B.J.; Crawford, S.G.; Field, C.J.; Simpson, J.S.A. Vitamins, minerals, and mood. *Psychol. Bull.* **2007**, *133*, 747–760. [CrossRef] [PubMed]

78. Saito, N.; Nishiyama, S. Aging and magnesium. *Clin. Calcium* **2005**, *15*, 29–36. [PubMed]

79. Altura, B.M.; Altura, B.T. Role of magnesium in patho-physiological processes and the clinical utility of magnesium ion selective electrodes. *Scand. J. Clin. Lab. Investig.* **1996**, *56*, 211–234. [CrossRef]

80. Malon, A.; Brockmann, C.; Fijalkowska-Morawska, J.; Rob, P.; Maj-Zurawska, M. Ionized magnesium in erythrocytes—The best magnesium parameter to observe hypo-or hypermagnesemia. *Clin. Chim. Acta* **2004**, *349*, 67–73. [CrossRef] [PubMed]

81. King, D.E.; Mainous, A.G., III; Geesey, M.E.; Woolson, R.F. Dietary magnesium and C-reactive protein levels. *J. Am. Coll. Nutr.* **2005**, *24*, 166–171. [CrossRef] [PubMed]

82. Gröber, U.; Schmidt, J.; Kisters, K. Magnesium in prevention and therapy. *Nutrients* **2015**, *7*, 8199–8226. [CrossRef] [PubMed]

83. Eby, G.A.; Eby, K.L. Rapid recovery from major depression using magnesium treatment. *Med. Hypotheses* **2006**, *67*, 362–370. [CrossRef] [PubMed]

84. Młyniec, K.; Davies, C.L.; de Agueero Sanchez, I.G.; Pytka, K.; Budziszewska, B.; Nowak, G. Essential elements in depression and anxiety. Part I. *Pharmacol. Rep.* **2014**, *66*, 534–544. [CrossRef] [PubMed]

85. Singewald, N.; Sinner, C.; Hetzenauer, A.; Sartori, S.B.; Murck, H. Magnesium-deficient diet alters depression-and anxiety-related behavior in mice—Influence of desipramine and Hypericum perforatum extract. *Neuropharmacology* **2004**, *47*, 1189–1197. [CrossRef] [PubMed]

86. Winther, G.; Jørgensen, B.M.P.; Elfving, B.; Nielsen, D.S.; Kihl, P.; Lund, S.; Sørensen, D.B.; Wegener, G. Dietary magnesium deficiency alters gut microbiota and leads to depressive-like behaviour. *Acta Neuropsychiatr.* **2015**, *27*, 168–176. [CrossRef] [PubMed]

87. Gu, Y.; Zhao, K.; Luan, X.; Liu, Z.; Cai, Y.; Wang, Q.; Zhu, B.; He, J. Association between serum magnesium levels and depression in stroke patients. *Aging Dis.* **2016**, *7*, 687–690. [CrossRef] [PubMed]

88. Jacka, F.N.; Overland, S.; Stewart, R.; Tell, G.S.; Bjelland, I.; Mykletun, A. Association between magnesium intake and depression and anxiety in community-dwelling adults: The Hordaland Health Study. *Aust. N. Z. J. Psychiatry* **2009**, *43*, 45–52. [CrossRef] [PubMed]

89. Tarleton, E.K.; Littenberg, B. Magnesium intake and depression in adults. *J. Am. Board Fam. Med.* **2015**, *28*, 249–256. [CrossRef] [PubMed]

90. Martínez-González, M.Á.; Sánchez-Villegas, A. Magnesium intake and depression: The SUN cohort. *Magnes. Res.* **2016**, *29*, 102–111. [PubMed]

91. Derom, M.-L.; Martínez-González, M.A.; Sayón-Orea, M.C.; Bes-Rastrollo, M.; Beunza, J.J.; Sánchez-Villegas, A. Magnesium Intake Is Not Related to Depression Risk in Spanish University Graduates. *J. Nutr.* **2012**, *142*, 1053–1059. [CrossRef] [PubMed]

92. Rajizadeh, A.; Mozaffari-Khosravi, H.; Yassini-Ardakani, M.; Dehghani, A. Effect of magnesium supplementation on depression status in depressed patients with magnesium deficiency: A randomized, double-blind, placebo-controlled trial. *Nutrition* **2017**, *35*, 56–60. [CrossRef] [PubMed]

93. Tarleton, E.K.; Littenberg, B.; MacLean, C.D.; Kennedy, A.G.; Daley, C. Role of magnesium supplementation in the treatment of depression: A randomized clinical trial. *PLoS ONE* **2017**, *12*, e0180067. [CrossRef] [PubMed]

94. Barragán-Rodríguez, L.; Rodríguez-Morán, M.; Guerrero-Romero, F. Efficacy and safety of oral magnesium supplementation in the treatment of depression in the elderly with type 2 diabetes: A randomized, equivalent trial. *Magnes. Res.* **2008**, *21*, 218–223. [PubMed]

95. Fard, F.E.; Mirghafourvand, M.; Mohammad-Alizadeh Charandabi, S.; Farshbaf-Khalili, A.; Javadzadeh, Y.; Asgharian, H. Effects of zinc and magnesium supplements on postpartum depression and anxiety: A randomized controlled clinical trial. *Women Health* **2017**, *57*, 1115–1128. [CrossRef] [PubMed]

96. Mayberg, H.S. Limbic-cortical dysregulation: A proposed model of depression. *J. Neuropsychiatr. Clin. Neurosci.* **1997**, *9*, 471–481.

97. Redlich, R.; Opel, N.; Bürger, C.; Dohm, K.; Grotegerd, D.; Förster, K.; Zaremba, D.; Meinert, S.; Repple, J.; Enneking, V. The limbic system in youth depression: Brain structural and functional alterations in adolescent in-patients with severe depression. *Neuropsychopharmacology* **2018**, *43*, 546–554. [CrossRef] [PubMed]

98. Peng, D.; Shi, F.; Li, G.; Fralick, D.; Shen, T.; Qiu, M.; Liu, J.; Jiang, K.; Shen, D.; Fang, Y. Surface vulnerability of cerebral cortex to major depressive disorder. *PLoS ONE* **2015**, *10*, e0120704. [CrossRef] [PubMed]

99. Collingridge, G. The role of NMDA receptors in learning and memory. *Nature* **1987**, *330*, 604–605. [CrossRef] [PubMed]

100. Coan, E.; Collingridge, G. Magnesium ions block an N-methyl-D-aspartate receptor-mediated component of synaptic transmission in rat hippocampus. *Neurosci. Lett.* **1985**, *53*, 21–26. [CrossRef]

101. Ghafari, M.; Whittle, N.; Miklósi, A.G.; Kotlowsky, C.; Schmuckermair, C.; Berger, J.; Bennett, K.L.; Singewald, N.; Lubec, G. Dietary magnesium restriction reduces amygdala–hypothalamic GluN1 receptor complex levels in mice. *Brain Struct. Funct.* **2015**, *220*, 2209–2221. [CrossRef] [PubMed]

102. Pochwat, B.; Szewczyk, B.; Sowa-Kucma, M.; Siwek, A.; Doboszewska, U.; Piekoszewski, W.; Gruca, P.; Papp, M.; Nowak, G. Antidepressant-like activity of magnesium in the chronic mild stress model in rats: Alterations in the NMDA receptor subunits. *Int. J. Neuropsychopharmacol.* **2014**, *17*, 393–405. [CrossRef] [PubMed]

103. Murck, H. Ketamine, magnesium and major depression–From pharmacology to pathophysiology and back. *J. Psychiatr. Res.* **2013**, *47*, 955–965. [CrossRef] [PubMed]

104. Mark, L.P.; Prost, R.W.; Ulmer, J.L.; Smith, M.M.; Daniels, D.L.; Strottmann, J.M.; Brown, W.D.; Hacein-Bey, L. Pictorial review of glutamate excitotoxicity: Fundamental concepts for neuroimaging. *Am. J. Neuroradiol.* **2001**, *22*, 1813–1824. [PubMed]

105. Durlach, J.; Bac, P. Mechanisms of action on the nervous system in magnesium deficiency and dementia. In *Mineral and Metal Neurotoxicology*; CRC Press: Boca Raton, FL, USA; New York, NY, USA; London, UK; Tokyo, Japan, 1997.

106. Poleszak, E.; Wlaź, P.; Kędzierska, E.; Nieoczym, D.; Wróbel, A.; Fidecka, S.; Pilc, A.; Nowak, G. NMDA/glutamate mechanism of antidepressant-like action of magnesium in forced swim test in mice. *Pharmacol. Biochem. Behav.* **2007**, *88*, 158–164. [CrossRef] [PubMed]

107. Ehlert, U.; Gaab, J.; Heinrichs, M. Psychoneuroendocrinological contributions to the etiology of depression, posttraumatic stress disorder, and stress-related bodily disorders: The role of the hypothalamus-pituitary-adrenal axis. *Biol. Psychol.* **2001**, *57*, 141–152. [CrossRef]

108. Guerry, J.D.; Hastings, P.D. In search of HPA axis dysregulation in child and adolescent depression. *Clin. Child Fam. Psychol. Rev.* **2011**, *14*, 135–160. [CrossRef] [PubMed]

109. Lee, A.L.; Ogle, W.O.; Sapolsky, R.M. Stress and depression: Possible links to neuron death in the hippocampus. *Bipolar Disord.* **2002**, *4*, 117–128. [CrossRef] [PubMed]

110. Uno, H.; Eisele, S.; Sakai, A.; Shelton, S.; Baker, E.; DeJesus, O.; Holden, J. Neurotoxicity of glucocorticoids in the primate brain. *Horm. Behav.* **1994**, *28*, 336–348. [CrossRef] [PubMed]

111. Kelly, J.R.; Borre, Y.; O'Brien, C.; Patterson, E.; El Aidy, S.; Deane, J.; Kennedy, P.J.; Beers, S.; Scott, K.; Moloney, G. Transferring the blues: Depression-associated gut microbiota induces neurobehavioural changes in the rat. *J. Psychiatr. Res.* **2016**, *82*, 109–118. [CrossRef] [PubMed]

112. Dinan, T.G.; Cryan, J.F. Melancholic microbes: A link between gut microbiota and depression? *Neurogastroenterol. Motil.* **2013**, *25*, 713–719. [CrossRef] [PubMed]

113. Pachikian, B.D.; Neyrinck, A.M.; Deldicque, L.; De Backer, F.C.; Catry, E.; Dewulf, E.M.; Sohet, F.M.; Bindels, L.B.; Everard, A.; Francaux, M. Changes in Intestinal Bifidobacteria Levels Are Associated with the Inflammatory Response in Magnesium-Deficient Mice. *J. Nutr.* **2010**, *140*, 509–514. [CrossRef] [PubMed]

114. Dibaba, D.T.; Xun, P.; He, K. Dietary magnesium intake is inversely associated with serum C-reactive protein levels: Meta-analysis and systematic review. *Eur. J. Clin. Nutr.* **2014**, *68*, 510–516. [CrossRef] [PubMed]

115. Chacko, S.A.; Song, Y.; Nathan, L.; Tinker, L.; De Boer, I.H.; Tylavsky, F.; Wallace, R.; Liu, S. Relations of dietary magnesium intake to biomarkers of inflammation and endothelial dysfunctions in an ethnically diverse cohort of postmenopausal women. *Diabetes Care* **2010**, *33*, 304–310. [CrossRef] [PubMed]

116. Miller, A.H.; Maletic, V.; Raison, C.L. Inflammation and its discontents: The role of cytokines in the pathophysiology of major depression. *Biol. Psychiatry* **2009**, *65*, 732–741. [CrossRef] [PubMed]

117. Miller, A.H.; Raison, C.L. The role of inflammation in depression: From evolutionary imperative to modern treatment target. *Nat. Rev. Immunol.* **2016**, *16*, 22–34. [CrossRef] [PubMed]

118. Kiecolt-Glaser, J.K.; Derry, H.M.; Fagundes, C.P. Inflammation: Depression fans the flames and feasts on the heat. *Am. J. Psychiatry* **2015**, *172*, 1075–1091. [CrossRef] [PubMed]

119. Cardoso, C.C.; Lobato, K.R.; Binfaré, R.W.; Ferreira, P.K.; Rosa, A.O.; Santos, A.R.S.; Rodrigues, A.L.S. Evidence for the involvement of the monoaminergic system in the antidepressant-like effect of magnesium. *Prog. Neuro-Psychopharmacol. Biol. Psychiatry* **2009**, *33*, 235–242. [CrossRef] [PubMed]

120. Poleszak, E. Modulation of antidepressant-like activity of magnesium by serotonergic system. *J. Neural Transm.* **2007**, *114*, 1129–1134. [CrossRef] [PubMed]

121. Pochwat, B.; Sowa-Kucma, M.; Kotarska, K.; Misztak, P.; Nowak, G.; Szewczyk, B. Antidepressant-like activity of magnesium in the olfactory bulbectomy model is associated with the AMPA/BDNF pathway. *Psychopharmacology* **2015**, *232*, 355–367. [CrossRef] [PubMed]

122. Billyard, A.J.; Eggett, D.L.; Franz, K.B. Dietary magnesium deficiency decreases plasma melatonin in rats. *Magnes. Res.* **2006**, *19*, 157–161. [PubMed]

123. Elin, R.J. Assessment of magnesium status. *Clin. Chem.* **1987**, *33*, 1965–1970. [PubMed]

124. Assadi, F. Hypomagnesemia: An evidence-based approach to clinical cases. *Iran. J. Kidney Dis.* **2010**, *4*, 13–19. [PubMed]

125. Jahnen-Dechent, W.; Ketteler, M. Magnesium basics. *Clin. Kidney J.* **2012**, *5*, i3–i14. [CrossRef] [PubMed]

126. Deng, X.; Song, Y.; Manson, J.E.; Signorello, L.B.; Zhang, S.M.; Shrubsole, M.J.; Ness, R.M.; Seidner, D.L.; Dai, Q. Magnesium, vitamin D status and mortality: Results from US National Health and Nutrition Examination Survey (NHANES) 2001 to 2006 and NHANES III. *BMC Med.* **2013**, *11*, 187. [CrossRef] [PubMed]

127. Anglin, R.E.; Samaan, Z.; Walter, S.D.; McDonald, S.D. Vitamin D deficiency and depression in adults: Systematic review and meta-analysis. *Br. J. Psychiatry* **2013**, *202*, 100–107. [CrossRef] [PubMed]

128. Dittman, J.S.; Kreitzer, A.C.; Regehr, W.G. Interplay between facilitation, depression, and residual calcium at three presynaptic terminals. *J. Neurosci.* **2000**, *20*, 1374–1385. [CrossRef] [PubMed]

129. Holben, D.H.; Smith, A.M. The diverse role of selenium within selenoproteins: A review. *J. Acad. Nutr. Dietet.* **1999**, *99*, 836–843. [CrossRef]

130. Rayman, M.P. The importance of selenium to human health. *Lancet* **2000**, *356*, 233–241. [CrossRef]

131. Rotruck, J.T.; Pope, A.L.; Ganther, H.; Swanson, A.; Hafeman, D.G.; Hoekstra, W. Selenium: Biochemical role as a component of glutathione peroxidase. *Science* **1973**, *179*, 588–590. [CrossRef] [PubMed]

132. Council, N.R.; Council, N.R. *Dietary Reference Intakes for Vitamin C, Vitamin E, Selenium, and Carotenoids*; National Academy Press: Washington, DC, USA, 2000.

133. Bleys, J.; Navas-Acien, A.; Guallar, E. Serum selenium levels and all-cause, cancer, and cardiovascular mortality among US adults. *Arch. Intern. Med.* **2008**, *168*, 404–410. [CrossRef] [PubMed]

134. UNICEF; Micronutrient Initiative. Vitamin and Mineral Deficiency: A Global Progress Report. Available online: https://www.unicef.org/media/files/vmd.pdf (accessed on 1 June 2017).

135. Iglesias, P.; Selgas, R.; Romero, S.; Díez, J.J. Selenium and kidney disease. *J. Nephrol.* **2013**, *26*, 266–272. [CrossRef] [PubMed]

136. Alasfar, F.; Ben-Nakhi, M.; Khoursheed, M.; Kehinde, E.O.; Alsaleh, M. Selenium is significantly depleted among morbidly obese female patients seeking bariatric surgery. *Obesity Surg.* **2011**, *21*, 1710–1713. [CrossRef] [PubMed]

137. Gao, S.; Jin, Y.; Unverzagt, F.W.; Liang, C.; Hall, K.S.; Cao, J.; Ma, F.; Murrell, J.R.; Cheng, Y.; Li, P. Selenium level and depressive symptoms in a rural elderly Chinese cohort. *BMC Psychiatry* **2012**, *12*, 72. [CrossRef] [PubMed]

138. Mokhber, N.; Namjoo, M.; Tara, F.; Boskabadi, H.; Rayman, M.P.; Ghayour-Mobarhan, M.; Sahebkar, A.; Majdi, M.R.; Tavallaie, S.; Azimi-Nezhad, M. Effect of supplementation with selenium on postpartum depression: A randomized double-blind placebo-controlled trial. *J. Matern. Fetal Neonatal Med.* **2011**, *24*, 104–108. [CrossRef] [PubMed]

139. Pasco, J.A.; Jacka, F.N.; Williams, L.J.; Evans-Cleverdon, M.; Brennan, S.L.; Kotowicz, M.A.; Nicholson, G.C.; Ball, M.J.; Berk, M. Dietary selenium and major depression: A nested case-control study. *Complement. Ther. Med.* **2012**, *20*, 119–123. [CrossRef] [PubMed]

140. Mitchell, J.; Nicol, F.; Beckett, G. Selenoprotein expression and brain development in preweanling selenium-and iodine-deficient rats. *J. Mol. Endocrinol.* **1998**, *20*, 203–210. [CrossRef] [PubMed]

141. Shimizu, E.; Hashimoto, K.; Okamura, N.; Koike, K.; Komatsu, N.; Kumakiri, C.; Nakazato, M.; Watanabe, H.; Shinoda, N.; Okada, S.; et al. Alterations of serum levels of brain-derived neurotrophic factor (BDNF) in depressed patients with or without antidepressants. *Biol. Psychiatry* **2003**, *54*, 70–75. [CrossRef]

142. Björkholm, C.; Monteggia, L.M. BDNF—a key transducer of antidepressant effects. *Neuropharmacology* **2016**, *102*, 72–79. [CrossRef] [PubMed]

143. Brüning, C.A.; Souza, A.C.G.; Gai, B.M.; Zeni, G.; Nogueira, C.W. Antidepressant-like effect of m-trifluoromethyl-diphenyl diselenide in the mouse forced swimming test involves opioid and serotonergic systems. *Eur. J. Pharmacol.* **2011**, *658*, 145–149. [CrossRef] [PubMed]

144. Johnson, L.A.; Phillips, J.A.; Mauer, C.; Edwards, M.; Balldin, V.H.; Hall, J.R.; Barber, R.; Conger, T.L.; Ho, E.J.; O'Bryant, S.E. The impact of GPX1 on the association of groundwater selenium and depression: A project FRONTIER study. *BMC Psychiatry* **2013**, *13*. [CrossRef] [PubMed]

145. Ekramzadeh, M.; Mazloom, Z.; Sagheb, M. Association of Depression With Selenium Deficiency and Nutritional Markers in the Patients With End-Stage Renal Disease on Hemodialysis. *J. Ren. Nutr.* **2015**, *25*, 381–387. [CrossRef] [PubMed]

146. Colangelo, L.A.; He, K.; Whooley, M.A.; Daviglus, M.L.; Morris, S.; Liu, K. Selenium exposure and depressive symptoms: The coronary artery risk development in young adults trace element study. *Neurotoxicology* **2014**, *41*, 167–174. [CrossRef] [PubMed]

147. Conner, T.S.; Richardson, A.C.; Miller, J.C. Optimal Serum Selenium Concentrations Are Associated with Lower Depressive Symptoms and Negative Mood among Young Adults. *J. Nutr.* **2014**, *145*, 59–65. [CrossRef] [PubMed]

148. Rayman, M.; Thompson, A.; Warren-Perry, M.; Galassini, R.; Catterick, J.; Hall, E.; Lawrence, D.; Bliss, J. Impact of selenium on mood and quality of life: A randomized, controlled trial. *Biol. Psychiatry* **2006**, *59*, 147–154. [CrossRef] [PubMed]

149. Młyniec, K.; Gaweł, M.; Doboszewska, U.; Starowicz, G.; Pytka, K.; Davies, C.L.; Budziszewska, B. Essential elements in depression and anxiety. Part II. *Pharmacol. Rep.* **2015**, *67*, 187–194. [CrossRef] [PubMed]

150. Kohrle, J.; Jakob, F.; Contempre, B.; Dumont, J.E. Selenium, the thyroid, and the endocrine system. *Endocr. Rev.* **2005**, *26*, 944–984. [CrossRef] [PubMed]

151. Mertens, K.; Lowes, D.; Webster, N.; Talib, J.; Hall, L.; Davies, M.J.; Beattie, J.; Galley, H. Low zinc and selenium concentrations in sepsis are associated with oxidative damage and inflammation. *Br. J. Anaesth.* **2015**, *114*, 990–999. [CrossRef] [PubMed]

152. Prystupa, A.; Kiciński, P.; Luchowska-Kocot, D.; Błażewicz, A.; Niedziałek, J.; Mizerski, G.; Jojczuk, M.; Ochal, A.; Sak, J.J.; Załuska, W. Association between Serum Selenium Concentrations and Levels of Proinflammatory and Profibrotic Cytokines—Interleukin-6 and Growth Differentiation Factor-15, in Patients with Alcoholic Liver Cirrhosis. *Int. J. Environ. Res. Public Health* **2017**, *14*, 437. [CrossRef] [PubMed]

153. Duntas, L. Selenium and inflammation: Underlying anti-inflammatory mechanisms. *Horm. Metab. Res.* **2009**, *41*, 443–447. [CrossRef] [PubMed]

154. De Berardis, D.; Marini, S.; Piersanti, M.; Cavuto, M.; Perna, G.; Valchera, A.; Mazza, M.; Fornaro, M.; Iasevoli, F.; Martinotti, G. The relationships between cholesterol and suicide: An update. *ISRN Psychiatry* **2012**, *2012*. [CrossRef] [PubMed]

155. Spallholz, J.E. On the nature of selenium toxicity and carcinostatic activity. *Free Radic. Biol. Med.* **1994**, *17*, 45–64. [CrossRef]

156. Castaño, A.; Ayala, A.; Rodríguez-Gómez, J.A.; Herrera, A.J.; Cano, J.; Machado, A. Low selenium diet increases the dopamine turnover in prefrontal cortex of the rat. *Neurochem. Int.* **1997**, *30*, 549–555. [CrossRef]

157. Nogueira, C.W.; Rocha, J.B. Toxicology and pharmacology of selenium: Emphasis on synthetic organoselenium compounds. *Arch. Toxicol.* **2011**, *85*, 1313–1359. [CrossRef] [PubMed]

158. Brüning, C.A.; Prigol, M.; Roehrs, J.A.; Nogueira, C.W.; Zeni, G. Involvement of the serotonergic system in the anxiolytic-like effect caused by m-trifluoromethyl-diphenyl diselenide in mice. *Behav. Brain Res.* **2009**, *205*, 511–517. [CrossRef] [PubMed]

159. Solovyev, N.D. Importance of selenium and selenoprotein for brain function: From antioxidant protection to neuronal signalling. *J. Inorg. Biochem.* **2015**, *153*, 1–12. [CrossRef] [PubMed]

160. Sher, L. Role of selenium depletion in the effects of dialysis on mood and behavior. *Med. Hypotheses* **2002**, *59*, 89–91. [CrossRef]

161. Carreras, O.; Ojeda, M.L.; Nogales, F. Selenium dietary supplementation and oxidative balance in alcoholism. In *Molecular Aspects of Alcohol and Nutrition*; Elsevier: New York, NY, USA, 2016; pp. 133–142.

162. Brière, F.N.; Rohde, P.; Seeley, J.R.; Klein, D.; Lewinsohn, P.M. Comorbidity between major depression and alcohol use disorder from adolescence to adulthood. *Compr. Psychiatry* **2014**, *55*, 526–533. [CrossRef] [PubMed]

163. Hasin, D.S.; Stinson, F.S.; Ogburn, E.; Grant, B.F. Prevalence, correlates, disability, and comorbidity of DSM-IV alcohol abuse and dependence in the United States: Results from the National Epidemiologic Survey on Alcohol and Related Conditions. *Arch. Gen. Psychiatry* **2007**, *64*, 830–842. [CrossRef] [PubMed]

164. Shariatpanaahi, M.V.; Shariatpanaahi, Z.V.; Moshtaaghi, M.; Shahbaazi, S.; Abadi, A. The relationship between depression and serum ferritin level. *Eur. J. Clin. Nutr.* **2007**, *61*, 532–535. [CrossRef] [PubMed]

165. House, W.A.; Welch, R.M. Bioavailability of and interactions between zinc and selenium in rats fed wheat grain intrinsically labeled with 65Zn and 75Se. *J. Nutr.* **1989**, *119*, 916–921. [CrossRef] [PubMed]

166. Burk, R.F.; Hill, K.E. Regulation of selenium metabolism and transport. *Annu. Rev. Nutr.* **2015**, *35*, 109–134. [CrossRef] [PubMed]

167. Behne, D.; Höfer-Bosse, T. Effects of a low selenium status on the distribution and retention of selenium in the rat. *J. Nutr.* **1984**, *114*, 1289–1296. [CrossRef] [PubMed]

168. Reid, M.E.; Stratton, M.S.; Lillico, A.J.; Fakih, M.; Natarajan, R.; Clark, L.C.; Marshall, J.R. A report of high-dose selenium supplementation: Response and toxicities. *J. Trace Elem. Med. Biol.* **2004**, *18*, 69–74. [CrossRef] [PubMed]

169. Jones, G.D.; Droz, B.; Greve, P.; Gottschalk, P.; Poffet, D.; McGrath, S.P.; Seneviratne, S.I.; Smith, P.; Winkel, L.H. Selenium deficiency risk predicted to increase under future climate change. *Proc. Natl. Acad. Sci. USA* **2017**, *114*, 2848–2853. [CrossRef] [PubMed]

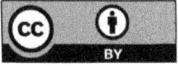

MDPI

St. Alban-Anlage 66

4052 Basel

Switzerland

Tel. +41 61 683 77 34

Fax +41 61 302 89 18

www.mdpi.com

Nutrients Editorial Office

E-mail: nutrients@mdpi.com

www.mdpi.com/journal/nutrients

www.ingramcontent.com/pod-product-compliance
Lightning Source LLC
Chambersburg PA
CBHW051840210326
41597CB00033B/5715